Introduction to Environmental Health

Second Edition

Daniel S. Blumenthal, MD, MPH, received his medical degree from the University of Chicago and his MPH from Emory University. He has served on the staff of the Centers for Disease Control and Prevention and on the faculty of Emory University. He is currently Professor and Chairman of the Department of Community Health and Preventive Medicine at Morehouse School of Medicine in Atlanta.

A. James Ruttenber, PhD, MD, received a doctorate in human ecology and an MD at Emory University. He was an officer in the Epidemic Intelligence Service and a medical epidemiologist at the Centers for Disease Control, and an adjunct faculty member in both the School of Public Health and the Human and Natural Ecology Program at Emory University. He specializes in occupational and environmental epidemiology and is an associate professor in the Department of Preventive Medicine and Biometrics at the University of Colorado School of Medicine.

Introduction to

Environmental Health

Second Edition

Daniel S. Blumenthal, MD, MPH

A. James Ruttenber, PhD, MD

with contributions by

Herman T. Blumenthal, MD, PhD

Andrew Robert Green, JD

Renate D. Kimbrough, MD

Linda R. Murray, MD, MPH

Harvey L. Ragsdale, PhD

S SPRINGER PUBLISHING COMPANY

Copyright © 1995 by Springer Publishing Company, Inc.

Springer Publishing Company, Inc.
536 Broadway
New York, NY 10012-3955

The first edition of *Introduction to Environmental Health* was published by Springer Publishing Company in 1985.

Cover design by Tom Yabut
Production Editor: Pamela Lankas

95 96 97 98 99 / 5 4 3 2 1

Library of Congress Cataloging in Publication Data

Introduction to environmental health/Daniel S. Blumenthal, A. James
Ruttenber, editors.—2nd ed.
  p. cm.
  Includes bibliographical references and index.
  ISBN 0-8261-3901-0
  1. Environmental health, I. Blumenthal, Daniel S.
II. Ruttenber, A. James.
  [DNLM: 1. Environmental Health. WA 30 I613 1994]
  RA565.I58 1994
  616.9'8—DC20
  DNLM/DLC
  for Library of Congress   93-38205
                                                                    CIP

Printed in the United States of America

DSB: *To Janet*

AJR: *To Joan, Annie, and Marya and in memory of Tim (aka Deacon Lunchbox)*

Permissions

- Figure 1.7A is reprinted with permission from Mackay, D. & S. Paterson (1993), *Mathematical Models of Transport and Fate*, p. 131, in G.W. Suter (Ed.), *Ecological Risk Assessment*. Boca Raton, FL: Lewis Publishers, an imprint of CRC Press. Copyright©1993.

- Figure 1.7B is reprinted with permission from *Beyond the Limits* by Meadows, Meadows, & Randers. Copyright © 1992 by Chelsea Green Publishing Co., White River Junction, VT.

- Figure 5.1 is reprinted with permission from Glaser, Z.R. (1992), *Organization and Management of a Nonionizing Radiation Safety Program*, pp. 44–45 in K.L. Miller (Ed.), *CRC Handbook of Management of Radiation Programs, 2nd Ed.* Boca Raton, FL: CRC Press. Copyright©1992.

- Figure 5.2 is adapted with permission from Shimizu, Y., W.J. Schull, & H. Kato (1990), "Studies of the mortality of A-bomb survivors. 9. Mortality, 1950—1985: Part 2. Cancer mortality based on the recently rervised doses (DS86)." *Radiation Research,* 121, pp. 120–141.

- Figure 10.3 is reprinted with permission from Schulte, P.A. & F.P. Perera (1993), *Molecular Epidemiology.* San Diego: Academic Press. Copyright©1993.

- Table 5.2 is reprinted with permission from *The Effects on Populations of Exposure to Low Levels of Ionizing Radiation.* Copyright©1990 by the National Academy of Sciences. Courtesy of the National Academy Press, Washington, DC.

- Table 7.1 is reprinted with permission from *State of the World 1993*, edited by L. R. Brown et al., with the permission of W.W. Norton Co., Inc. Copyright©1993 by Worldwatch Institute.

- Table 7.2 is reprinted with permission from Meybeck, M., D.V. Chapman, & R. Helmer (1989), *Global Freshwater Quality.* Oxford, UK: Blackwell. Copyright©1989.

- Table 7.3 is reprinted with permission from Cotruvo, J.A. & M. Regelski (1989), "Overview of the current national primary drinking water regulations and regulation development process," 20 in E.J. Calabrese, C.E. Gilbert, & H. Pastides (Eds.), *Safe Drinking Water Act: Amendments, Regulations, and Standards.* Boca Raton, FL: Lewis Publishers, an imprint of CRC Press. Copyright©1989.

- Table 9.2 is reprinted from Smith, T.J., & T. Schneider (1995), "Occupational hygiene" (pp. 125–144) in D.S. Levy & D.H. Wegman (Eds.), *Occupational Health: Recognizing and Preventing Work-Related Disease, 3rd Ed.* Boston: Little, Brown, & Co. Copyright©1995.

- Table 9.6 is reprinted from Baker & Schottenfeld (1995), "Disorders of the nervous system" (pp. 519–541) in D.S. Levy & D.H. Wegman (Eds.), *Occupational Health: Recognizing and Preventing Work-Related Disease, 3rd Ed.* Boston: Little, Brown, & Co. Copyright©1995.

Contents

Contributors

Herman T. Blumenthal, MD, PhD, received his medical degree and his doctorate in pathology from Washington University in St. Louis. He has served as laboratory director at Jewish Hospital, Jefferson Barracks Veterans Administration Hospital, and Midwest Medical Laboratories, all in St. Louis. He is an adjunct professor in the Department of Family and Community Medicine, St. Louis School of Medicine, and research professor of gerontology at Washington University.

Andrew Robert Greene, JD, is a partner with Bradley, Arant, Rose & White in Birmingham, Alabama. He specializes in federal and state environmental law and serves as the representative of the firm's environmental practice group. He is a former Deputy Regional Counsel at the U.S. Environmental Protection Agency Region IV Office in Atlanta, Georgia. Mr. Green received a JD degree from Catholic University.

Renate D. Kimbrough, MD, received a medical degree from Ernst August University, Gottigen, Germany and has residency training in pathology. She is a specialist in clinical toxicology and has been a researcher in toxicology and environmental health at the Centers for Disease Control and Prevention and the U.S. Environmental

Protection Agency. She is currently a Senior Medical Associate at the Institute for Evaluating Health Risks in Washington, DC.

Linda Rae Murray, MD, MPH, received her MD and MPH degrees from the University of Illinois, where she also trained in both internal and occupational medicine. She has served with the Manitoba Federation of Labour Occupational Health Centre in Winnipeg, with the Chicago Health Department, and on the faculty of Meharry Medical College. She is currently medical director for the Near North Health Service Corporation in Chicago.

Harvey L. Ragsdale, MS, PhD, is Professor and Director of the Human and Natural Ecology Program at Emory University. He received MS and PhD degrees from the University of Tennessee as an Oak Ridge Associated Universities Fellow. He joined the Emory University faculty in 1968 and initiated Emory's interdisciplinary program in human and natural ecology in 1988. He currently is a Fellow of the Carter Presidential Center.

Introduction

ENVIRONMENTAL HEALTH DEFINED

Environmental health focuses on the relation between the environment and human health, encompasses many areas of specialization in the sciences, and in one way or another depends on most academic disciplines. According to the medical definition, a disease is caused by genetic factors, environmental agents, or a combination of the two. Though most diseases are caused in part by environmental factors, the majority of these are lifestyle, dietary, or social factors unrelated to toxic agents in the environment. Because the environment is so broadly defined with regard to disease causation, the field of environmental health is usually restricted to the study of those diseases caused by toxic agents in air, water, soil, and food and the methods used to diagnose and prevent such diseases.

To date there is no well-defined body of knowledge that students master to become experts in environmental health. Many universities throughout the world have undergraduate degree programs in environmental health, and graduate students can concentrate in this area in masters- and doctoral-level programs in epidemiology, public health, engineering, and the environmental sciences. In Great Britain, the academic preparation for a career in environmental health is more specifically defined and over 6,000 environmental health officers, trained in well-defined 4-year college programs, are employed by local governments.

Because it includes many well-established scientific disciplines, environmental health does not have a history of its own. Rather, the histories of disciplines such as civil engineering, environmental engineering, industrial hygiene, toxicology, sanitary engineering, and epidemiology contribute to the history of this field.

The field of environmental health has also been influenced by the evolution of the field of public health. In the eighteenth and nineteenth centuries, environmental health was practiced by public health sanitarians under the supervision of physicians. Because little was known about the biological agents responsible for the diseases of public health concern, environmental health was based on common-sense approaches to sanitation.

The American Public Health Association was founded in 1872, and helped to place new emphasis on hygienic reform and sanitary science. In the early 1900s, major improvements were made in rural sanitation and state and local health departments were established with sanitarians on their staffs. Some trace the origin of the field of environmental health to the studies of water pollution and water and sewage treatment that were launched by the U. S. Public Health Service during this period. This research was performed by teams of medical officers, sanitary engineers, and bacteriologists who employed the techniques of epidemiology and biostatistics in their studies (Mullan, 1989).

In the nineteenth century, the discovery that microorganisms were responsible for the majority of morbidity and mortality transformed environmental health into a field that emphasized microbiology and the clinical field of infectious disease medicine. In the modern era, the field has been profoundly impacted by the development of scientific approaches to the study of the environment—approaches that rely heavily on measurements made with sophisticated equipment and computer analyses of large sets of environmental data. Sanitarians and sanitary engineers have been joined by environmental scientists trained in such disciplines as hydrology, atmospheric and marine sciences, ecology, and epidemiology.

In order to take advantage of the "information explosion" in the environmental sciences, environmental health professionals must be well trained in the natural and physical sciences, and know how to work across disciplinary boundaries. Educators in medicine and the health sciences have also recognized the importance of training in environmental health for clinicians, who should be able to diagnose and treat diseases caused by exposure to toxic agents in the environment and the workplace and to discuss intelligently health risks from environmental agents with their patients and citizens in their communities (Institute of Medicine, 1993).

A SYSTEMS APPROACH TO ENVIRONMENTAL HEALTH

We emphasize a systems approach in presenting the material in this book because it is the most effective way to connect ideas from diverse disciplines, because it provides methods that can be used to solve new problems in environmental health, and because we have seen it work year after year in the training of our students. This perspective is not new; it is the foundation of modern ecology (E.P. Odum, 1993; H.T. Odum, 1994) and is the unifying theory for the field of human ecology—a field that overlaps substantially with environmental health.

A systems-based perspective is different from those commonly used in teaching most subjects in the health sciences, where it is common for graduate and professional students to spend much of their time memorizing facts from various subject areas. The field of environmental health encompasses too much information to be taught this way—just imagine having to memorize all the relevant facts in medicine, toxicology, epidemiology, and the environmental and social sciences!

A systems approach stresses understanding of the basic principles governing the behavior of toxic agents in the environment and their effects on humans. It also stresses managing information rather than rotely memorizing facts. After all, the revolution in information technology has created computers to store these data—we just have to learn how to access them, and it is getting easier and easier to do this all the time.

The systems perspective also recognizes time as an important variable. Often, activities that are not current health risks become ones in the future. Measurable effects of global warming and ozone-

depleting gases are not easily observed today but, according to projections, will be evident in the future. Other examples of environmental damage that impact public health include air and water pollution,
soil erosion, wetland destruction, and deforestation.

Scientists in the fields of ecology and other environmental sciences have developed predictive models that help forecast the long-
term consequences of changes in the environment, whether natural or
man-induced (H.T. Odum, 1994). Ecologists can now interpret the
impact of human activities and help prevent the destruction of
ecosystems that support all life and are necessary for the survival of
the human species (E.P. Odum, 1993).

Predictive analyses are also used in the field of public health,
where the primary goal is preventing disease and promoting the
health of humans. Altering the environment or behavior of people to
prevent disease has usually involved a systematic grasp of scientific
data. The more sophisticated techniques used by systems ecologists
have only recently been recognized by public health practitioners,
however.

A systems approach to environmental health problems also
encompasses disciplines outside the physical and biological sciences.
To develop environmental health policy without assessing social and
economic consequences is impractical in a world strongly influenced
by values defined by money. For example, strategies for promoting
economic "growth" are usually recommended for poor countries, but
such growth can destroy the natural resources that have helped protect public heath. Combining techniques from the fields of systems
ecology, environmental engineering, human ecology, and economics
is now recognized to be important for environmental protection
(Costanza, 1991), and will play an important role in the future of public health. In many instances there *are* solutions that protect public
health, maintain ecosystems, and support healthy economies.

Those who have difficulty viewing the environment as a system
of interconnected processes can learn the systems perspective from
introductory texts in ecology and environmental sciences that are listed at the end of Chapter 1. Readers who find the systems approach to
be obvious and, perhaps, overly simplistic can delve more deeply into
papers and texts on systems theory and modeling in ecology, hydrology, physiology, toxicology, and the atmospheric, marine, and computer sciences.

EDUCATIONAL OBJECTIVES

This book is designed to give an overview of environmental health for students in the biological and health sciences. Although we assume that readers are familiar with the material covered in the core curriculum of public health training programs, those with strong backgrounds in the biological sciences should have little trouble understanding the material we cover. We're sorry there is not enough room in this text to cover the areas of environmental engineering, economics, urban and regional planning, and demography. An understanding of the ideas in these fields is also important to the practice of environmental health. We hope that the perspective provided in this text will stimulate the further study in these areas and help students integrate these disciplines with those of public health.

After reading this text, the student should be able to:

1. Identify the pathways through which humans are exposed to toxic agents and trace an agent of interest from its origin to the sites of damage in the human body;
2. Classify toxic agents by their physical, chemical, and biological properties and, for each type of agent, be able to describe the routes of environmental transport and mechanisms of human toxicity for representative agents;
3. Describe the activities of humans and the effects of ecotoxicants that can damage ecosystems to the point that the health of humans and other species are jeopardized. Discuss approaches to altering these activities to avoid or minimize such damage;
4. Describe the ways by which toxic agents contaminate food and identify the natural processes that impact food-chain transport;
5. List the major air pollutants and the factors that influence doses to humans from atmospheric routes;
6. Describe the hydrologic cycle, the important water pollutants, the problems we face in supplying water for human populations, and the problems associated with insuring adequate water for ecosystem health;

7. Describe the themes or philosophies on which environmental laws are based and list the major U.S. laws used to protect the environment and human health;
8. List the leading causes of occupational morbidity and mortality and discuss the ways practitioners of occupational health try to improve the health of workers; and
9. Describe the techniques used to assess the potential for human toxicity from toxic agents in the environment.

WILL THIS TEXT BE OUT OF DATE BY THE TIME YOU READ IT?

It is often said that the information in any new book is around 4 years out of date from the day it is published. This is an accurate reflection of the time lags involved in writing, editing, and publishing a textbook. Because the field of environmental health is an extremely active one, new articles and books with relevant information appear daily. For the following reasons, we think the second edition will be an exception to the "4 -year" principle.

1. We have tried hard to obtain the latest data for the topics we present. Many sources were updated two or more times during the preparation of this edition.
2. We have limited the material we present to methods and findings that have been generally accepted by the scientific community. In areas that are still controversial, we have tried to present the evidence on both sides and not jump to conclusions. Information presented in this way will be less susceptible to replacement by new studies. In addition, the systems approach we used to help link the facts is "state-of-the-art" and unlikely to become dated.

Although textbooks are not really good for providing the latest information, readers need not despair. An on-line computer information system, which includes a computer, modem, telephone, and an Internet connection, will allow you to access the latest data in every subject area. New information sources and user-friendly interfaces are always being developed and provided via modem through the 'net' and other modem-accessible sources, such as the National Library of

Medicine. The guides prepared by Hane (1992) and Rittner (1992) will get you started. Recent articles can also be found in the environmental health journals that are cited in the reference section of each chapter; the tables of contents of many of these can be browsed "online."

REFERENCES

Costanza, R. (1991). *Ecological economics: The science and management of sustainability.* New York: Columbia University Press.

Hane, P. (Ed.). (1992). *Environment online: The greening of databases.* Wilton, CT: Eight Bit Books.

Institute of Medicine. (1993). *Environmental medicine and the medical school curriculum.* Washington, DC: National Academy Press.

Mullan, F. (1989). *Plagues and politics: The story of the United States Public Health Service.* New York: Basic Books.

Odum, E. P. (1993). *Ecology and our endangered life-support systems* (2nd ed.). Sunderland, MA: Sinauer Associates.

Odum, H. T. (1994). *Ecological and general systems: An introduction to systems ecology* (Rev. ed.). Niwot, CO: University Press of Colorado.

Rittner, D. (1992). *Ecolinking: Everyone's guide to online environmental information.* Berkeley, CA: Peachpit Press.

Part I

Principles of Environmental Health

Chapter 1

The Ecologic Basis of Health and Disease

A. James Ruttenber and Harvey L. Ragsdale

ENVIRONMENT AND DISEASE

The prevalence of diseases induced by environmental factors varies geographically and with the economic status of individual countries. In the heavily industrialized and economically strong "developed" countries, pollution control, changes in technology, and environmental legislation have substantially reduced human exposures to toxic agents over the past 20 years. On the other hand, new environmental problems have emerged as urban areas continue to expand. For instance, "transboundary" air quality in many regions of the United States and Europe continues to deteriorate from the combined impact of increasing automobile traffic in contiguous urban areas. Furthermore, there is good evidence that air pollution levels in many North American and European cities, although within regulatory limits, will increase the risk for death from cardiovascular and chronic pulmonary disease.

Though many developed countries have reduced the direct health risks from environmental agents, all are experiencing problems with fresh water availability that stem from high rates of consumption without regard for the capacity of regional hydrologic cycles to maintain these rates. Fossil fuel use and generation of ozone-depleting gases in industrialized countries have contributed to the "greenhouse effect" and stratospheric ozone depletion to a degree far in excess of the per capita average for the planet. Reduced availability of fresh water, the "greenhouse effect," and ozone depletion each have important indirect effects on public health.

In many of the developed countries, scientists have studied the distribution of environmental contaminants and their effects on human health and used the results from these studies to reduce dangerous environmental exposures. Governments and private agencies have funded this research and specialists in environmental health and epidemiology are employed in governments at local, state, and national levels as well as in universities and private research groups.

Common environmental diseases in the developed world are lung cancer from radon and its decay products, skin cancer from solar radiation, unintentional injuries from automobiles, intentional injuries from weapons, and allergic reactions to natural and synthetic compounds. Since the 1980s, large outbreaks of gastrointestinal illness from poorly treated drinking water have begun to occur more frequently in developed countries—due in part to the scarcity of clean drinking water sources for large populations and increased dependence on complex treatment strategies for water of marginal quality.

In the Third World many environmentally based diseases—both infectious and noninfectious—are endemic. Although diseases from environmental chemicals account for only a small portion of total morbidity and mortality in these countries, exposures to toxic agents are far higher than in Europe, North America, and in most areas in the former Soviet Union. Furthermore, urban centers in Third World countries are now experiencing the same health risks from air and water pollution as cities in heavily industrialized nations.

In Third World countries, scientific studies of the effects of toxic chemicals are rare, in part because preventing common environmental diseases involves implementing known public health measures and in part because scarce resources are allocated to health problems with more severe societal impacts. Recently, Third World governmental agencies have expressed more interest in reducing the health risks from industrial and agricultural chemicals, and scientists from other nations are beginning to assist in such efforts. Without opportunities for economic improvement, however, long-term success will not be realized.

Countries that are emerging from Third World status (South Korea and Taiwan, for example) have environmental problems common to both industrialized and Third World countries. Circumstances are similar for the East European and the other former Communist Bloc nations. These countries have air pollution levels that are among the highest in the world because the push for rapid economic growth has outpaced and "out-prioritized" the use of appropriate pollution control technology and environmental planning. There are similar problems with surface and ground water pollution. To some extent rapidly developing countries have conquered the Third World problems of sewage disposal and fresh water distribution and their environmental diseases now have longer latent periods than those for infectious diseases.

With the end of the Cold War and expanding global trade, it is getting harder to place countries in the traditional categories for development status. It is also clear that development can be defined with a variety of terms that are related to a fairly wide spectrum of environmental quality and, consequently, environmental health problems. Choucri and North (1992) have developed a "growth profile" that ranks countries according to population, natural resources, and technological development, and note that the rates of change for these categories are also important to consider.

The People's Republic of China, for instance, has one of the world's largest gross national products and is one of the largest generators of the greenhouse gas CO_2 but, because it also has the world's largest population, its per capita gross national product is similar to small Third World countries (Choucri & North, 1992). Because of extensive foreign investment in China, the level of industrial development and standard of living is rapidly expanding. As a result, air pollution from industry and coal burning (not automobiles!) is the greatest environmental health problem (Hricko, 1994).

Workers and the general public in all countries, regardless of their levels of development, are at risk for diseases caused by industrial accidents. The health effects from such accidents can vary widely, as evidenced by the explosions at chemical plants in Bhopal, India (Koplan, Falk, & Green, 1990; Mehta, Mehta, Mehta, & Makhijani, 1990), and Seveso, Italy (Bertazzi, Pesatori, Guericilena, Sanarico, &

Radice, 1992), and by the Chernobyl nuclear reactor accident in Ukraine (Ahearne, 1992; Goldman, 1992; Wilson, 1992).

Just as the risks from environmental exposures are strongly correlated with the development status of countries, they also are related to the socio-economic status of individuals and communities. The poor are almost always afforded less protection from environmental risks than the rich, whether the risks are from factories, hazardous waste sites, urban atmospheres, contaminated drinking water, or indoor environments. This is true in cities, suburbs, and rural areas as well as in the workplace, regardless of the development status of a country. Minority races and ethnic groups that have been discriminated against economically are also at increased risk for the toxic effects of environmental exposures. Just as Third World countries find it difficult to devote scarce resources to environmental health, under most economic systems the poor and minorities are also faced with prioritizing their resources. Food, housing, and the health of children are deemed more important than protection from the more abstract risks posed by environmental agents.

Although some would argue that minority groups are not consciously placed at risk from environmental hazards, there is evidence that this has happened (Commission for Racial Justice, United Church of Christ, 1987). Exposure to such risk is highest in communities with the least political power, and this lack of power is associated with either lower economic status or minority racial status, or both. Many feel that change will depend on a greatly heightened awareness of this issue. Recently in the United States, groups have begun to organize around the issue of environmental racism and make demands for environmental justice (Bullard, 1993, 1994).

It may be just as difficult to improve the environmental quality and reduce risks from environmental agents for the poor without first improving their opportunities for economic equity as it will be for Third World countries to focus on environmental health without first improving economically. On the other hand, substantial improvements in the environments of humans could be made in tandem with efforts to correct economic and racial inequities. We believe that all too often scientists working in the field of environmental health become mesmerized by the technical issues of environmental problems and lose sight of the important social aspects.

ECOSYSTEM STABILITY: THE BASIS FOR HUMAN HEALTH

Environmental health problems are not confined to the direct impact of pollutants that are inhaled, ingested, or absorbed through the skin. Toxic agents also affect human health indirectly by damaging stable ecosystems, thereby reducing their productivity and making them more hospitable to agents that pose risk to human health.

For instance, clear-cutting forests to sell timber, provide firewood for cooking or land for cattle grazing enhances the runoff of rainwater into streams and rivers. During the past few years in Bangladesh and the Philippines, severe flooding and mud slides resulted from such practices. The flooding has decreased agricultural productivity and caused the loss of many human lives through drowning and trauma. Flooding also destroyed sewage and water treatment plants, causing the spread of infectious diseases. In less developed areas where communities depend exclusively on river water, the human health impact from severely degraded surface water is immediate and difficult to correct. Destruction of tropical forests has also increased the spread of malaria and other parasitic diseases by increasing the number of stagnant water pools around partly cleared forests and the new roads constructed for logging (Shapiro, 1993).

In developed countries, deforestation and extensive urbanization in watersheds have increased concentrations of sediments and other pollutants in rivers used for public drinking water, requiring expensive water treatment to protect human health. Urban runoff laden with chemical fertilizers has increased the frequency of blooms of microorganisms in rivers and shallow coastal waters, which, in turn, have depleted oxygen concentrations and resulted in fatal anoxia in fish and other organisms.

Regardless of the development status of a country, deforestation impacts both regional and global atmospheric conditions. Destruction of forests alters patterns of regional rainfall (Myers, 1988; Shulka, 1990) and enhances global warming by removing trees and other plant species that absorb CO_2 from the atmosphere and convert it into plant biomass. Burning trees and plants also releases CO_2 to the atmosphere.

Although it may be surprising to some, the impact of deforestation on human health is not a modern problem. Throughout history, degradation of soil and surface water and flooding have followed deforestation. In the past, this practice was used to provide land for agriculture to feed expanding populations. The resulting ecological damage has been linked to the decline of civilizations in the Mediterranean region, Mesoamerica, China, and the Nile valley (Ponting, 1991).

Damage to regional and global hydrologic and atmospheric systems also produces indirect health risks. The halogenated hydrocarbons released to the atmosphere by automobile air conditioners, refrigerators, and factories are not particularly toxic to humans (unless they are exposed in an occupational setting), but they accumulate in the stratosphere and destroy the protective ozone layer. A direct result for humans is an elevated risk for skin cancer from the increased flux of ultraviolet radiation to the earth's surface.

Increased ultraviolet radiation also causes crop damage, thereby reducing farm productivity. To offset this damage farmers may try to use more fertilizers and pesticides. This strategy increases costs, fossil fuel consumption, and the potential for contaminating drinking water supplies. These public health risks, though indirect and not immediately apparent, could be more serious than the increased risk for skin cancer.

Correcting the problems from damaged ecosystems, altered global atmospheric dynamics, or contaminated regional aquifers is far more difficult than reducing concentrations of pollutants in the atmosphere of urban areas. Moreover, it may take decades to restore damaged watersheds and aquifers.

ECOSYSTEMS: MODELS FOR ENVIRONMENTAL PROCESSES

One of the simplest ways to "organize" the environment is along spatial lines, by dividing the distance between the center of the earth and the outer reaches of the atmosphere into different zones (Figure 1.1). The *lithosphere* includes the solid portion of our planet, from its center to the highest mountain; in the *hydrosphere* are bodies of water (lakes, rivers, estuaries, coastal wetlands, bays, reefs, and oceans) as

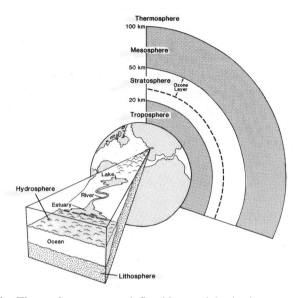

Figure 1.1   The environment, as defined by spatial criteria.

well as water stored in the ground (*groundwater*). As this figure illustrates, the *biosphere* is a zone that encompasses all life on our planet in an amazingly thin layer compared with the diameter of the earth and the thickness of its atmosphere.

The atmosphere can be divided into the *troposphere* (which includes the air near the ground) where most air pollutants from industry and automobiles are released and deposited, and the *stratosphere*, where industrial gases such as methane and chlorofluorocarbons (CFCs) accumulate and contribute to "greenhouse" warming. The outer layers are the *mesosphere* and *thermosphere*.

Although dividing the planet and its atmosphere into zones helps to locate toxic agents, this perspective does not describe the processes that lead to environmental degradation or cause humans to be exposed to toxic agents. Alternately, the environment can be viewed as a network of ecosystems (biotic communities and their physical environment functioning as systems), which are all directly or indirectly influenced by human activities. This perspective stresses the function of natural processes rather than their location. Most importantly, ecosystems can be described with diagrams (*conceptual models*) that stress how physical and chemical energy, nutrients, and water are transported and stored in the environment, and the way organisms utilize these resources for survival (Odum, 1971, 1994).

Food chains or webs (Figure 1.2) are conceptual models that describe the pathways by which energy from sunlight is converted to plant biomass by producers and then transferred to herbivores, carnivores, and humans (primary, secondary, and tertiary consumers, respectively). Beyond describing how energy is transferred in ecosystems, food webs depict the transfer and cycling of chemical nutrients. Chemicals are transferred with energy along the same pathways, but unlike energy, they are recycled within ecosystems by decomposers. Toxic chemicals from industry and other sources (Chapter 4) can enter food webs from any point and move with the flow of energy and nutrients between producers and consumers and ultimately expose humans who ingest contaminated food. Chemicals move through food webs at different rates, depending on such factors as solubility in water and lipids and the ability to form compounds with other chemicals.

The movement of toxic substances through food chains is influenced by the same natural processes and human activities that affect nutrient cycling in ecosystems. In terrestrial ecosystems, toxic chemicals are deposited from air on the leaves and other edible parts of plants where they can be ingested by consumers. Chemicals are also actively absorbed from the soil by plant roots. In aquatic ecosystems, organisms at the bases of food chains can filter large volumes of water and concentrate a variety of agents—including microbes, metals, and organic compounds. If toxic chemicals are soluble in fat (dichlorodiphenyltrichloroethane [DDT] and polychlorinated

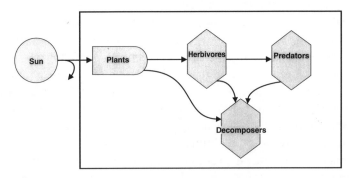

Figure 1.2   Food chain model describing general pathways for the transport of energy and toxic agents.

biphenyls [PCBs], for instance), they can be progressively concentrated at each successive level of a food chain (a process termed *bioaccumulation* or *bioamplification*).

As mentioned before, microbes that decompose the organisms in food webs also play an important role in the dynamics of toxic chemicals, releasing them to the air, soil, and water, and by converting them to new compounds that may be more or less toxic than the parent compounds.

In Figure 1.3, the atmosphere is connected to the food web, illustrating the pathways through which atmospheric contaminants can damage organisms and expose humans. Toxic agents in the atmosphere (Chapter 6) travel between its layers (Figure 1.1). The physical energy embodied in wind and heat and the chemical nature of atmospheric particles strongly influence the dynamics of air pollutants.

The distribution of an atmospheric contaminant is influenced by winds and a complexity of local climatic conditions. The production, distribution, and degradation of one toxic agent can be influenced by concentrations of other contaminants in the air. For example, photochemical smog, which contains high concentrations of ozone, is produced by a reaction between sunlight, natural oxygen, oxides of nitrogen, and organic molecules. The exhaust of motor vehicles is the main source of oxides of nitrogen; vehicles, industry, and terrestrial vegetation are the sources of organic compounds in the atmosphere.

The hydrosphere is added to the ecosystem model in Figure 1.4, and discussed in detail in Chapter 7. The cycling of water between the atmosphere, surface water, and ground water (the *hydrologic*

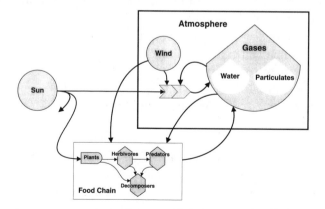

Figure 1.3 A model combining food chain and atmospheric pathways for the transport of energy and toxic agents.

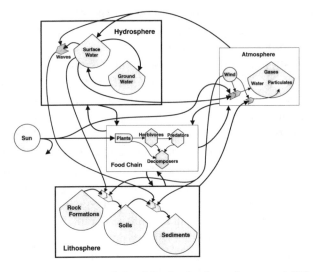

Figure 1.4 Ecosystem model with the hydrosphere and lithosphere emphasized.

cycle) maintains the water supply for all ecosystems and determines the availability of large quantities of fresh water for use by human communities. Waves and tides are the physical energies that influence the distribution of toxic agents in the hydrosphere.

Aquifers are confined zones of water in the ground that provide an important source of fresh water for human and industrial consumption. Toxic agents leached from the soil can contaminate ground water in aquifers, or can be diluted to safe concentrations by the large volumes of water. The dynamics of water in aquifers are strongly influenced by regional geology.

The distribution of toxic agents in surface water is determined by: (1) their chemical characteristics; (2) the different types of physical energy (streamflow, winds, waves, tides) associated with each aquatic ecosystem; (3) the biota in aquatic and wetland ecosystems; and (4) the particle size distribution and location of sediments within these systems.

In the lithosphere (Figure 1.4), soil in terrestrial ecosystems and sediment in aquatic ecosystems are often contaminated by industrial wastes; they are also the sites of nutrient release by decomposers. Toxic chemicals are transferred between the hydrosphere and lithosphere in aquifers and sediments. Contaminants in the lithosphere expose humans through a number of pathways, including ingestion, resuspension and subsequent inhalation, transfer to the hydrologic cycle, and ingestion of contaminated water or aquatic organisms such as fish or shellfish.

When water moves through soil, it exchanges chemicals with the soil by a process called *leaching*. Physical and chemical processes in the environment and the physical and chemical properties of the agents themselves influence the rate of leaching. The size distribution of soil particles strongly influences the rate at which toxic agents leach into ground water—small particles retard movement, larger ones increase the leaching rate.

Leaching is also affected by the chemical properties of soil, which determine whether elements or compounds will be chemically bound or physically adsorbed to soil particles. In addition, leaching is affected by both the volume and rate of water movement through soil and by the structural characteristics of soil, such as the presence of pores that enhance water flow. Although the term *leaching* is usually applied to chemicals, it also can be used to describe the movement of biologic agents such as bacteria and viruses.

In Figure 1.5, the interactions between ecosystems and industrial society are depicted. This model shows the many ways toxic agents can be introduced to natural ecosystems, and serves as the foundation for more detailed models of toxic agents in the environment.

THE NITROGEN CYCLE: A MODEL FOR THE DYNAMICS OF CHEMICALS IN ECOSYSTEMS

The illustrative models in Figures 1.2–1.5 are simple and not designed to trace specific chemicals through complex ecosystems. But general models can be expanded to provide as much detail as needed to depict the transport of toxic agents. Ecologists commonly use complex models to describe mineral or biogeochemical cycles— the systems of nutrient transfers within specific ecosystems and between all ecosystems on the planet.

The nitrogen cycle (Figure 1.6) is an example of a more complex model. The pathways in this model are similar to the ones that would be used to describe the dynamics of toxic chemicals. In fact, the techniques now used to study the dynamics of toxic chemicals in

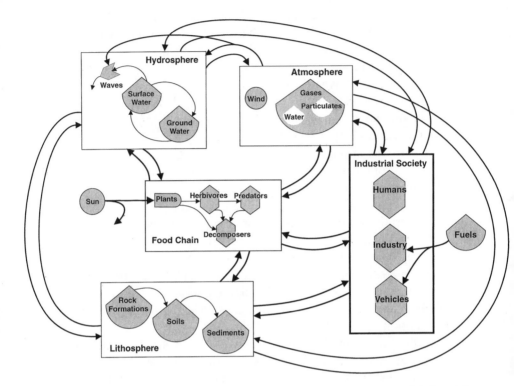

Figure 1.5   A model of the interactions between ecosystems and industrial society.

the environment have evolved from ecological studies of natural bio-geochemical cycles.

As described in Figure 1.6, nitrogen is transferred from the atmosphere, the largest reservoir of this element in the biosphere, to terrestrial and aquatic ecosystems by a variety of processes (the numbers in the following discussion correspond to pathway numbers in the model): (1) in nitrogen fixation; nitrogen gas is converted to nitrates by microorganisms and then absorbed by plant roots (the major pathway of transfer from atmospheric nitrogen to terrestrial and aquatic nitrogen compounds); (2) lightning also converts atmospheric nitrogen to nitrates, which are then transferred to terrestrial ecosystems in rain; (3) ammonia is converted to nitrates by microorganisms in a process called nitrification; (4) nitrates are converted to nitrogen by microbes in the soil (denitrification); (5) microbes decompose plants to ammonia; (6) animals excrete nitrogen com-

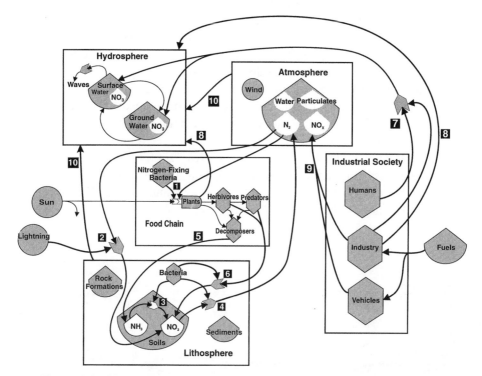

Figure 1.6   The nitrogen cycle: A model for pathways of toxic exposure.

pounds as metabolic wastes which are then converted to nitrates by microbes; (7) human metabolic wastes are converted to nitrates by microbes in sewage treatment facilities or septic tanks and released to surface or ground water; (8) industry and agriculture release nitrogen-containing compounds as liquid wastes and as runoff from fertilized fields; (9) oxides of nitrogen are released to the atmosphere by industry and motor vehicles; (10) nitrates move from soil and the atmosphere to ground and surface water.

Because the dynamics of toxic substances in the environment are similar to those of the nitrogen cycle, they can be described with conceptual models similar to the one in Figure 1.6. These diagrams depict how and where toxic agents are introduced into ecosystems, where they go, how quickly they move, and how they reach humans. A general model such as that for nitrogen is a useful template to use for constructing a new model; but ultimately a more specific model evolves—one that captures the unique dynamics of a chemical in the ecosystem to which it is released.

Figure 1.7 illustrates other conceptual models used in the field of environmental health. Notice that the symbols of each model are different and each illustrates a different level of detail. In spite of the different model styles, each can be understood after just a little practice. In this text, we use the modeling style developed by the ecologist Howard T. Odum (1971, 1994), which can be easily translated to any other style.

Models similar to the ones in Figures 1.2–1.7 are also used to organize environmental measurement data and to construct mathematical equations for analysis and computer simulation (Hall & Day, 1990; Hannon & Ruth, 1994; Odum, 1994; Roberts, Andersen, Deal,

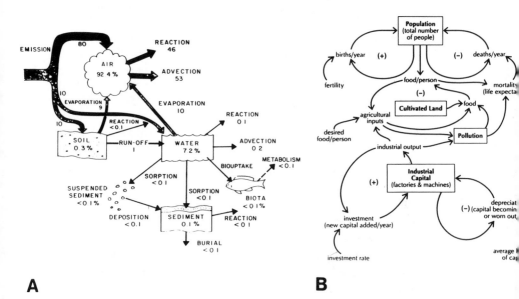

A   **B**

Figure 1.7   Other types of models used in environmental health. (A) A mass-balance model illustrating the fate (in percentages) of all trichloroethylene (TCE) released to the environment (from Mackay & Paterson [1993], with permission), and showing how quantities of toxic agents can be displayed with models. (B) A model showing the interconnections between the human population, agriculture, industrial investment, and pollution, with positive and negative signs identifying positive and negative feedback loops (from Meadows, Meadows, & Randers [1992], with permission).

Garet, & Shaffer, 1994). Such analytical approaches can be used, for instance, to predict the amount of nitrogen that enters rivers from agricultural runoff under different levels of rainfall or to compute the quantity of nitrate compounds consumed by an infant who drank well water from a contaminated aquifer. Models are also used to simulate the atmospheric dynamics associated with global warming or the depletion of ozone in the stratosphere (Charlson et al., 1992) and the deposition of toxic environmental contaminants such as radioactive isotopes from the Chernobyl nuclear power plant accident.

Both conceptual and simulation models help us answer "what if" questions and think about the presently unseen consequences of human activities. Results from analysis and simulation of environmental models have produced new insights into the magnitude of public health risks as well as ways to prevent or reduce these risks. Today, environmental health cannot be practiced without understanding and using these models — they are the tools of the modern environmental scientist.

WHERE DO TOXIC SUBSTANCES COME FROM?
WHERE DO THEY GO?

Toxic substances occur naturally and are also by-products of industry, transportation, and other human activities. When diagnosing a problem of exposure to a toxic agent in the environment, it helps to know where it comes from—how and where it was made and when it was first released to the environment. Some representative chemical and biologic agents and their sources are listed in Table 1.1. Whether toxic agents pose health risks to humans depends on their distribution in the environment—which can be predicted using the previously described ecosystem models and knowledge of the factors that influence transport within ecosystems.

The movement of a toxic substance through the environment is influenced substantially by its chemical and physical properties (Grisham, 1986). These include water solubility, ionization potential, solubility in lipids and nonaqueous solvents, and susceptibility to decomposition by light (photolysis). Such properties can increase or decrease the reactivity and toxicity of environmental agents. Metals that form ionic compounds, for example, are adsorbed on particles of clay in soil and effectively prevented from entering ground water,

Table 1.1 Environmental Pathways For Selected Toxic Agents

Toxic Agent	Disease	Source	Environmental Pathway
Biological			
Legionella pneumophila	Legionnaires' Disease	Soil, Cooling Towers	Air, Building Ventilation Systems
Giardia lamblia	Giardiasis (Chronic Diarrhea)	Human or Animal Feces	Water, Food
Salmonella species	Acute Diarrhea	Human or Animal Feces	Water, Meat, Eggs
Chemical			
Pesticides	Central and Peripheral Nervous System Disease	Agriculture	Food, Drinking Water
Dioxins	Chloracne and Soft Tissue Tumors	Herbicides, Paper Mills, Incinerators	Air, Water, Food
Polychlorinated Biphenyls (PCBs)	Chloracne, Liver Disfunction	Electrical Transformers	Air, Water, Food
Physical			
Radon-222	Lung Cancer	Rock Formations	Air, Water
Iodine-131	Thyroid Nodules and Cancer	Nuclear Power Plants and Weapons Production Facilities	Air, Dairy Products, Vegetables
Asbestos	Asbestosis, Lung Cancer	Insulation, Auto Brakes	Air, Water

whereas an organic solvent such as trichloroethylene moves easily through the same clay.

Physical properties such as density, particle size, and vapor pressure also determine the environmental distribution of toxic agents. Uranium dust is released to the atmosphere from processing uranium oxides in the production of nuclear weapons. The distance the dust travels is strongly influenced by the size of the particles. Large particles fall close to ventilation stacks and smaller particles are transported greater distances.

The location of toxic agents within an ecosystem also determines whether they pose health risks to humans. Many industries contaminate air, water, and soil with the same toxic compound, but the degree of human exposure may vary for each environmental medium. Lead from a smelter, for example, vaporizes in the atmosphere and can be inhaled. It also adsorbs to atmospheric particles that can be inhaled if they are small enough. Particles in air eventually settle on vegetation or soil where they may be ingested by humans or resuspended by vehicles or animals and then inhaled.

Lead can move from soil to ground or surface water and provide exposure by contaminating water used for irrigation or drinking. Foodchain exposure is possible if humans ingest leafy vegetables contaminated by lead from the atmosphere. Although lead in soil is not absorbed by plant roots, it can contaminate food crops if it is resuspended and deposited on vegetation. Soil can also be ingested directly— especially by children playing in contaminated areas.

In the above example, persons living a great distance from the smelter would not be exposed to as much vapor as those nearby, but persons further away may be at greater risk from exposure to contaminated drinking water or to road dust than those who live closer.

The major physical forces that influence the movement and deposition of toxic agents in ecosystems are also important. In coastal ecosystems, waves, tides, and wind help determine the distribution of water pollutants (Mitsch & Gosselink, 1993). Wind is also a major factor in the movement and deposition of dry toxic particles. Rainfall causes contaminants in the atmosphere to be deposited on land and water. This happened after the Chernobyl nuclear power plant accident when terrestrial contamination from radioactive iodine and cesium was correlated with rainfall patterns.

EVALUATING ENVIRONMENTAL EXPOSURES TO TOXIC SUBSTANCES

When human exposure to toxic substances is suspected, three critical questions must be answered before attempting to quantify human exposure and to predict disease risk. The first is: *What is the suspected toxic agent?* Often a specific agent has been identified in the effluent from an industry or in environmental samples, or has been linked to illness in an exposed community. Other times only general information is available for an agent or a disease suspected to have been caused by an environmental agent. For example, all that may be known is that the liquid effluent of an industry has contaminated pathways that could expose humans and that the effluent is suspected to contain a toxic chemical.

In many instances two or more toxic agents might be implicated. Although the following discussion does not explicitly address multiple toxic agents, the principles that apply to assessing a single toxic substance also apply to multiple agents. The only difference between assessing single and multiple agents is the need to evaluate the potential interactions between multiple agents, as some increase or decrease the toxicity of others (Yang, 1994).

The next important question is: *What is the source of the toxic material?* Sources of toxic agents in the environment can be identified through analysis of environmental monitoring data collected in the past for compliance with government regulations. These historical data can be examined for concentration gradients that may help locate sources of contamination. Environmental samples taken at increasing distances from an industrial site can also help quantify its contribution to regional pollution.

When there are many possible sources of the same toxic agent, the isolation of the major ones may be difficult, as evidenced in the Woburn, Massachusetts community exposed to municipal drinking water contaminated by trichloroethylene (DiPerna, 1985; Lagakos, Wessen, & Zelen, 1986). In this particular case, several industries near the city's drinking water wells used this chemical, and extensive environmental monitoring and investigations of production records were required to pinpoint the major source.

Once the toxic agent and its suspected source are identified, then the third question should be asked: *What are the possible routes of human exposure?* The answer requires a detailed analysis of the ways by which humans could be exposed and the quantities of toxic agents associated with the different modes of exposure. Usually it is necessary to diagram the important exposure pathways with a conceptual model to identify relevant ecosystem dynamics and to keep track of environmental data. Although simple models are our best approximations at the time we draw them, they are often revised as new information becomes available.

Identifying exposure routes from an ecological perspective pinpoints important natural influences on environmental concentrations that may not have been considered when the original environmental samples were taken. Moreover, environmental measurements made for determining compliance with governmental regulations may not be adequate for making quantitative estimates of exposures to humans, as many regulations have required only cursory monitoring with inadequate sampling strategies and inappropriate detection limits for chemical analyses.

Computer simulation models are commonly used to calculate concentrations of an agent in environmental media and to describe its movement over time among components of an ecosystem. These mathematical models are particularly useful for predicting concentrations of agents in environmental media for which monitoring data are unavailable. Models for environmental transport have been used extensively in describing and predicting the environmental transport of radionuclides (Moskowitz, Pardi, DePhillips & Meinhold, 1992; Till & Meyer, 1983; Whicker & Schultz, 1982), and are becoming increasingly popular in analyses of toxic chemicals in the environment (Calabrese & Kostecki, 1992).

Models for assessing environmental movement of toxic substances depend on data that accurately reflect their release, transport, and accumulation—particularly for pathways that result in exposure to humans. In the case of chemicals contaminating ground water, measured concentrations in water samples provide the most accurate index of human exposure. This exposure could also be estimated with a model that describes the input and distribution of the contaminant from its source to an aquifer and the distribution within the aquifer.

For dairy products contaminated with a toxic chemical, measurements of concentrations in milk are the best data for estimating human exposure. When concentrations of toxic agents in milk are unavailable, chemical concentrations in vegetation samples can be multiplied by *uptake factors* to estimate concentrations in dairy products. Uptake factors are determined by experiment or from studies of other incidents of environmental contamination and are available in the scientific literature (Petron, 1993; Suter, 1993).

If there are no environmental measurements available, environmental concentrations can be approximated with transport models that estimate environmental concentrations based on the quantity of an agent released to the environment from its source. This quantity, usually expressed as mass (for chemicals) number of organisms (for microbes), or activity (for radionuclides) per unit time, is called the *source term*. It can be measured with instruments placed in the exhaust or ventilation stacks of a facility releasing toxic substances to the atmosphere, or in effluent lines from an industry that releases wastes to a body of water. Source terms can also be estimated indirectly from a factory's production records.

QUANTIFYING EXPOSURE TO TOXIC AGENTS IN THE ENVIRONMENT

Tracing toxic agents through environmental pathways will not tell us much about risks for disease. To predict disease risk, we must first estimate the amount of an agent that enters the body, the amount that is actually deposited in particular tissues or organs, and the risk for disease that would result from this deposition. To perform these analyses, certain terms must first be understood.

Exposure is the term used to describe the quantity of a toxic agent at the interface between the environment and the human body. It is a measure of the quantity of an agent that *could* enter the body, as opposed to the quantity that *does* enter the body. There are at least five different definitions for exposure to toxic agents in the environment: (1) the concentration of an agent in an environmental medium; (2) the amount of an agent available at the exchange boundaries (i.e., the lungs, gut, skin) during a specified time period (EPA, 1989); (3) the rate at which a toxic agent is released to the environment; (4) the rate per unit body weight at which the agent is taken into the body (EPA, 1988); and (5) the product of the environmental concentration and time (National Research Council, 1991; EPA, 1992).

Because the term *exposure* has been assigned conflicting definitions and units, we prefer to use it as a general, descriptive term when dealing with chemicals and biologic agents. When quantitatively describing exposure to a toxic agent in the environment, we recommend using the *environmental concentration*, measured in units of mass, activity (for radionuclides), or the number of organisms per unit volume or mass of environmental medium. Environmental concentrations can be expressed as: (1) percentage by weight, volume, or mass; (2) the quantity of an agent (mass or volume) per unit of environmental medium (measured with the same unit)—commonly expressed as parts per million (ppm) or parts per billion (ppb); or (3) units of radioactivity or number of organisms per unit area.

The concentration of sulfur dioxide (SO_2) in the atmosphere, for instance, can be expressed as micrograms per cubic meter ($\mu g/m^3$) or ppm (with *parts* having units of mass, volume, or number of molecules). The concentration of cadmium in soil might be expressed in the same units, or as percent by weight (%[wt]). Examples of these units are provided in Table 1.2.

Assigning a time dimension to exposure—as recommended by many scientists—can cause confusion, particularly in assessing exposures that are ongoing or that may occur in the future. Such conditions exist in emergency responses to accidental or purposeful releases of toxic agents to the environment. A chlorine gas release is one example that could occur anywhere. Imagine trying to quantify the exposure to a cloud of chlorine gas in units of ppm-hours. An exposure of 500 ppm-hours could occur after contact with 5,000 ppm for 0.1 hours, or after contact with 5 ppm for 100 hours—two entirely different situations with regard to public health risk. The first exposure would be lethal and the second would only irritate the upper airway. Furthermore, some would confuse the term 500 ppm-hour with the release rate of 500 ppm per hour—an entirely different circumstance.

In the above example, we suggest reporting exposure as the environmental concentration in air in units of ppm, and then estimating duration of exposure for different scenarios as needed. Coupling environmental concentration with duration of exposure is most useful when reconstructing historical exposures to environmental agents. Where possible, however, we recommend combining environmental concentration with the time dimension by computing *intake* and *dose*, as defined in the next section.

When exposures are determined by measuring concentrations in environmental media, one should be careful to obtain samples that represent actual exposures to humans. Lead, for example, is deposited on soil surfaces and accumulates there. Soil samples taken to depths of 5 or 10 cm would provide underestimates of exposure for children inhaling resuspended surface dust and ingesting soil from the first few millimeters of the soil surface.

Many different techniques can be employed to quantify exposure in the environment and alternatives should be considered in light of their detection limits, accuracy, precision, and cost. Before new measurements are made, the number of environmental samples needed to accurately characterize an exposure should first be determined (Gilbert, 1987). Preliminary estimates of exposure can be made with a limited set of measurements and these data can help determine the scope of additional data collection efforts.

INTAKE AND DOSE

In order to quantify the disease risk to humans from an environmental agent—whether a chemical, a type of radiation, or a biologic agent such as a bacterium or virus—we must first estimate how much of the agent actually enters the body or the amount that is deposited in specific tissues or organs. As was the case with quantifying exposure, there are conflicting definitions for the terms used to specify the amount of an agent that enters the body. *Intake* is defined as the quantity of an agent entering the body per unit time (µg/hr of particulate lead, for instance). Often, it is expressed as a function of the mass of the organism—µg/hr-kg, for instance. The term *uptake* is used interchangeably with intake by some; others define it differently.

Dose is the best term for quantifying the accumulation of a toxic agent in a specific tissue or organ—the site where the agent actually produces biologic damage. It is computed by multiplying intake by one or more predetermined constants (termed absorption factors or absorption efficiencies [EPA, 1989]) that account for the distribution of the agent to different tissues within the body and its deposition in these tissues. To accurately predict the dose of an agent in a specific tissue, a variety of physiologic conditions must be determined (Chapter 2). Dose, like the term intake, can be expressed as the mass of a toxic chemical deposited in a tissue, an organ, or in the entire body. Dose can also be measured on a per unit mass basis such as the mass of a toxic chemical per unit mass of a specific tissue or organ, or per unit total body mass.

It is also useful to express dose as a function of time. *Dose rate* is measured in units of mass per unit time (μg/day for particulate cadmium deposited in the lung, for instance). Like the terms dose and intake, dose rate can be expressed per unit mass of the tissue or organ in which an agent is deposited, or per unit mass of the entire body.

Although dose rate and intake are quantified with the same units, they are quite different measures. Intake describes the movement of an agent across the theoretical boundary between the environment and the exposed organism. Imagine a filter placed over your nose and mouth—everything passing through the filter in a specified time period would be considered intake.

Intake is not a measure of the deposition of an agent in tissue— dose is. If a child drank all the metallic mercury in an old-fashioned thermometer, the intake would be considered large compared with other possible environmental exposures to mercury. Such intake would result in only a small dose to the brain, however, as metallic mercury is poorly absorbed by the gastrointestinal tract and does not pass readily through the blood–brain barrier.

For estimating exposure to toxic agents in the environment we cannot overemphasize how important it is to both describe the pathways of exposure and to quantify environmental concentrations and doses. Such analyses are termed, respectively, *exposure* and *dose assessments*. When made for exposures that occurred in the past, they are called exposure or dose *reconstructions*. Both types of analysis can be performed for individuals, groups, or for theoretical persons who represent individuals with particular exposure conditions. Their data help determine the health risks associated with environmental exposure—a process termed *risk assessment* (Chapter 10).

DETERMINING EXPOSURE FOR INDIVIDUALS

Just as exposure and dose assessments are crucial for interpreting community exposures, the environmental exposure history is necessary to a clinician who is interested in evaluating exposures to an individual patient (Goldman & Peters, 1981). A good exposure history begins with clarifying whether the patient has a disease possibly caused by an environmental agent, or whether the patient is concerned about the disease risk from a specific exposure. Though a patient may be worried about both an exposure and a disease, these concerns are best separated in the first stages of the history.

If the patient has a disease, then it should be properly diagnosed before proceeding to questions of etiology. This approach helps reduce bias in both making the diagnosis and linking the disease to an environmental cause.

When a diagnosis has been made, then the search for possible causes can begin. The search should start with asking the patient what he or she thinks caused the disease. For acute diseases or symptoms, the patient can be asked about the situations that preceded their onset. Although lists of the environmental agents known to cause the disease can be obtained from textbooks, journal articles, and on-line databases, knowledge of common environmental and occupational diseases and their causes helps focus this search (Kipen & Craner, 1992; Landrigan & Baker, 1991). The patient is then asked in detail about possible exposures to the suspect environmental agents.

Although there are many preprinted forms available to clinicians for taking exposure histories, most are too general to be of much use. We recommend structuring the interview around a timeline that organizes the dates of exposure along with the dates of first symptoms of the disease. Detailed notes can be recorded for each exposure period, and should include any information that could help in making quantitative estimates of exposure, intake, or dose. Notations should include specific locations of exposure sources, reasons for suspecting exposure (e.g., odors, symptoms, visual evidence, or environmental measurements), estimated duration of exposure, and an indication of whether the patient took any precautions to prevent exposure.

If a patient presents with a question about an environmental exposure but does not suspect disease, then the exposure can be assessed by first identifying the specific agent or agents of concern, the pathways of possible exposure, and the data necessary for estimating intake and dose. This information can help guide the clinician in identifying diagnostic procedures that are appropriate for detecting evidence of biological damage from the exposure. If there is no evidence of disease, these data can be used in the process of risk assessment (Chapter 10) to determine the probability of developing disease in the future.

REFERENCES

Ahearne, J. F. (1992). Nuclear power after Chernobyl. *Science, 236*, 673-679.

Bertazzi, P. A., Zocchetti, C., Pesatori, A. C., Guercilena, S., Sanarico, M., & Radice, L. (1992). Ten-year mortality study of the population involved in the Seveso incident in 1976. *American Journal of Epidemiology, 129*, 1187-1200.

Bullard, R. D. (Ed.). (1993). *Confronting environmental racism: Voices from the grassroots*. Boston: South End Press.

Bullard, R. D. (1994). *Dumping in Dixie: Race, class, and environmental quality* (2nd ed.). Boulder, CO: Westview Press.

Calabrese, E. J., & Kostecki, P. T. (1992). *Risk assessment and environmental fate methodologies*. Boca Raton, FL: Lewis.

Charlson, R. J., Schwartz, S. E., Hales, J. M., Cess, R. D., Coakley, J. A., Hansen, J. E., & Hofmann, D. J. (1992). Climate forcing by anthropogenic aerosols. *Science, 255*, 423-430.

Choucri, N., & North, R.C. (1993). *Growth, development and environmental sustainability: Profiles and paradox*. In N. Choucri (Ed.), *Global accord: Environmental challenges and international responses*. Cambridge, MA: MIT Press.

Commission for Racial Justice, United Church of Christ. (1987). *Toxic wastes and race in the United States: A national report on the racial and socio-economic characteristics of communities with hazardous waste sites*. New York: United Church of Christ.

DiPerna, P. (1985). *Cluster mystery: Epidemic and the children of Woburn, Mass*. St. Louis: C. V. Mosby.

Environmental Protection Agency. (1988). *Superfund exposure assessment manual* (EPA/540/1-88/001). Washington, DC: U.S. Environmental Protection Agency.

Environmental Protection Agency. (1989). *Risk assessment guidance for superfund. Volume II: Environmental evaluation manual, interim final* (EPA/540/1-89/001). Springfield, VA: National Technical Information Service.

Environmental Protection Agency. (1992). Guidelines for exposure assessment; notice. *Federal Register, 57*, 22888-22938.

Gilbert, R. O. (1987). *Statistical methods for environmental pollution monitoring*. New York: Van Nostrand Reinhold.

Goldman, M. (1992). Chernobyl: A radiobiological perspective. *Science, 238*, 622-623.

Goldman, R. H., & Peters, J. M. (1981). The occupational and environmental health history. *JAMA, 246*, 2831-2836.

Grisham, J. W. (Ed.). (1986). *Health aspects of the disposal of waste chemicals*. New York: Pergamon Press.

Hall, C. A. S., & Day, J. W. (Eds.). (1990). *Ecosystem modeling in theory and practice: An introduction with case histories*. Niwot, CO: University Press of Colorado.

Hannon, B., & Ruth, M. (1994). *Dynamic modeling*. New York: Springer-Verlag.

Hricko, A. (1994). Environmental problems behind the Great Wall. *Environmental Health Perspectives, 102*, 154-159.

Kipen & Craner. (1992). Sentinel pathophysiologic conditions: An adjunct to teaching occupational and environmental disease recognition and history taking. *Environmental Research, 59*, 93-100.

Koplan, J. P., Falk, H., & Green, G. (1990). Public health lessons from the Bhopal chemical disaster. *Journal of the American Medical Association, 264*, 2795-2796.

Landrigan, P. J., & Baker, D. B. (1991). The recognition and control of occupational disease. *JAMA, 266*, 676-680.

Lagakos, S. W., Wessen, B. J., & Zelen, M. (1986). An analysis of contaminated well water and health effects in Woburn, Massachusetts. *Journal of the American Statistical Association, 81*, 583-596.

MacKay, D., & Paterson, S. (1993). Mathematical models of transport and fate. In G.W. Suter (ed.), *Ecological risk assessment*. Boca Raton, FL: Lewis.

Meadows, D.H., Meadows, D.L., & Randers, J. (1992). *Beyond the limits: Confronting global collapse, envisioning a sustainable future*. Post Mills, VT: Chelsea Green.

Mehta, P. S., Mehta, A. S., Mehta, S. J., & Makhijani, A. B. (1990). Bhopal tragedy's health effects: A review of methyl isocyanate toxicity. *JAMA, 264*, 2781-2787.

Miller, G. T. (1994). *Living in the environment: Principles, connections, and solutions* (8th ed.). Belmont, CA: Wadsworth.

Mitsch, W. J., & Gosselink, J. G. (1993). *Wetlands* (2nd ed.). New York: Van Nostrand Reinhold.

Moskowitz, P. D., Pardi, R., DePhillips, M. P., & Meinhold, A. F. (1992). Computer models used to support cleanup decision-making at hazardous and radioactive waste sites. *Risk Analysis, 12*, 591-621.

Myers, N. (1988). Tropical deforestation and climatic change. *Environmental Conservation, 15*, 293-297.

National Research Council. (1991). *Human exposure assessment for airborne pollutants: Advances and opportunities.* Washington, DC: National Academy Press.

National Institute of Radiation Protection (Sweden). (1991). *BIOMOVS (Biosphere model validation study)* (Tech. Rep. Nos. 8, 11 & 13). Stockholm, Sweden: National Institute of Radiation Protection.

Odum, H. T. (1971). *Environment, power, and society.* New York: Wiley-Interscience.

Petron, S. E. (1993). Biological transfer of contaminants in terrestrial ecosystems. In J. T. Maughan (Ed.), *Ecological assessment of hazardous waste sites.* New York: Van Nostrand Reinhold.

Ponting, C. (1991). *A green history of the world: The environment and the collapse of great civilizations.* New York: Penguin.

Raven, P. H., Berg, L. R., & Johnson, G. B. (1993). *Environment.* New York: Sunders College Publishing.

Roberts, N., Andersen, D. F., Deal, R.M., Garet, M.S., & Shaffer, W. A. (1994). *Introduction to computer simulation: The system dynamics approach.* Portland, OR: Productivity Press.

Shapiro, R. L. (1993). The effects of tropical deforestation on human health. *PSR Quarterly, 3*, 126-135.

Shulka, J. (1990). Amazon deforestation and climate change. *Science, 247*, 1322-1325.

Suter, G. W. (1993). *Ecological risk assessment.* Boca Raton, FL: Lewis.

Till, J. E., & Meyer, R. H. (Eds.). (1983). *Radiological assessment: A textbook on environmental dose analysis.* Washington, DC: U.S. Government Printing Office.

Whicker, F. W., & Schultz, V. (1982). *Radioecology: Nuclear energy and the environment* (Vols. 1-2). Boca Raton, FL: CRC Press.

Wilson, R. (1992). A visit to Chernobyl. *Science, 236*, 1636-1640.

Yang, R. S. H. (1994). *Toxicology of chemical mixtures: Case studies, mechanisms, and novel approaches.* San Diego: Academic Press.

SUGGESTED READINGS

Bartell, S. M., Gardner, R. H., & O'Neill, R. V. (Eds.). (1992). *Ecological risk estimation.* Boca Raton, FL: Lewis.

Brown, L. R. (1994). *State of the world. 1995.* New York: Norton.

Brown, L. R., Lenssen, N. S., & Kane, H. (1995). *Vital signs 1995: The trends that are shaping our future.* New York: Norton.

Bullard, R. D. (Ed.). (1993). *Confronting environmental racism: Voices from the grassroots.* Boston: South End Press.

Butcher, S. S., Charlson, R. J., Orians, G. H., & Wolfe, G. V. (1992). *Global biochemical cycles.* New York: Harcourt, Brace, & Jovanovich.

Chivian, E., McCally, M., Hu, H., & Haines, A. (Eds.). (1993). *Critical condition: Human health and the environment.* Cambridge, MA: MIT Press.

Christopherson, R. W. (1992). *Geosystems: An introduction to physical geography.* New York: Macmillan.

Cook, J. R., Doyle, K., & Sharp, B. (1993). *The new complete guide to environmental careers.* Washington, DC: Island Press.

Costanza, R. (Ed.). (1991). *Ecological economics: The science and management of sustainability.* New York: Columbia University Press.

Costanza, R., Norton, B. G., & Haskell, B. D. (Eds.). (1992). *Ecosystem health: New goals for environmental management.* Washington, DC: Island Press.

Ellis, D. (1989). *Environments at risk: Case histories of impact assessment.* New York: Springer-Verlag.

Gilbert, R. O. (1987). *Statistical methods for environmental pollution monitoring.* New York: Van Nostrand Reinhold.

Golley, F. B. (1993). *A history of the ecosystem concept in ecology: More than the sum of the parts.* New Haven, CT: Yale University Press.

Goude, A. (1994). *The human impact on the natural environment* (4th ed.). Cambridge, MA: MIT Press.

Groffman, P. R. & Likens, G. E. (1994). *Integrated regional model: Interactions between humans and their environment.* New York: Chapman and Hall.

Hall, C. A. S., & Day, J. W. (Eds.). (1990). *Ecosystem modeling in theory and practice: An introduction with case histories.* Niwot, CO: University Press of Colorado.

Hannon, B., & Ruth, M. (1994). *Dynamic modeling.* New York: Springer-Verlag.

High Performance Systems, Inc. (1993). *Stella II technical documentation.* Hanover, NH: Author (Computer software).

Imagine That, Inc. (1994). *Extend: Performance modeling for decision support* (Version 3). San Jose, CA: Author (Computer software).

Jackson, M. H., Morris, G. P., Smith, P. G., & Crawford, J. F. (1989). *Environmental health reference book.* London: Butterworths.

Keith, L. H. (Ed.). (1988). *Principles of environmental sampling.* Washington, DC: American Chemical Society.

Keller, E. A. (1992). *Environmental geology* (6th ed.). New York: Macmillan.

Lake, J. V., Bock, G. R., & Ackrill (Eds). (1993). *Environmental change and human health.* Chichester: Wiley.

Last, J. M. (1987). *Public health and human ecology.* East Norwalk, CT: Appleton & Lange.

Maughan, J. T. (Eds.). (1993). *Ecological assessment of hazardous waste sites.* New York: Van Nostrand Reinhold.

Meadows, D. H., Meadows, D. L., & Randers, J. (1992). *Beyond the limits: Confronting global collapse, envisioning a sustainable future.* Post Mills, VT: Chelsea Green.

Miller, J. A., Friedman, S. M., Grigsby, D. C., & Huddle, A. (Eds.). (1993). *Bibliography of environmental literature.* Washington, DC: Island Press.

Mitsch, W. J., & Jorgensen, S. E. (Eds.). (1989). *Ecological engineering.* New York: Wiley-Interscience.

Mitsch, W. J., & Gosselink, J. G. (1993). *Wetlands* (2nd ed.). New York: Van Nostrand Reinhold.

Moeller, D. W. (1992). *Environmental health.* Cambridge, MA: Harvard University Press.

Myers, N. (1993). *Gaia, an atlas of planet management* (Rev. ed.). New York: Anchor Books.

Myers, N. (1994). *Scarcity or abundance?: A debate on the environment.* New York: Norton.

Myers, N. (1994). *Ultimate security: The environmental basis of political stability.* New York : Norton.

Odum, E. P. (1983). *Basic ecology.* Philadelphia: Saunders.

Odum, E. P. (1993). *Ecology and our endangered life-support systems* (2nd ed.). Sunderland, MA: Sinauer Associates.

Odum, H. T. (1994). *Ecological and general systems: An introduction to systems ecology* (Rev. ed.). Niwot, CO: University Press of Colorado.

Organization for Economic Cooperation and Development. (1991). *Environmental data compendium 1991.* Paris: Author.

Roberts, N., Andersen, D. F., Deal, R. M., Garet, M. S., & Shaffer, W. A. (1994). *Introduction to computer simulation: The system dynamics approach.* Portland, OR: Productivity Press.

Schlesinger, W. H. (1991). *Biogeochemistry—an analysis of global change.* San Diego: Academic Press.

Suter, G. W. (1993). *Ecological risk assessment.* Boca Raton, FL: Lewis.

Turner, B. L. (1990). *The earth as transformed by human action.* Cambridge: Cambridge University Press.

Weeks, J. R. (1992). *Population: An introduction to concepts and issues* (5th ed.). Belmont, CA: Wadsworth.

White, I. D., Mottershead, D. N., & Harrison, S. J. (1992). *Environmental systems: An introductory text* (2nd ed.). London: Chapman & Hall.

World Bank. (1994). *World development report 1994.* New York: Oxford.

World Health Organization Commission on Health and the Environment. (1992). *Our planet, our health: Report of the WHO Commission on Health & the Environment.* Geneva, Switzerland: WHO.

World Resources Institute. (1994). *World Resources 1994-95.* New York: Oxford University Press.

World Resources Institute. (1994). *The 1994 information please environmental almanac.* New York: Houghton Mifflin.

Chapter 2

The Pathophysiology of Environmental Diseases

A. James Ruttenber and Renate D. Kimbrough

The study of diseases related to environmental exposures involves many disciplines in the health sciences, including toxicology, pathology, physiology, as well as various clinical specialties, particularly occupational and environmental medicine. In order to predict the health effects from environmental toxicants, a basic understanding of the mechanisms of toxicity is required. The issues discussed generally in this chapter provide such a foundation—particularly for those without training in medicine or the biological sciences; they can be explored more thoroughly in texts from the forementioned disciplines, some of which are listed at the end of this chapter.

THE INTAKE OF TOXIC AGENTS

Chemical agents in the environment gain access to living cells by inhalation, ingestion, or dermal absorption, whereas physical agents such as ionizing and nonionizing radiation pass through the body as electromagnetic radiation. Evaluating exposure to a toxic substance begins with describing the way it enters the body. As discussed in Chapter 1, the quantity of a toxicant that reaches a specific tissue depends on the chemical and physical properties of the agent, its location in the environment, its concentration in environmental media, and many different physiological factors.

The Respiratory System

The respiratory system (Figure 2.1) is commonly affected by environmental agents and is often the body's first line of defense against them. The nasopharynx, larynx, trachea, and the main bronchi compose the upper airway. The middle and lower airways comprise the network of smaller bronchi, bronchioles and alveoli. The surface area of the respiratory tract ranges between 80 and 100 m^2, approximately the size of a tennis court, and the highly compartmentalized surface area of the terminal airways comprises some 300 million tiny alveoli. An individual inspires about 10,000 to 20,000 L of air per day, and each liter may contain several million suspended particles and a variety of inorganic and organic gases.

Neuroreceptors located throughout the respiratory system provide the first line of defense against inspired toxic gases. Stimulation of different receptors leads to coughing, sneezing, laryngospasm, bronchoconstriction, or tachypnea.

Material deposited in the upper airways is absorbed through the epithelium or cleared by different processes at three distinct levels within the respiratory tract. In the nasopharynx, inspired particles are deposited on fine hairs and the epithelium of the narrow and tortuous passages of the nose. Clearance is accomplished by nose blowing, sneezing, coughing, mucociliary action, and swallowing. Relatively insoluble particles that impact the ciliated regions of the nasopharynx are deposited on a mucous blanket that moves particles toward the pharynx where they mix with saliva and are swallowed. The mucous blanket is critically important to clearance in this region of the respiratory tract. Intrinsic and extrinsic factors that affect ciliary action also modify the rate at which an irritant is cleared.

In the tracheobronchial tree, inspired particles are removed from the air stream by sedimentation and diffusion. Once a particle is deposited, it is cleared by coughing or mucociliary action or it is absorbed by blood. The lower alveolar zone of the respiratory tract is not ciliated and particles deposited there may be phagocytized and moved toward the ciliated epithelium by alveolar macrophages. These cells help prevent particles from penetrating the alveolar wall.

Injured or dying macrophages leak proteolytic enzymes—a process that has been implicated in the pathogenesis of emphysema. In addition, macrophages tend to concentrate irritants and toxins into

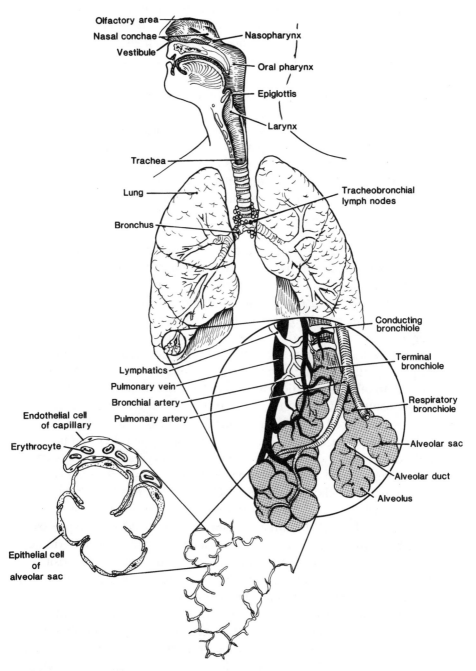

Figure 2.1   Anatomy of the human respiratory tract.

"hot spots," thereby magnifying their pathogenic effects. Particles not otherwise cleared may be transported across the respiratory epithelium to the lymphatic and circulatory systems. Although removed from the respiratory tissues, these particles may cause damage elsewhere in the body.

How well particles deposit at epithelial surfaces depends on three factors: (1) the anatomy of the respiratory tract; (2) the aerodynamic diameters of the inspired particles, and (3) the pattern of breathing. Because inspired particles are usually irregularly shaped, their size is more accurately measured with units that account for their effective aerodynamic diameter as determined by size, shape, and density. Inertia and sedimentation primarily influence the rate at which large particles deposit; Brownian diffusion acts chiefly on the smallest particles.

Anatomic factors affecting deposition include airway diameter, the number and size of the angles an inspired particle encounters, and the distance a particle travels to reach the alveolar walls. The air stream velocity is also important and can vary with a switch from nose to mouth breathing and with any change in the volume of the lungs, whether from aging or disease. Breathing patterns also help determine the air-flow velocity and, to a degree, the number of inspired particles. The volume and frequency of inspiration affects the length of time a particle resides in the respiratory tract and hence the probability it will be deposited due to gravitation and diffusion.

As described in Chapter 6, substances in the atmosphere occur in many different chemical and physical forms, and these properties help determine the location of damage in the respiratory system. Gases, vapors, and aerosols (suspensions of fine solids or liquids in a gas) move throughout the system. On the other hand, the size of a solid particle or liquid droplet determines how far into the respiratory system it will travel (Figure 2.2). Gravity and impaction (the process by which a particle is trapped at a bend in an airway) determine where particles greater than 1 micron (μm) in diameter are deposited. For particles less than 0.5 μm in diameter and for gases, retention in pulmonary tissue is determined by diffusion.

Particles between 5 and 20 μm in diameter—road sand and wood dust, for example—are deposited in the nose and pharynx; those between 1 and 5 μm reach the bronchioles and alveoli. Fibers like asbestos and fiberglass have high ratios of length to diameter,

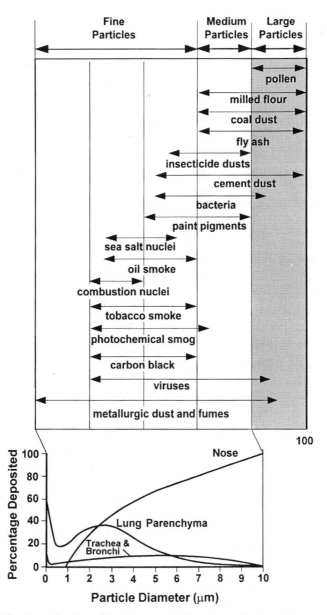

Figure 2.2 Particle sizes for common environmental contaminants and the sites of their deposition within the respiratory tract, assuming a respiratory rate of 15 per minute and a tidal volume of 700 to 750 mL. (Based on data from Frumkin, 1995; Miller, 1994; Task Group on Lung Dynamics, Committee II, International Commission on Radiological Protection, 1966.)

which allow them to be trapped in small airways. Particles smaller than 0.5 μm are usually exhaled.

The rates of absorption of inspired gases are determined by their solubility and chemical reactivity as well as by the rate and depth of respiration. Soluble gases such as sulfur dioxide (SO_2) are largely absorbed in the upper airway. There they may be buffered or detoxified and then diffuse into the circulatory system. Gases in ambient air can also produce local damage. SO_2 from automobile exhaust and other sources is adsorbed onto particulates and the two pollutants act synergistically to cause damage, especially if the particles are less than 1 μm in diameter. Less soluble gases such as nitrogen dioxide (NO_2) and ozone move more deeply into the respiratory tract. Despite the relatively low solubility of these gases, the large alveolar surface area of the lung enables fairly efficient absorption. Nonirritant gases such as carbon monoxide (CO) bypass the defense mechanisms of the upper airway and are efficiently absorbed in the lower respiratory tract.

Solubility in physiologic fluids determines the extent to which a chemical enters the bloodstream from the lungs. Soluble compounds pass through alveolar cell membranes into adjoining capillaries, whereas insoluble particles are trapped and either exhaled, deposited in connective tissue, engulfed by macrophages and moved to regional lymph nodes, or expelled in sputum. The mere presence of a toxic substance in air does not necessarily mean it will damage the respiratory system or enter the bloodstream and thereby damage other tissues.

The Gastrointestinal Tract

Ingestion is another common mode of intake, which exposes the epithelium of the gastrointestinal tract to chemicals as they are absorbed in the stomach and small intestine and transported to the bloodstream. Vomiting and diarrhea are effective responses for removing toxicants from the gastrointestinal tract, as are stomach acids that hydrolyze toxic compounds and digestive enzymes that destroy toxic molecules such as snake venom.

On the other hand, the relatively low acidity of the infant's stomach is an excellent environment for bacteria to convert nitrates to nitrites. Fetal hemoglobin, the predominant form of hemoglobin in the blood of infants less than three months old, is much more rapidly oxidized by nitrites than adult hemoglobin, making them more susceptible than adults to methemoglobinemia.

Chemicals in the intestines are also diluted by secreted fluids and metabolized by resident bacteria. The mucosa of the gastrointestinal tract protects against many chemical and biological agents, preferentially allowing lipid-soluble compounds to pass into the bloodstream. The pH in the stomach and small intestine also affects the solubility of many chemicals and thus their absorption. Chemicals that are not absorbed by the upper gastrointestinal tract can damage the lining of the large intestine.

The Skin

The skin is an important site of intake, particularly for nonpolar chemicals that are soluble in lipids. For many polar compounds and biologic agents, the skin is an effective barrier to intake. Cuts, abrasions, burns, and skin diseases permit local absorption of chemicals and microorganisms. Nuclear workers, for example, have received internal radiation doses from radioactive materials that contaminated wounds from occupational injuries. The scrotum of males of all ages and the skin of neonates (especially premature infants) are more easily penetrated by nonpolar chemicals.

Metabolism and Distribution of Chemicals

With the possible exception of chemicals that elicit immune responses, chemical toxicity is related to dose, regardless of the route of exposure. Therefore, quantitative estimates of dose, intake, or exposure are necessary to predict the extent of damage from a toxicant. The frequency with which doses are received also influences toxicity—a dose administered at one time is usually more toxic than if the same amount is administered in small increments over a longer time period. The characteristics of specific toxic agents must also be understood before interpreting their health risks. Such information is available in many reference texts and computerized databases that list chemical and toxicologic data in a retrievable and understandable fashion.

Once inside the body, chemicals are distributed locally by active or passive diffusion and throughout the body by the circulatory and lymphatic systems. They may cause damage at the site of entry, or at other locations as they are distributed in the body. Chemicals can be metabolized to compounds that are either more or less toxic than the parent compounds. Figure 2.3 is a conceptual model describing many of the tissues commonly affected by toxic substances and the routes of transfer for these substances.

Like the models of environmental processes illustrated in Chapter 1, the general conceptual model in Figure 2.3 can be modified to describe in detail the dynamics of any toxicant. Mathematical equations can then be developed for predicting the dynamics of toxicants. The models and equations can also be simulated by computer to extend predictive capabilities over a wide range of conditions. Such physiologically-based pharmacokinetic models are now used extensively to estimate doses and health risks from exposures to toxic chemicals (Cox, 1990; Johannsen, 1990; Tuler & Hattis, 1990; Krishnan, Andersen, Clewell, & Yang, 1994). Before using such models for predictive purposes, however, they must be validated with laboratory measurements of the absorption, metabolism, and excretion of the specific chemical compound of interest.

Cells in the liver and kidney play major roles in metabolizing toxic chemicals; concentrations of many chemicals are high in these organs soon after exposure. Specific chemicals are also preferentially concentrated in other organs. Nonpolar lipid-soluble compounds such as dichlorodiphenyltrichloroethane (DDT) and polychlorinated biphenyls (PCBs) pass through cell membranes easily, are preferentially stored in body fat, and may be excreted in breast milk. Lead enters the cytoplasm of red blood cells and is deposited in the endosteum of bone. Iodine, including its radioactive isotopes, is preferentially concentrated in the thyroid gland. Other tissues, such as those in the placenta and brain, retard the transfer of chemicals. For example, the blood–brain barrier is virtually impermeable to those chemicals that are ionized or bound to proteins.

Toxic chemicals are also bound to plasma proteins, other proteins, and other molecules; this binding affects both their distribution

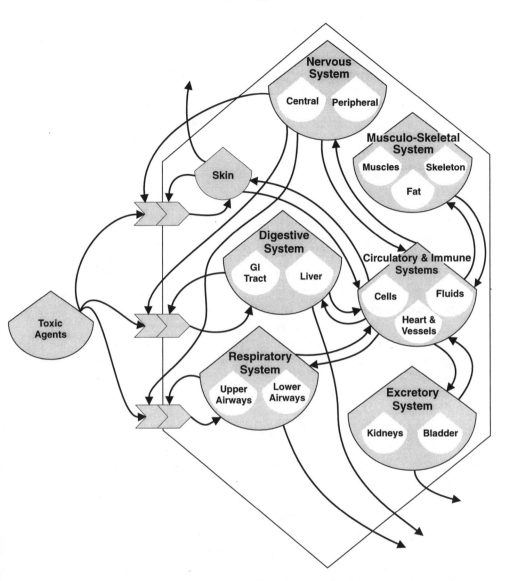

Figure 2.3   A model of the routes of intake, distribution, excretion, and elimination of toxic agents in the body.

and elimination. Although the immune system is best known for destroying invading microorganisms, it also modifies the toxicity of some chemicals—particularly toxins produced by bacteria.

At the cellular level toxic chemicals are eliminated by active transport, filtration, and diffusion. They are then exhaled through the lungs, excreted in urine by the kidneys, secreted in sweat, saliva, or sputum, or further metabolized in the digestive system, and then eliminated. A measure of the residence time for a toxic chemical is its *biological half-life*, the time it takes to eliminate half the quantity of the chemical that was originally taken into the body.

Quantifying Toxicity

Toxicologists often assess the toxicity of chemicals by administering them to animals and studying their effects. Toxic effects, however, are not constant within a single species and may vary widely between different species. This is because toxicity is influenced by many genetic, behavioral, and environmental factors. One of the crudest measures of toxicity is the median lethal dose or LD_{50}—the dose that produces death in 50% of exposed organisms. Other measures are the *Lowest Observed Effect Level* (*LOEL*), and the *No Observed Effect Level* (*NOEL*). These are defined, respectively, as the lowest dose producing a toxic effect and the highest dose producing no toxic effects.

These two measures are used to judge both acute and chronic toxicity from chemicals. For systemic toxicity other than cancer, regulatory agencies in the United States presently employ an uncertainty factor when they extrapolate results from animal experiments to humans. To estimate an acceptable lifetime dose for humans from agents that do not cause cancer, the NOEL (usually computed as the weight of the toxic chemical per unit body weight) from studies that assess toxic effects in animals over their entire lifetime is divided by an uncertainty factor of 100. This adjusts for the possibility that humans may be up to ten times more susceptible than animals to the toxic effects of chemicals and that the variability within the human population to chemical toxicity is no more than a factor of ten. The product of these two factors provides an estimate that probably errs on the side of safety. In cases where data for lifetime animal studies are not available, larger uncertainty factors may be applied.

Toxicity is also assessed by quantifying tissue damage or disease over a wide range of doses and constructing a dose–response curve. This approach is used to regulate exposures to carcinogens. The shapes of these curves can be defined by various mathematical expressions, including simple linear, supralinear, and linear-quadratic functions, linear and quadratic functions with terms that account for cell death, or quadratic and logistic functions without such terms (Figure 2.4). To protect the public health, a linear dose–response curve is assumed if a toxic agent produces tumors in laboratory animals or humans. This choice is based on the assumptions that any exposure to a carcinogen increases the risk for cancer and that, for carcinogens, there is no threshold dose (the dose below which no toxic effect is seen). These assumptions may be erroneous, however. The mechanisms by which chemicals induce cancer vary for different chemicals and there is evidence to suggest that a threshold may exist for certain carcinogens (Aldridge, 1986; Butterworth, 1990; Carlson-Lynch, Beck, & Boardman, 1994).

For some chemical and physical agents, such as noise, dose–response curves clearly exhibit a threshold. Regulations for these agents are supposed to be set below these thresholds, and risks for below-threshold exposures are considered to be zero, or much smaller than those predicted by a linear dose–response model.

Linear models do not always produce the best descriptions of dose–response relations. Logistic and quadratic functions more accurately describe the effects of agents that appear to be only slightly toxic at doses below a certain level. The more complex dose–response models also account for the effects of toxic agents at high doses, which often produce cell death without increasing the frequency of a particular disease. For instance, if radiation doses to the thyroid are high enough, all endocrine cells are killed, and none are left to become malignant.

Studies of dose–response relations in the laboratory usually do not consider the combined toxicity from exposure to multiple agents—a condition which is likely when humans are exposed in their environment. Therefore, dose-response data for a single agent must be interpreted cautiously when extrapolating the combined effects of toxic agents. Furthermore, previous exposure to an agent may reduce or enhance the severity of subsequent exposures. The toxic effects of chemicals in mixtures may be additive, synergistic, potentiating, or antagonistic. The relative concentrations of chemicals in a mixture may also influence the combined effect of the individual chemicals.

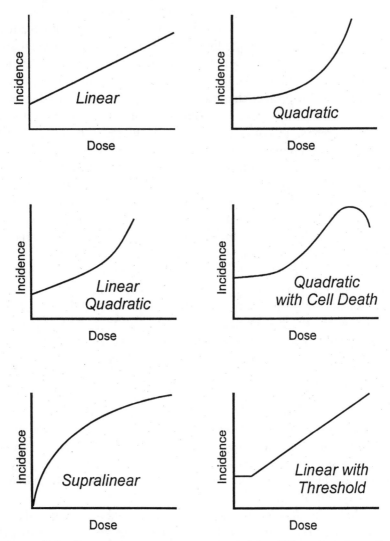

Figure 2.4   Dose–response curves generated by different mathematical models for the relation between cancer incidence and dose of a carcinogin. (See Upton, 1988 for additional information.)

Classifying Toxic Effects

The effects of toxic agents in the environment include known diseases as well as biologic effects that are not associated with recognized diseases or that may represent the early changes that precede disease. Such effects may be acute or chronic. Acute effects quickly follow exposure to precipitating agents; the pathology of these diseases commonly involves sudden changes in structure or function, which are usually transient but may be irreversible. Often, these changes are readily apparent and the responsible agents are easily identified.

Chronic effects last for long time periods, are often caused by multiple exposures, and may be irreversible. They also may follow a latent period between exposure and the first appearance of disease. For this reason, it may be difficult to identify the agents responsible for chronic toxicity.

Toxic effects can have both acute and chronic phases. For instance, gastrointestinal and neurologic disturbances occur early in the course of mercury vapor poisoning and may be followed by chronic, irreversible pulmonary fibrosis.

Hematopoietic and Immune Systems

Toxic agents in the bloodstream can damage developing and mature blood cells and induce illness by activating the immune system. Benzene interferes with the production of red and white blood cells and causes *aplastic anemia*, a disease of the bone marrow that can be irreversible. A high dose of ionizing radiation also causes transient depression of blood cell production and raises the risk for severe infections and hemorrhage. In mature red blood cells, lead inhibits enzymes and alters cell metabolism, thereby impairing heme synthesis and shortening red blood cell lifespan. Both effects contribute to anemia in victims of lead poisoning.

The immune system effectively eliminates molecules that are toxic to the host and destroys tumor cells. It comprises the bone marrow and thymus, where lymphocytes are produced and differentiate, and the lymph nodes, spleen, and lymphoid tissue of the mucosa, where lymphocytes concentrate. Damage to the immune system from toxic agents can result in *immunopotentiation,* characterized by allergic and hypersensitivity reactions, *immunosuppression,* which results in increased susceptibility to infection and cancer, or *autoimmunity,* the stimulation of an immune response to tissue of the host precipitated by *xenobiotic* agents (biologically active molecules that originate from outside the body).

There are two major types of immune response: *cell-mediated*, which involves sensitized T-lymphocytes, and *humoral*, which is implemented by antibodies in the cell-free portions of the blood. Xenobiotic agents commonly stimulate allergic reactions, which can be grouped into six categories (Gell & Coombs, 1963; Roitt, 1994):

Immediate hypersensitivity reactions (also called *allergic, anaphylactic* or *Type I* reactions) involve antigen-antibody responses that induce production of immunoglobulin E (IgE) and the release of histamine and other compounds which produce vasodilation, urticaria, and edema. Such responses usually occur in the organs where antigens from the environment are introduced: the gastrointestinal tract for antigens in food, the circulatory system for those that reach the bloodstream, and the respiratory system for inhaled antigens. *Asthma, seasonal rhinitis, and atopic dermatitis* (eczema) are examples of immediate hypersensitivity reactions to environmental substances. Asthma is induced by bioaerosols in the environment (Chapter 6) and by many different industrial chemicals such as isocyanates, formaldehyde, metals, and metal salts.

Cytotoxic (Type II) reactions are antibody-mediated responses that ultimately destroy antigen-carrying bacteria and viruses. Antibodies produced in response to an antigen may also react with cell membrane proteins in the host organism, resulting in damage to tissues such as blood cells, platelets, the glomeruli of the kidneys, and the delicate vasculature of the lung.

Arthus (Type III) reactions deposit antigen–antibody complexes in different tissues, thereby obstructing fluid transport and producing localized tissue damage. Common sites for deposition are blood vessels, skin, joints, and renal glomeruli. The acute phase of *Hypersensitivity pneumonitis*, an important environmental and occupational lung disease, involves the deposition of antigen–antibody complexes in the interstitial tissue of the lungs following exposure to a variety of organic and inorganic dusts (Rose & Newman, 1993). Heavy metals such as gold and mercury also elicit Type III responses, resulting in membranous glomerulonephritis.

In *delayed hypersensitivity (Type IV)* reactions, antigens in the skin elicit responses from T lymphocytes. As in immediate hypersensitivity reactions, delayed hypersensitivity reactions follow a previous exposure—or *sensitization*—to a chemical or a toxin (a complex chemical molecule produced by an organism). Compared with immediate hypersensitivity, the response time for delayed hypersensitivity is longer. An example of delayed hypersensitivity is contact dermatitis—an allergic response to organic chemicals or heavy metals in natural and manufactured substances—as evidenced by the rash and urticaria from poison ivy and by nickel dermatitis.

Type V or *stimulatory hypersensitivity* reactions and *innate hypersensitivity* are additional types of allergic reactions (Roitt, 1994). The former occurs when antibodies react with cell surface receptors and disrupt cell function. In the latter, excessive release of immune system components that are not associated with acquired immune responses can lead to conditions such as the adult respiratory distress syndrome.

Chemicals and biologic agents can induce other acute changes in the immune system, which can be detected as altered ratios of different types of white blood cells. Inflammation—the reaction of vascularized tissue to local damage—involves both the circulatory and immune systems and is caused by a variety of environmental agents including bacteria, viruses, chemical irritants, and both ionizing and non-ionizing radiation. Inflammatory responses can destroy, dilute, or isolate toxic agents and are also involved in hypersensitivity reactions. Acute inflammation is characterized by the build-up of fluid and plasma proteins and a local increase in the concentration of neutrophils, lymphocytes, and macrophages. Acute inflammation can resolve completely, lead to scarring or abscess formation, or progress to chronic inflammation. The features of chronic inflammation include increased concentrations of a variety of different white blood cells, proliferation of fibroblasts resulting in fibrosis, and tissue destruction. Exposures to silica and beryllium induce chronic granulomatous inflammation—characterized by clusters of macrophages, fibroblasts, and neutrophils (granulomas) that are usually surrounded by lymphocytes.

Immunosuppression from exposure to environmental agents is not well understood, and most evidence comes from animal studies. Polychlorinated biphenyls, dibenzodioxins, and certain pesticides and metals have been shown to depress the immune response in animals; similar effects, however, have not been convincingly demonstrated in humans.

Disorders of immunity sometimes present with complex clinical features that may not signal a pathophysiology that is readily traced to the immune system. The toxic oil syndrome—caused by rapeseed oil that was denatured with aniline for industrial use, but was marketed as cooking oil in Spanish villages in 1981—began with pulmonary signs and symptoms which were followed by eosinophilia and a gastrointestinal syndrome (Kilbourne et al., 1983, 1988). Some of the exposed persons then developed myalgia and muscle atrophy, skin thickening reminiscent of scleroderma, pulmonary hypertension, and vasculitis—features more consistent with an immune system disorder than those noted at the onset of disease. The causative agent in the rapeseed oil and the pathophysiology of this disease have yet to be specified.

Another progressive, multisystem disease with features of immune system damage is the eosinophilia–myalgia syndrome, which occurred as an epidemic in the United States in 1989 (Hertzman et al., 1990). This syndrome followed use of the amino acid food supplement L-tryptophan and presented with flu–like symptoms, myalgias, shortness of breath, pulmonary interstitial infiltrates, fatigue, and skin rash. Some patients later developed scleroderma-like skin thickening and rheumatoid symptoms. Other features included pulmonary hypertension, neuropathy, myocarditis, and cardiac arrhythmias. Many of these signs and symptoms are similar to those of the toxic oil syndrome. The cause of this syndrome has been narrowed to one or more contaminants of L-tryptophan and has been linked to changes in the bioengineering process used to produce L-tryptophan from bacteria (Hill et al., 1993; Philen et al., 1993).

Nervous System

Neurotoxins cause damage in both central and peripheral neurons. Not all tissues are equally vulnerable. The blood–brain barrier, for instance, restricts access to the brain for polar chemical compounds. It is maintained by tight junctions between the endothelial cells—junctions that are present throughout the nervous system. To enter the brain and other nerve tissue, molecules usually must pass through the membranes of endothelial cells, rather than between them as in other tissues. In children, the tight junctions are poorly developed and they are more susceptible than adults to central nervous system damage from certain chemicals.

The exact location of neuronal damage determines the clinical effects produced by neurotoxins. The physical and chemical properties of neurotoxins help determine where they are distributed, and thus where damage can occur. Neurotoxins compromise sensory, motor, and integrative functions. Loss or distortion of sensation may follow damage to either peripheral or central neurons, as exemplified by peripheral sensory loss in lower extremities following arsenic poisoning and visual field constriction and tremor caused by central nervous system damage from organic mercury.

Damage to motor function is characterized by weakness and paralysis and is produced by exposure to such chemicals as triethyl tin and hexachlorophene. Integrative functions of the central nervous system include coordination of sensation and movement, symbolic reasoning, and emotional responses. Organic solvents, including ethanol, commonly affect the integration of sensory and motor function (Arlien-Soborg, 1991). Inorganic lead and both the inorganic and organic forms of mercury can affect all three processes.

Neurotoxins produce both acute and chronic damage, which may be reversible or permanent. Acute irreversible central nervous system disease is caused by destruction of cells in the brain and spinal column following exposure to chemical neurotoxins, or from the bacteria and viruses that cause encephalitis and meningitis. Chronic exposure to high concentrations of manganese and acute exposure to 1,2,4,6-methylphenyl-tetrahydropyridine (MPTP)—a contaminant of an analog of the synthetic narcotic meperidine—have produced irreversible parkinsonism by destroying cells in the substantia nigra in manganese miners (Mena, Marin, Fuenzalida, & Cotzias, 1967; Cook, Fahn, & Brart, 1974) and narcotics abusers (Langston, Ballard, Tetrud, & Irwin, 1983), respectively. It is possible that chronic exposures to many chemicals in the environment are underrecognized causes of neurologic disease (Spencer, Kisby, & Ludolph, 1991).

Cell death does not always lead to irreversible neurologic disease—the remaining healthy cells can alter their function and compensate for neurons that are destroyed or damaged. Neurons can also develop tolerance to the effects of toxic agents.

Damage to the central nervous system can also reversibly alter consciousness, as evidenced by the transient intoxication produced by many organic solvents. Recovery from such exposures usually occurs when the exposure stops. A reversible form of parkinsonism following environmental exposures to CO has been observed.

A number of chronic neurologic diseases have been associated with environmental exposures: Aluminum has been hypothesized to cause Alzheimer's disease, but concentrations of this metal in tissue samples could result from but not cause Alzheimer's disease, or be due to aluminum in the chemicals used to stain brain tissue. Multiple sclerosis (a disease with pathology in both central and peripheral neurons) has occurred in clusters that suggest a viral etiology (Helmick et al., 1989), but little evidence has been developed to support this theory. Poliomyelitis is a well-known acute infection produced by a virus found in sewage-contaminated water. This infection may permanently damage peripheral nerves. Aggressive environmental monitoring for the polio virus has been suggested for Third World countries, where this disease is still a public health problem.

Cardiovascular System

Toxic agents can damage both the heart and blood vessels. Disruption of the coordinated signals in the neuronal conducting system is the most common and dangerous effect produced by toxic agents in the heart. Such damage results in *arrhythmias,* which may lead to *cardiac arrest.* Many different chemicals and drugs—nonhalogenated and halogenated industrial solvents, hydrogen sulfide, and CO, for instance—directly induce arrhythmias. Gases such as NO_2 can produce the same effect indirectly by displacing oxygen in the lung and producing anoxia in heart tissue.

Cardiac function can also be compromised by agents that induce structural damage to heart muscle (*cardiomyopathy*), which acutely or chronically disrupts the contraction of heart muscle, leading to reduced pumping ability (*congestive heart failure*), as well as to depressed circulation of blood to the entire body (*shock*). Cobalt has been linked to cardiomyopathy in beer drinkers who consumed beer that contained this element as a foam stabilizer (Morin, Foley, Martineau, & Roussel, 1967).

Hypertensive cardiac disease results from an increase in the rate and strength of cardiac contractility and from the constriction of peripheral vasculature. Chronic exposure to lead has been linked to hypertension in a number of studies (Chapter 4). Although cadmium may elevate blood pressure and cause renal damage, it has not been shown to cause hypertension in exposed workers (Fine, 1992). Some natural constituents of foods such as glycyrrhizin in licorice also induce hypertension.

Exposures to industrial chemicals have also been associated with coronary artery disease, although the mechanisms for such damage are still not clear. For example, workers exposed to carbon disulfide during the production of rayon have been shown to have increased mortality from arteriosclerotic heart disease (MacMahon & Monson, 1988). Cadmium and CO are chemicals that may damage the endothelium of blood vessels and produce atherosclerosis —deposits of lipids and fibrous tissue that can occlude the vessels and cause anoxic damage to cardiac muscle leading to *myocardial infarction.*

Coronary arteries can be occluded by acute vasospastic constriction caused by chemicals such as nicotine, cocaine, and nitrates. Studies of workers exposed to nitroglycerin, ethylene glycol dinitrate, and other aliphatic nitrates used in the manufacture of explosives and pharmaceuticals have identified increased risks for coronary vasospasm, myocardial infarction, angina, and arrhythmias on the withdrawal of exposure to these vasoactive compounds (Daum, 1992). Chronic exposure to arsenic-contaminated well water has been linked to atherosclerosis and peripheral vascular disease (blackfoot disease) in Taiwan (Chen et al., 1988; Chen et al., 1994).

Chemicals and ionizing radiation produce hemorrhage at sites throughout the body by damaging the lining of blood vessels or by disrupting the complex biochemical system responsible for blood clotting. The yellow fever virus produces gastrointestinal hemorrhage by damaging blood vessels that supply the mucosa. Hypersensitivity reactions can acutely damage the smooth muscle lining of blood vessels and produce hemorrhage. Toxic agents also disrupt the vascular membranes that maintain the blood–brain barrier and thereby enter the brain.

Digestive System

Environmental exposures to viruses, bacteria, and parasites commonly cause acute damage to the digestive system. These infections usually inflame the mucosa and result in localized fluid loss. Vomiting and failure to replace fluid by oral intake may lead to generalized fluid loss, dehydration, and, if not treated, cardiac arrest. Infants and children in Third World countries frequently die as a result of this series of events. Gastrointestinal parasites compete with their human hosts for nutrients, induce chronic inflammation and diarrhea, and may physically obstruct the intestinal tract.

The liver is an important site for metabolizing chemicals and may produce metabolites that are more toxic than their parent compounds. Acute and chronic *hepatitis* may follow exposure to many organic chemicals, including carbon tetrachloride, *aflatoxins* (organic toxins produced by a species of the fungus *Aspergilus flavus* that contaminates grains and nuts), and viruses. Hepatitis A is caused by exposure to feces-contaminated water, shellfish, and other contaminated food. Hepatitis B, hepatitis C, and non-A, non-B hepatitis are primarily transmitted by blood and body secretions, though several epidemics of non-A, non-B hepatitis have been linked to contaminated water (Gust & Purcell, 1987).

In the early stages of disease, the liver accumulates lipids. Such *fatty change* follows excessive exposure to many different chemicals, including ethanol and carbon tetrachloride. Liver necrosis may follow. Chronic exposure to toxic agents can lead to *cirrhosis*—a serious stage of liver damage, characterized by disrupted liver architecture and proliferating fibrous tissue. Cirrhosis can follow exposures to both chemical and biologic agents. Chemicals can also acutely damage the liver by altering or obstructing blood flow and producing hemorrhage and necrosis. Some drugs cause bile to accumulate in the liver, which can damage hepatocytes.

Respiratory System

The chemical, physical, and biologic properties of toxic agents, such as pH, solubility, reactivity, fibrogenicity, and immunogenicity determine the extent to which they damage the respiratory system. The physiologic status of the respiratory system and unique metabolic conditions also modify toxicity.

Substances in air, particularly in enclosed spaces, may produce acute damage by: (1) *asphyxiation* (the displacement of oxygen by other gases, resulting in death by a combination of cardiac and respiratory processes); (2) alteration of respiratory enzyme function; (3) irritation or necrosis of lung tissue; (4) constriction or obstruction of airways; (5) production of *pulmonary edema* (accumulation of fluid in the airways); (6) hemorrhage or inflammation of vascular tissue; and (7) allergic responses.

Pneumonia is another example of an acute disease that can follow exposure to bacteria, viruses, parasites, or aspirated chemicals such as petroleum products. It is characterized by inflammation and fluid secretion in the small airways and, in severe cases, cardio-respiratory failure that may be fatal.

Damage in the upper airways produces throat inflammation, dry cough, and hoarseness. In the middle airways, irritant and reactive chemicals cause inflammation, constriction of bronchi and bronchioles, bronchospasm, and asthma-like responses by a non-allergic mechanism. *Asthma* is an allergic response to chemicals and toxins that involves antibody production, airway constriction, and mucous plugging of bronchioles.

In the lower airways, toxic agents produce pulmonary edema, bronchiolar obstruction, and fibrosis. *Emphysema,* a disease most commonly caused by cigarette smoking, has also been associated with air pollution. Its pathogenesis involves the disruption of the network of elastic fibers surrounding the alveoli, producing extensive enlargement of lower airways.

Diffuse alveolar damage with edema and hemorrhage is produced by toxic agents in the epithelium of the lower airways. Alveolar damage can be caused by reactive chemicals such as oxygen in high concentrations, ammonia, and cadmium and by bacteria, viruses, and ionizing radiation. This disorder can be acute or chronic, depending on the intensity and duration of exposure. In chronic alveolar damage, the respiratory epithelium and adjoining tissue are replaced by fibrous tissue. Acute pulmonary edema produced by chemicals such as mercury vapor, chlorine, or phosgene can be fatal.

Hypersensitivity pneumonitis is a group of diseases induced by organic toxins and some reactive chemicals (Rose & Newman, 1993). This term encompasses the true allergic responses as well as pathologic effects not associated with antibody production. Farmer's lung is the classic form of hypersensitivity pneumonitis. Acute hypersensitivity pneumonitis usually resolves, but can be fatal. Prolonged responses can result in chronic disease as well as damage that is less severe and not clinically evident.

Pneumoconioses comprise a group of chronic pulmonary diseases caused by inhaled inorganic dusts. The term has also been used to describe chronic pulmonary disease associated with other agents. The damage is produced by particles less than 5 μm in diameter that deposit in the terminal bronchioles and alveoli. The pathology of these diseases is characterized by local or diffuse fibrosis; their severity depends on the intensity and duration of exposure. Common environmental pneumoconioses are asbestosis and silicosis.

Excretory System

The kidneys excrete metabolic wastes and exogenous chemicals, regulate the concentrations of salt in body fluids, and help control blood pressure. The pathophysiology of toxic exposure to the kidney is best understood by regarding the organ as a collection of *nephrons.* Each nephron comprises three important structures: (1) the glomerulus, which serves as a blood filtration unit; (2) the arterioles that carry blood to and from the glomerulus; and (3) the collecting tubule, which receives the material filtered from the glomerulus, exchanges chemical compounds, ions, and water with surrounding renal tissue, and collects the liquid wastes that are released as urine through the ureters and bladder.

The kidneys are perfused by the circulatory system and are vulnerable to blood-borne chemical and infectious agents. The capillary walls of the glomerulus can be damaged by many different chemicals, resulting in reduced filtration and release of proteins and other large molecules to the urine. Heavy metals and organic chemicals usually damage the collecting tubules near the glomerulus by inducing vasoconstriction.

Some chemicals selectively damage the epithelium of the collecting tubules, causing toxic nephropathy. These chemicals include carbon tetrachloride, ethylene glycol (antifreeze), mercuric chloride, and phosphorus. Toxic nephropathy may also result from idiosyncratic reactions to drugs and from antibiotics administered to infants.

Skin and Sensory Organs

The skin is a common site of deposition and intake for toxic agents in water, air, and soil. Reactive chemicals produce inflammation (contact dermatitis) and necrosis (chemical burns) in the epidermal, dermal, and subcutaneous layers of the skin. Parasites, bacteria, and viruses also produce inflammation, irritation, and necrosis. In addition, acute and chronic damage can be caused by nonionizing radiation from the sun, microwaves, and lasers. Such radiation can cause burns and destroy collagen in the connective tissue below the dermal layer. All forms of ionizing radiation except alpha particles, which cannot penetrate the skin's epidermal layer, cause erythema, irritation, and necrosis.

Some chemicals may discolor the skin and skin diseases may be part of a systemic reaction, such as pink disease (acrodynia) in small children poisoned by inorganic and organic forms of mercury (Warkany & Hubbard, 1951; Agocs et al., 1990), and argyria, which is caused by exposure to silver. *Chloracne,* an acneiform skin disease with comedones, hyperpigmentation, and yellow cysts, follows local or systemic exposure to polyhalogenated organic compounds, including chlorinated naphthalenes, PCBs, chlorinated dibenzofurans, and 2,3,7,8-tetrachloro-p-dioxin (TCDD).

Environmental exposures to the eye involve four regions: the cornea, the anterior chamber which contains the lens, the retina, and the optic nerve. The most common serious environmental eye injury is scarring of the cornea by chemicals, physical trauma, or electromagnetic radiation. Acute reversible contraction of the iris is a sign of toxicity from organophosphate insecticides and other chemicals that inhibit the metabolism of the neurotransmitter acetylcholine. Methanol damages the optic nerve in humans and monkeys by interfering with folic acid-dependent pathways that metabolize methanol to carbon dioxide, resulting in the accumulation of toxic concentrations of formic acid.

Cataracts can be induced by most forms of electromagnetic energy, including heat, microwaves, and X-rays, and by chemicals such as 2,4-dinitrophenol and naphthalene. Lasers and other sources of intense light can also scar the retina. Conjunctivitis is caused by a variety of chemicals, bacteria, and viruses.

The external ear, comprising the external auditory meatus, the ear canal, and the tympanic membrane (ear drum), is the site of entry for chemicals, biologic agents, and the build up of air pressure. Infection and inflammation are the most common damages, but are usually not related to air or water pollution (Calderon & Mood, 1982). The middle ear houses the delicate bones that transmit sound to the sensory cells in the inner ear. Most damage to the inner ear occurs in the sensory cells from noise and infection, though the auditory nerve can also be damaged by chemicals, including antibiotics.

An increased air pressure differential between the inner and outer ear can rupture the tympanic membrane and damage structures of the middle ear. Persons who survive lightening strikes often have damage to structures in the external, middle, and inner ear (Bergstrom, 1974).

Cancer

No other environmentally related disease has received as much attention as cancer. Cancer is the malignant variety of *neoplasia*—the process of uncontrolled and undifferentiated cell growth. It results from damage to chromosomal DNA and from the failure of the immune system to destroy malignant cells—a process called *immune surveillance*. The term *malignant* refers to both the appearance and the behavior of neoplastic cells. Compared with cells of benign neoplasms, malignant cells have enlarged nuclei, divide more frequently, and infiltrate surrounding tissues.

Genotoxic agents can induce cancer in the developing fetus by inducing mutations in DNA, and breaks and sister chromatid exchange in chromosomes. For instance, exposure to ionizing radiation in utero has been associated with induction of acute lymphocytic leukemia (Stewart, Webb, Giles & Hewitt, 1956; Stewart, Webb, & Hewitt, 1958; Stewart, 1971). Wilm's tumor of the kidney, neuroblastoma, and primary carcinoma of the liver are other cancers induced prenatally. The etiology of these tumors has not been well established, though inherited genetic damage and in utero exposure to environmental agents, such as ionizing radiation, have been suggested.

Some cancers respond to medical treatment, but many are ultimately fatal, causing death by damaging crucial organs or physiologic processes. Cancer cells can also separate from the original tumor mass or neoplasm and *metastasize* to other locations through the circulatory or lymphatic systems. At these distant sites they form new implants of the tumor.

Cancers are classified according to the type of cells from which they arise: *carcinoma* for epithelial cells, *adenocarcinoma* for secretory epithelium, *germ cell cancer* for reproductive tissue, *sarcoma* for tissue of mesenchymal (connective tissue and bone) origin, *lymphoma* for lymphatic tissue, and *leukemia* for hemopoietic tissue in the bone marrow. The etiology of many cancers is unknown. Based on results from animal studies, it is now presumed that cancer is caused or promoted by many different factors, including viral infection, diet, and physical and chemical agents.

Initiators (genotoxic agents) are carcinogens that produce mutations in DNA at different functional sites on chromosomes. They are thought to operate by activating oncogenes, interfering with the functions of tumor suppressor genes, and through mechanisms that have yet to be identified. *Promoters* (epigenetic agents) are carcinogens that stimulate cell division—thereby increasing the probability that a mutation will survive and proliferate. Some promoters are thought to stimulate tumor growth by deleting gap junctions between cells, thereby disrupting communication between them. Others, such as TCDD, act through a specific receptor molecule. Recently, a number of additional processes have been recognized to play important roles in the development of cancer. Tumor suppressor genes have been identified and shown to regulate division of cancer cells, repair of damaged DNA, and stimulation of apoptosis—the process of cell death that plays an important role in removing cells with damaged genomes and structural defects. Mutations in DNA repair genes have also been linked to hereditary cancers.

Because not all exposures to carcinogens result in cancer, the effects of carcinogens are best described as stochastic or probabilistic processes. Some exposures produce no damage, whereas others cause damage that is either repaired or results in cell death. The probability of developing cancer, however, increases with the magnitude and duration of exposure to a carcinogen.

Cancers do not appear immediately after the initial damage to cellular DNA. In humans it usually takes many years for a cancer to be recognized, though some have short *latent periods* ranging from a few months (leukemia induced by *in utero* exposure to ionizing radiation) to a few years (leukemia in adults exposed to ionizing radiation and hepatic angiosarcoma from vinyl chloride exposure). Factors such as age at tumor initiation and dose (cumulative dose as well as dose rate) of a carcinogen influence the length of the latent period.

Adverse Reproductive Outcomes and Infertility

Environmental agents affect reproduction by damaging the gametes of one or both parents, the somatic (nonreproductive) tissues of the fetus, or by altering the fertility of one or both parents. Diseases of the mother may also be deleterious to the fetus.

Genetic damage includes gains or losses of complete chromosomes, additions, rearrangements or deletions of sections of chromosomes, and mutations. Such damage can be caused by a variety of environmental agents. It is currently thought that most genetic damage is repaired by biochemical processes in the nucleus. Ova and zygotes with mutations that have not been repaired are also at risk for failing to implant in the uterus or for being spontaneously aborted following implantation. The extent of genetically induced damage in the fetus is determined by the particular enzyme systems and other physiologic processes that are under the control of the damaged DNA and the degree to which the altered DNA code is actually expressed.

Approximately 30% of implanted ova result in spontaneous abortions, with most occurring during the first trimester (Kline, Stein, & Susser, 1989). Usually, the products of conception consist of the placenta only, or the placenta and a severely deformed and nonviable fetus. In most cases a logical explanation can not be given for why a pregnancy results in miscarriage. Exposures to environmental agents have been suggested as possible causes, but these have been hard to prove.

A number of physiologic changes in pregnancy enhance the toxicity of chemicals to the fetus. Transport of digested food in the small intestine is delayed, thereby enhancing the uptake of toxic compounds. In the maternal lung, tidal volume is decreased and residual lung volume is increased, leading to increased absorption of volatile and soluble compounds.

Pregnancy also increases total body water and fat and decreases both the protein concentration in plasma and the total plasma volume.

Expanding the volume of extracellular fluid (exhibited as maternal edema) can increase the distribution of chemicals throughout the mother, and enhance transport through the placenta. The placenta has enzymes for transforming toxic chemicals. It also permits transport of non-polar compounds and blocks passage of charged molecules. Toxic chemicals can also be concentrated in amniotic fluid; from there they can penetrate the developing skin and digestive tract of the fetus.

Teratogens are agents that cause fetal abnormalities or birth defects without damaging the DNA of the fetus. They stop or retard cell replication and cause cell death. The time at which a teratogen begins to exert its effects on the fetus has a strong influence on the type of damage that results. Toxic effects can occur in the embryo before implantation, during organogenesis in the implanted embryo, and in the fetal and perinatal phases of development. The critical period for teratogenicity is from the third to the ninth week of gestation (Figure 2.5).

Birth defects are classified by structure and function, and are divided into major defects, which cause severe medical or cosmetic consequences, and minor defects, which are less significant (Jones, 1988). Examples of environmental teratogenicity include: (1) fetal rubella syndrome, which causes eye, heart, and hearing abnormalities as well as mental retardation; (2) methyl mercury poisoning or Minamata Disease which causes growth deficiency, microcephaly and neurologic damage (Chapter 4); (3) fetal iodine deficiency, which leads to mental retardation (cretinism) and neurologic damage to the eyes and ears; (4) hyperthermia—from maternal fever and, reportedly, from exposure in saunas and hot tubs—which can retard fetal growth and neurologic development; (5) maternal malnutrition, caloric restriction, and protein deficiency, which lead to growth retardation, thyroid deficiencies, and delayed maturation of the central nervous system in the fetus; (6) vitamin A and folic acid deficiencies, which cause malformations, growth retardation, and embryonic death; and (7) maternal exposure to high doses of vitamin A during pregnancy, which produces major fetal abnormalities (Lammer et al., 1985; Werler, Lammer, Rosenberg, & Mitchell, 1990).

Toxic agents impair fertility by causing mutations in sperm and ova, which often lead to cell death. Other causes of infertility from toxic exposures include damage to reproductive processes under the control of the endocrine system—spermatogenesis and ejaculation in men and oogenesis, ovulation, fertilization, and implantation in women.

Environmental agents that cause infertility include heat, which decreases sperm count and motility (Levine et al., 1990); metals such as lead, arsenic, and mercury; pesticides such as dibromochloropropane (DBCP) and kepone (chlordecone), the fumigant ethylene dibromide (EDB), and solvents (Gold & Tomich, 1994). Most cases of infertility caused by exposures to these agents have occurred in workers who were exposed to comparatively high concentrations— not in the general public.

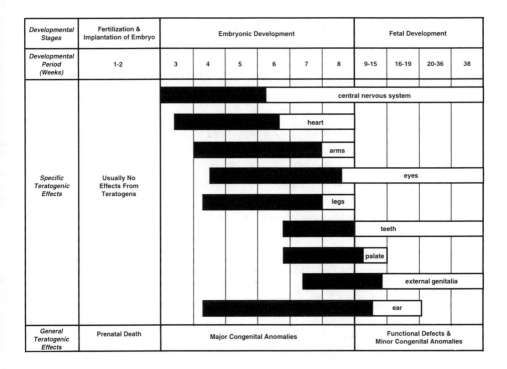

Figure 2.5   Critical periods of development for human organs and organ systems: The dark portions of the bars are the periods during which the developing embryo or fetus is highly sensitive to teratogens. (Based on data from Moore & Persaud [1993].)

Endocrine System

Little is known about the effects of environmental agents on the endocrine system of humans. Compounds such as chlorinated hydrocarbons (DDT, chlordecone, PCBs, dioxins, atrazine, and kepone), and polycyclic aromatic hydrocarbons affect estrogen production and metabolism (Davis et al., 1993; Soto, Chung, & Sonnenschein, 1994). These "xenoestrogens" have been shown to disrupt endocrine system development in a variety of wildlife species and laboratory animals (Colborn, vomSaal, & Soto, 1993; Soto, Chung, & Sonnenschein, 1994).

Because estrogens and progestins play important roles in the development of breast cancer, some have theorized that xenoestrogens may be responsible for the steady increases in breast cancer in the United States (Davis et al., 1993). Recent epidemiologic evidence is contradictory on this point for DDT and PCBs (Chapter 4). So far, there is no evidence that the effects of xenoestrogens noted in animals are found in exposed humans, but such effects would be difficult to evaluate in epidemiologic studies.

Multiple Chemical Sensitivities

After seeing patients with a variety of complaints relating to exposure to one or more chemicals and not being able to explain these findings, allergists and occupational physicians began using the term *multiple chemical sensitivities* (MCS) to describe disorders characterized by recurrent symptoms in multiple organ systems that follow exposure to many different unrelated chemicals at concentrations lower than those usually associated with disease (Cullen, 1987). Although disorders of the immune system may explain some complaints, many are not consistent with these mechanisms. Some believe that the majority of complaints have psychological origins and others postulate interactions between the immune and nervous systems.

The consistent appearance of patients with complaints more compatible with MCS than with other diagnoses has made it difficult for the medical community to disregard this complex problem. Physicians in traditional clinical specialties as well as the less-traditional clinical ecologists and environmental physicians diagnose and treat patients with MCS and related problems. The clinical ecologists have developed a variety of definitions, theories, diagnostic strategies, and treatments that rely on abnormalities in the immune system to help explain and treat MCS and other "environmental" or "ecologic" illnesses (Ashford & Miller, 1991). Many argue, however, that their theories have not been adequately tested (Terr, 1987), and recent data suggest that MCS are more closely related to psychological symptoms than to immune system dysfunction (Simon et al., 1993).

REFERENCES

Agocs, M. M., Etzel, R. A., Parrish, R. G., Paschal, D. C., Campagna, P. R., Cohen, D. S., Kilbourne, E. M., & Hesse, J. L. (1990). Mercury exposure from interior latex paint. *New England Journal of Medicine, 323,* 1096-1101.

Aldridge, W. N. (1986). The biological basis and measurement of thresholds. *Annual Review of Pharmacology and Toxicology, 26,* 39-58.

Arlien-Soborg, P. (1991). *Solvent neurotoxicity.* Boca Raton, FL: CRC Press.

Ashford, N. A., & Miller, C. S. (1991). *Chemical exposures: Low levels and high stakes.* New York: Van Nostrand Reinhold.

Bergstrom, L. (1974). The lightning-damaged ear. *Archives of Otolaryngology, 100,* 117-121.

Brodsky, C. M. (1987). Multiple chemical sensitivities and other "environmental illness": A psychiatrist's views. *Occupational Medicine: State of the Art Reviews, 2,* 695-704.

Butterworth, B. E. (1990). Consideration of both genotoxic and nongenotoxic mechanisms in predicting carcinogenic potential. *Mutation Research, 239,* 117-132.

Calderon, R.. & Mood, E. W. (1982). An epidemiological assessment of water quality and "swimmers ear." *Archives of Environmental Health, 37,* 300-305.

Carlson-Lynch, H., Beck, B. D., & Boardman, P. D. (1994). Arsenic risk assessment. *Environmental Health Perspectives, 102,* 354-356.

Chen, C-J, Wu, M-M, Lee, S-S, Wand, J-D, Cheng, S-H, & Wu, S-Y. (1988). Atherogenicity and carcinogenicity of high-arsenic artesian well water. *Atherosclerosis, 8,* 452-460.

Chen, S-L, Dzeng, S. R., Yang, M-H, Chlu, K-H, Shieh, G-M, & Wai, C. M. (1994). Arsenic species in groundwaters of the blackfoot disease area, Taiwan. *Environmental Science and Technology, 28,* 877-881.

Colborn, T., vom Saal, F. S., & Soto, A. M. (1993). Developmental effects of endocrine-disrupting chemicals in wildlife and humans. *Environmental Health Perspectives, 101,* 378-384.

Cook, D. G., Fahn, S., & Brart, K. A. (1974). Chronic manganese intoxication. *Archives of Neurology, 30,* 59-64.

Cox, L. A. (1990). Assessing cancer risks: From statistical to biological models. *Journal of Energy Engineering, 116,* 189-210.

Cullen, M. R. (1987). The worker with multiple chemical sensitivities: An overview. *Occupational Medicine: State of the Art Reviews, 2,* 655-661.

Daum, S. M. (1992). Nitroglycerin and alkyl nitrates. In W. Rom (Ed.), *Environmental and occupational medicine* (2nd ed.) (pp. 269-291). Boston: Little, Brown.

Davis, D. L., Bradlow, H. L., Wolff, M., Woodruff, T., Hoel, D. G., & Anton-Culver, H. (1993). Medical hypothesis: Xenoestrogens as preventable causes of breast cancer. *Environmental Health Perspectives, 101,* 372-377.

Fine, L. J. (1992). Occupational heart disease. In W. Rom (Ed.), *Environmental and occupational medicine* (2nd ed.) (pp. 269-291). Boston: Little, Brown.

Frumkin, H. (1995). Toxins and their effects. In B. S. Levy & D. H. Wegman (Eds.), *Occupational health: Recognizing and preventing work-related disease* (3rd ed., pp. 261-285). Boston: Little, Brown.

Gell, P. G. H., & Coombs, R. R. A. (Eds.). (1963). *Clinical aspects of immunology.* Philadelphia: Davis.

Gold, E. B., & Tomich, E. (1994). Occupational hazards to fertility and pregnancy outcome. *Occupational Medicine: State of the Art Reviews, 9,* 435-469.

Gust, I. D., & Purcell, R. H. (1987). Waterborne non-A, non-B hepatitis. *Journal of Infectious Diseases, 156,* 630-635.

Helmick, C. G., Wrigley, J. M., Zack, M. M., Bigler, W. J., Lehman, J. L., Janssen, R. ., Hartwig, E. C., & Witte, J. J. (1989). Multiple sclerosis in Key West, Florida. *American Journal of Epidemiology, 130,* 935-949.

Hertzman, P. A., Blevins, W. L., Mayer, J., Greenfield, B., Ting, M., Gleich, G. J. (1990). Association of the eosinophilia-myalgia syndrome with the ingestion of tryptophan. *New England Journal of Medicine, 322,* 869-873.

Hill, R. H., Caudill, S. P., Philen, R. M., Bailey, S. L., Flanders, W. D., Driskell, W. J., Kamb, M. L., Needham, L. L., & Sampson, E. J. (1993). Contaminants in L-tryptophan associated with eosinophilia myalgia syndrome. *Archives of Environmental Contamination and Toxicology, 25,* 134-142.

Johannsen, F. R. (1990). Risk assessment of carcinogenic and noncarcinogenic chemicals. *Critical Reviews in Toxicology, 20,* 341-367.

Jones, K. L. (1988). *Smith's recognizable patterns of human malformation.* (4th ed.) Philadelphia: Saunders.

Kilbourne, E. M., Rigau-Perez, J. G., Heath, C. W., Zack, M. M., Falk, H., Martin-Marcos, M., de Carlos, A. (1983). Clinical epidemiology of toxic-oil syndrome. Manifestation of a new illness. *New England Journal of Medicine, 309,* 1408-1414.

Kilbourne, E. M., Bernert, J. T., Posada de la Paz, M., Hill, R. H., Abaitua Borda, I., Kilbourne, B. W., & Zack, M. M. (1988). Chemical correlates of pathogenicity of oils related to the toxic oil syndrome of Spain. *American Journal of Epidemiology, 127,* 1210-1227.

Kline, J., Stein, Z., & Susser, M. (1989). *Conception to birth: Epidemiology of prenatal development* (p. 68). New York: Oxford University Press .

Krishnan, K., Andersen, M. E., Clewell, H. J., & Yang, R. S. H. (1994). Physiologically based pharmacokinetic modeling of chemical mixtures. In R. S. H. Yang *(Ed.), Toxicology of chemical mixtures: Case studies, mechanisms, and novel approaches* (pp. 399–437). San Diego: Academic Press.

Lammer, E. J., Chen, D. T., Hoar, R. M., Agnish, N. D., Benke, P. J., Braun, J. T., Curry, C. J., Fernhoff, P. M., Grix, A. W., & Lott, I. T. (1985). Retinoic acid embryopathy. *New England Journal of Medicine, 313,* 837-841.

Langston, J. W., Ballard, P., Tetrud, J. W., & Irwin, I. (1983). Chronic parkinsonism in humans due to a product of meperidine analog synthesis. *Science, 219,* 979-980.

Levine, R. J., Mathew, R. M., Chenault, C. B., Brown, M. H., Hurtt, M. E., Bentley, K. S., Mohr, K. L., & Working, P. K. (1990). Differences in the quality of semen in outdoor workers during summer and winter . *New England Journal of Medicine, 323,* 12-16 .

MacMahon, B., & Monson, R. (1988). Mortality in the U.S. rayon industry. *Journal of Occupational Medicine, 30,* 698-703.

Mena, I., Marin, O., Fuenzalida, S., & Cotzias, G. C. (1967). Chronic manganese poisoning: Clinical picture and manganese turnover. *Neurology, 17,* 128-136.

Miller, G. T. (1994). *Living in the environment: Principles, connections, and solutions* (8th ed.) Belmont, CA: Wadsworth.

Moore K. L., & Persaud, T. V. N. (1993). *The developing human: Clinically oriented embryology.* Philadelphia: Saunders.

Morin, Y. L., Foley, A. R., Martineau, G., & Roussel, J. (1967). Quebec beer-drinkers' cardiomyopathy: forty-eight cases. *Canadian Medical Association Journal, 97,* 881-883.

Philen, R. M., Hill, R. H., Flanders, W. D., Caudill, S. P., Needham, L., Sewell, L., Sampson, E. J., Falk, H., Kilbourne, E. M. (1993). Tryptophan contaminants associated with eosinophilia-myalgia syndrome. The eosinophilia-myalgia studies of Oregon, New York and New Mexico. *American Journal of Epidemiology, 138,* 154-159.

Roitt, I. (1994). *Essential immunology* (8th ed.). Oxford: Blackwell.

Rose, C. S., & Newman, L. S. (1993). Hypersensitivity pneumonitis and chronic beryllium disease. In M. I. Schwarz & T. E. King (Eds.), *Interstitial lung disease* (pp. 231–270). St. Louis: Mosby.

Simon, G. E., Daniell, W., Stockbridge, H., Claypoole, K., & Rosenstock, L. (1993). Immunologic, psychological, and neuropsychological factors in multiple chemical sensitivity. *Annals of Internal Medicine, 19*, 97-103.

Soto, A. M., Chung, K. L., & Sonnenschein, C. (1994). The pesticides endosulfan, toxaphene, and dieldrin have estrogenic effects on human estrogen-sensitive cells. *Environmental Health Perspectives, 102*, 380-383.

Spencer, P. S., Kisby, G. E., & Ludolph, A. C. (1991). Slow toxins, biologic markers, and long-latency neurodegenerative disease in the western Pacific region. *Neurology, 41*(Suppl 2), 62-66.

Stewart, A. M. (1971). Low dose radiation cancers in man. In J. P. Greenstein & A. Haddow (Eds.), *Advances in cancer research* (pp. 359-389). London: Academic Press.

Stewart, A. M., Webb, J., Giles, D., & Hewitt, D. (1956). Malignant disease in childhood and diagnostic irradiation in utero: Preliminary communication. *Lancet, 2*, 447.

Stewart, A. M., Webb, J., & Hewitt, D. (1958). A survey of childhood malignancies. *British Medical Journal, 1*, 1495-1508.

Task Group on Lung Dynamics, Committee II, International Commission on Radiological Protection, (1966). Deposition and retention models for internal dosimetry of the human respiratory tract. *Health Physics, 12*, 173-207.

Tedeschi, L. G. (1982). The Minamata disease. *American Journal of Forensic Medicine and Pathology, 3*, 335-338.

Terr, A. I. (1987). "Multiple chemical sensitivities": Immunologic critique of clinical ecology theories and practice. *Occupational Medicine: State of the Art Reviews, 2*, 683-694.

Tuler, S., & Hattis, D. (1990). Carcinogenesis risk assessment of two-carbon alkylating agents using dynamic simulation of absorption and metabolism. In L. A. Cox & P. F. Riddi (Eds.), *New risks: Issues and management* (pp. 701–709). New York: Plenum.

Upton, A. C. (1988). Epidemiology and risk assessment. In L. Gordis (Ed.), *Epidemiology and health risk assessment* (pp. 18–36). New York: Oxford University Press.

Warkany, J., & Hubbard, D. M. (1951). Adverse mercurial reactions in the form of acrodynia and related conditions. *American Journal of Diseases of Children, 81*, 335-373.

Werler, M. M., Lammer, E. J., Rosenberg, L., & Mitchell, A. A. (1990). Maternal vitamin A supplementation in relation to selected birth defects. *Teratology, 42,* 497-503.

SUGGESTED READINGS

Amdur, M. O., Doul, J. & Klaassen, C. D. (Eds.). (1991). *Casarett and Doull's toxicology: The basic science of poisons* (4th ed.). New York: Pergamon.

Cockerham, L. G., & Shane, B. S. (1994). *Basic environmental toxicology.* Boca Raton, FL: Lewis.

Cotran, R. S., Kumar, V., & Robbins, S. L. (1994). *Robbins pathologic basis of disease* (5th ed.). Philadelphia: W. B. Saunders.

Ellenhorn, M. J., & Barceloux, D. G. (1988). *Medical toxicology: Diagnosis and treatment of human poisoning.* New York: Elsevier.

Gilman, A. G., Rall, T., Nies, A. S., & Taylor, P. (Eds.). (1990). *Goodman and Gilman's the pharmacological basis of therapeutics* (8th ed.). New York: Pergamon Press.

Gold, E. B., Lasley, B. L., & Schenker, M. B. (Eds.). (1994). Reproductive hazards. *Occupational Medicine: State of the Art Reviews, 9,* Philadelphia: Hanley & Belfus.

Jones, K. L. (1988). *Smith's recognizable patterns of human malformation* (4th ed.). Philadelphia: Saunders.

Kimbrough, R. D., Mahaffey, K. R., Grandjean, P., Sandoe, S., & Rutstein, D. D. (1989). *Clinical effects of environmental chemicals.* New York: Hemisphere.

Kline, J., Stein, Z., & Susser, M. (1989). *Conception to birth: Epidemiology of prenatal development.* New York: Oxford University Press.

Lu, F. C. (1991). *Basic toxicology: Fundamentals, target organs, and risk assessment* (2nd ed.). Bristol, PA: Taylor & Francis.

Manahan, S. E. (1989). *Toxicological chemistry.* Chelsea, MI: Lewis.

Rosenstock, L., & Cullen, M. R. (Eds.). (1994). *Textbook of clinical occupational and environmental medicine.* Philadelphia: W. B. Saunders.

Smith, R. P. (1992). *A primer of environmental toxicology.* Philadelphia: Lea & Febiger.

Stacey, N. H. (1993). *Occupational toxicology.* Bristol, PA: Taylor & Francis.

Sullivan, J. B. & Krieger, G. R. (Eds.). (1992). *Hazardous materials toxicology: Clinical principles of environmental health.* Baltimore, MD: Williams and Wilkins.

Tarcher, A. B. (Ed.). (1992). *Principles and practice of environmental medicine.* New York: Plenum Medical.

Tardiff, R. G., & Rodricks, J. V. (Eds.). (1987). *Toxic substances and human risk*. New York: Plenum Press.

Timbrell, J. A. (1991). *Principles of biochemical toxicology* (2nd ed.). Bristol, PA: Taylor & Francis.

Wexler, P. (1988). *Information resources in toxicology* (2nd ed.). New York: Elsevier.

Williams, M. P. (Ed.). (1993). *Occupational and environmental reproductive hazards: A guide for clinicians*. Baltimore, MD: Williams and Wilkins.

Yang, R. S. H. (Ed.). (1994). *Toxicology of chemical mixtures: Case studies, mechanisms, and novel approaches*. San Diego: Academic Press.

Part II

Agents of Environmental Disease

Chapter 3

Infectious Agents in the Environment

Daniel S. Blumenthal

Environmentally transmitted infectious disease constitutes the oldest environmental health problem of humans. In the United States and other industrialized countries manufactured toxins and carcinogens are now generating widespread concern. In developing countries, however, infectious diseases transmitted by environmental routes remain the greatest cause of morbidity and mortality. In the United States, environmental spread of infectious disease has by no means been eliminated; thousands of cases of food- and water-borne illness—and even soil-borne parasitic infections—occur each year.

An infectious disease is considered to be environmentally transmitted when it is spread from a common source (usually food, water, or soil), by a vector, by fomites (inanimate objects), or through ventilation systems. Strictly speaking, infections transmitted from person-to-person by droplets or aerosols might be considered to be spread through the environment. Such illnesses usually cannot be controlled by environmental manipulations, however, and are thus not generally classified as environmental health concerns.

Infectious disease spread through the environment has been described in some of humanity's earliest writings. Schistosomiasis, a water-borne illness, was known in ancient Egypt. Plague, spread by an insect vector, appears in the writings of Dionysius in the third century; the first pandemic of this disease was documented in the sixth century.

The mode of transmission of these illnesses was not known until recent times. John Snow, the English physician, is credited with first documenting environmental spread of a disease when he demonstrated in the early 1850s that cholera in London was transmitted by contaminated drinking water. Snow, however, knew nothing of the microbial nature of infectious disease; he attributed cholera to the consumption of "water containing the sewage of London, and, amongst it, whatever might have come from the cholera patients..." (Snow, 1855, p. 201). Pasteur and Koch later demonstrated the role of microbes in the etiology of infectious disease.

Communicable disease control was the original mission of state and local health departments in the United States, and today infectious disease is the only environmental health hazard whose control is vested primarily with state and local officials. Regulation of toxic agents in the environment, carcinogens, and occupational health hazards is primarily the responsibility of the federal government; but the power to create and enforce sanitary codes remains in the hands of state and local health officers.

This chapter describes the most important infectious diseases spread by environmental routes. Knowledge of the pathology of these diseases, the biology of the organisms that cause them, and the mechanisms by which they are spread are important to their prevention and control. A detailed discussion of the mechanisms of spread and approaches to controlling water-borne disease appears in Chapter 7.

CLASSIFICATION OF INFECTIOUS ORGANISMS AND DISEASES

Infectious diseases may be classified (1) according to the organisms that cause them, which helps to define the approach to treatment; (2) according to their modes of transmission, which aids in environmental approaches to prevention and control; or (3) according to their characteristic signs and symptoms, which helps clarify the clinical diagnosis.

Causative Agents

Organisms infecting humans include viruses, bacteria, fungi, and parasites. The diagnosis of infectious disease involves identifying the infecting organism directly, or indirectly by immunologic or other evidence. Control of infectious disease involves both rapid identification of the infecting agent and notification of local health authorities. Requirements and recommendations for reporting diseases varies over political jurisdictions and between diseases (Benenson, 1990). Physicians and other practitioners are required to report individual cases of certain infections, and are encouraged to report outbreaks or epidemics of all infections.

Outbreaks of food- and water-borne disease caused by chemicals are often included in health department reports along with outbreaks caused by infectious agents. The chemicals may be produced in nature (as with ciguatera and scombroid fish poisoning) or by industry (Chapter 4).

Mode of Transmission

Food-borne infectious disease is transmitted when the causative organism (or a preformed toxin) is ingested by the host along with food. Organisms causing water-borne infectious disease are also usually ingested, but there are exceptions: microscopic schistosome larvae (metacercariae), for instance, penetrate the skin of individuals standing or bathing in contaminated water.

Vector-borne organisms are actively injected into the human host by an insect or other carrier. These organisms may be distinguished from those that have an intermediate host—that is, a nonhuman host that harbors the pathogen for part of its life cycle but does not transmit it actively. Examples of the former are the protozoan parasites *(Plasmodium* species) that cause malaria, which have a mosquito vector. An example of the latter are the schistosomes, the parasites that cause schistosomiasis, for which a snail is the intermediate host. If the infection is transmitted when the intermediate host is ingested by man (e.g., trichinosis, for which swine are intermediate hosts), the infection is considered food-borne.

Soil-borne parasites, such as *Ascaris lumbricoides* and hookworm, have eggs that must incubate in the soil before they become infectious. Air-borne infectious disease is sometimes considered an environmental health problem, particularly when "tight" buildings or ventilation systems play a role in transmission. Legionnaire's disease (caused by the bacteria *Legionella pneumophila*) and tuberculosis are prominent examples (Chapter 6).

Signs and Symptoms of Disease

Viruses and bacteria transmitted by food or water usually cause acute gastroenteritis, with vomiting, diarrhea, or both. There are exceptions to this rule: hepatitis A causes acute liver damage, and the *Clostridium* species that causes botulism produces a neurological syndrome.

The viruses, bacteria, and parasites that are transmitted by vectors—and that are therefore injected into the bloodstream—may cause disease in virtually any organ system, or in several at one time. Many parasites are able to migrate to various sites in the body and may cause a variety of clinical syndromes.

WATER-BORNE INFECTIOUS DISEASE

Providing sanitary water supplies to the world's population remains one of the great public health challenges. The annual death and disability of millions of people in the developing countries from water-borne infections such as diarrheal disease, schistosomiasis, and Guinea worm disease led the World Health Organization (WHO) to declare the 1980s the International Drinking Water Supply and Sanitation Decade. Only modest progress was made, however, toward the WHO goal of safe drinking water for all.

In the United States sanitary drinking water supplies often are taken for granted, yet over 30,000 rural communities (not including isolated single residences) do not have safe central water systems. During the 22-year period 1971–1992, 609 outbreaks of water-borne disease, affecting over 150,000 persons, were reported to the Centers for Disease Control and Prevention (CDC) (1993a). These numbers represent the proverbial tip of the iceberg, for the great majority of outbreaks went unreported. An outbreak of water-borne illness may or may not come to the attention of state or local health officials, depending on the size of the outbreak, the interest of local physicians, and the investigative resources of the health department.

The specific etiology of about half of all water-borne disease outbreaks reported in the United States is never identified. Most of the remainder are caused by a relatively small number of organisms and chemicals.

Parasites

In the United States a protozoa, *Giardia lamblia,* has been responsible for more reported outbreaks of water-borne disease and for more cases per outbreak than any other organism. This parasite caused over 20% of the outbreaks reported from 1971–1992 (CDC, 1988, 1990a, 1993a) and has been responsible for a number of major municipal outbreaks (Craun, 1979; Navin et al., 1985; Kent et al., 1988). It also is well-known to backpackers who drink untreated surface water in the wilderness.

Giardiasis, a nonfatal gastrointestinal illness, is characterized by intermittent diarrhea, bloating, and malabsorption. The disease is diagnosed by finding the organism in either its encysted or its motile (trophozoite) form on microscopic examination of the stool, but this may be difficult. The examination of numerous stools or even duodenal fluid may be required. For this reason, once the organism has been identified as responsible for an outbreak of illness, cases may be added to the total and patients may be treated on the basis of symptoms alone, without laboratory confirmation.

Giardia enters water supplies in the feces of humans and wild or domestic animals, which can also be infected by the parasite. *Giardia* cysts are destroyed by chlorinating water under proper conditions, but cysts may survive if the free chlorine concentration is too low or the contact time is too short. For this reason, additional treatments of flocculation, sedimentation, and filtration are recommended (Jakubowski, 1988).

Water-borne spread of the protozoan parasite *Cryptosporidium* has been documented with increasing frequency in the United States; major outbreaks with thousands of infected persons occurred in Georgia in 1987 (Hayes et al., 1989), Oregon in 1992, and Wisconsin in 1993 (CDC, 1993a). Water from large municipal drinking water systems was the source of infection in all three epidemics. Many outbreaks have been linked to suboptimal processing by flocculation, filtering, or chlorination, as well as to contamination of water by domestic sewage or animal wastes. Some argue that treatment according to current standards may not completely protect consumers from this infection (Hayes et al., 1989). In 1992, outbreaks linked to *Cryptosporidium* were equal in number to those linked to *Giardia,* and far more people developed cryptosporidiosis than giardiasis. Cryptosporidiosis is characterized by watery diarrhea, which may persist for weeks; in immunocompromised persons (such as those with AIDS), the infection may be life-threatening.

The pathogenic ameba *Entameba histolytica* causes disease ranging from nonspecific diarrhea to bloody dysentery as well as extraintestinal disease such as liver abscesses. Water-borne outbreaks of amebiasis in the United States are rare.

An estimated 200–300 million persons in Africa, Asia, and Latin America suffer from schistosomiasis (Katz, Despommier, & Gwadz, 1989). Three species of the cestode worm genus *Schistosoma* infect humans: *S. mansoni* (Africa and Latin America), *S. hematobium* (Africa), and *S. japonicum* (Asia). *Schistosoma hematobium* damages the bladder and may lead to bladder cancer; the other two species chiefly cause liver disease.

Humans become infected when wading or swimming in fresh water contaminated with feces or urine that contain schistosome eggs. The eggs hatch into free-swimming miracidia that invade certain snail species, which serve as intermediate hosts. For each species and geographic strain of schistosome, there is a specific snail species that serves as an intermediate host. Snails release cercaria into the water, and they infect humans by penetrating their skin. Schistosomiasis is not transmitted in the United States because the requisite snail species do not live here.

Dracunculis medinensis (Guinea worm), a parasitic nematode infecting an estimated 50 million persons in Pakistan and Africa, is transmitted through contaminated drinking water. A copepod—a tiny aquatic crustacean—serves as intermediate host and transmits the disease when ingested (Katz et al., 1989). The worm lives in the subcutaneous tissues of the host and causes painful disabling leg ulcers. When the human host stands in water, the adult female releases larvae through the ulcer; the larvae can then penetrate the copepods that inhabit the shallow fresh water ecosystem.

Guinea worm disease has been targeted by several United Nations component organizations for eradication by 1995, primarily through providing safe drinking water supplies to infected villages (Hopkins & Ruiz-Tiben, 1990).

Bacteria

Species of *Salmonella* and *Shigella* have long been recognized as agents of water-borne illness in the United States and reports of outbreaks continue to occur. Shigellosis is more commonly transmitted from person-to-person. In the United States between 1991–1992, it was responsible for 2 of 34 outbreaks associated with drinking water and for 3 out of 11 outbreaks associated with exposure to contaminated water during recreational activities. Salmonellosis is usually a food-borne disease (Benenson, 1990). Both salmonellosis and shigellosis are characterized by the acute onset of diarrhea, with stools that sometimes contain blood or mucus, and by fever. Both infections are generally self-limited, although asymptomatic carriage of *Salmonella* may persist for over a year.

Salmonella typhi is the agent of typhoid fever, a disease that is now uncommon in the United States; generally fewer than 600 cases per year have been reported since 1962 (CDC, 1994a). An outbreak of water-borne typhoid fever was reported in 1985 in the U.S. Virgin Islands; this was the first such report from the U.S. or its territories since 1974 (CDC, 1988).

Cholera, caused by *Vibrio cholerae*, usually is spread by contaminated water. The disease has a rapid onset with profuse watery diarrhea and dehydration. For untreated disease, the case fatality rate is about 50%, but with proper treatment, it is less than 1%.

Cholera was confined largely to Asia during the first half of the 20th century, but has spread into Africa and eastern Europe since 1961 (Benenson, 1990). It was totally absent from the United States between 1911 and 1973 but has since recurred along the Gulf Coast (Pavia et al., 1987). In 1991, an epidemic of cholera appeared in Peru and other South American countries for the first time in this century and spread rapidly to Central America and Mexico (CDC, 1993b). This epidemic and its spread has been associated with deteriorating water quality in the poor communities of these countries.

Enterotoxigenic *Escherichia coli* has long been suspected as a cause of many of the outbreaks of water-borne gastroenteritis for which no organism has been identified. It is known to be an important cause of travelers' diarrhea, which is often transmitted by drinking water. However, only very rare outbreaks of this pathogen have been documented in the U.S. (Rosenberg et al., 1977; Swerdlow et al., 1992).

Campylobacter species were not recognized as human pathogens until the mid–1970s, but in 1978 one was identified as the cause of an outbreak in Vermont affecting about 3,000 people (Haley, Gunn, Hughes, Lippy, & Craun, 1980). It now appears that members of this genus are some of the most common causes of water-borne bacterial disease in the U.S. Between 1980 and 1988 *Campylobacter* species were responsible for 13 (45%) of the 29 reported water-borne bacterial disease outbreaks (CDC, 1988, 1990a).

Viruses

Viruses known to cause water-borne disease outbreaks include Norwalk virus and related agents (Kaplan et al., 1982)—which cause gastroenteritis—and hepatitis A virus. Commercially distributed ice contaminated with a Norwalk-like virus caused over 5,000 cases of illness in three states in 1987 (CDC, 1990a). Other viruses, such as rotaviruses and enteroviruses, are suspected of causing some water-borne outbreaks. Viral outbreaks are often more difficult to identify than those caused by bacteria or parasites because relatively sophisticated laboratory techniques are needed and, in the case of hepatitis A, there is a relatively long incubation period (15–50 days).

Water Supplies

Water purification is discussed in Chapter 7. The Safe Drinking Water Act of 1974 defines three types of water systems in the United States. Community (municipal) systems serve large or small communities with at least 15 service connections or 25 year-round residents. Noncommunity (semipublic) systems are those in institutions, industries, camps, parks, or service stations that may be used by the gener-

Table 3.1   Outbreaks Associated with Water Intended for Drinking, by Etiologic Agent and Type of Water System—United States, 1991–1992 ($N = 34$)

| | Type of Water System | | | | | | | |
| | Community | | Noncommunity | | Individual | | Total | |
Agent	Outbreaks	Cases	Outbreaks	Cases	Outbreaks	Cases	Outbreaks	Cases
AGI[a]	3	10,077	19	3,252	1	38	23	13,367
Giardia	2	95	2	28	0	0	4	123
Cryptosporidium	2	3,000	1	551	0	0	3	3,551
Hepatitis A	0	0	0	0	0	0	1	10
Shigella sonnei	0	0	1	150	0	0	1	150
Nitrate	0	0	0	0	1	1	1	1
Fluoride	1	262	0		0	0	1	262
Total	**8**	**13,434**	**23**	**3,981**	**3**	**49**	**34**	**17,464**
(Percent[b])	(24)	(77)	(68)	(23)	(9)	(<1)	(100)	(100)

[a] AGI = acute gastrointestinal illness of unknown etiology.

[b] The percentage of 34 outbreaks or of 17,464 cases.

From CDC (1993c).

al public. Individual systems (generally wells and springs) are those used by single or several residences or by persons traveling outside populated areas, such as backpackers.

Over the last 20 years about 45% of water-borne disease outbreaks involved community systems and another 45% involved noncommunity systems. More recently, noncommunity systems have accounted for the majority of outbreaks but municipal systems, which serve greater numbers of people, have accounted for the great majority of cases (Table 3.1). The greatest number of outbreaks occurred during the summer and were attributed to water treatment deficiencies (Table 3.2) (CDC, 1993a). The concentration of outbreaks in summer months is largely due to the stress placed on small water treatment units in campgrounds and parks by large influxes of visitors.

Recreational Water Use

Illness caused by swimming or bathing in contaminated water is not reported systematically; hence, the magnitude of this problem is essentially unknown. Most reported outbreaks originate in swimming pools, hot tubs, or whirlpool baths, but fresh water lakes and ocean beaches have also been implicated.

Table 3.2   Outbreaks Associated with Water Intended for Drinking, by Type of Deficiency and Type of Water System—United States, 1991–1992 ($N = 34$) (From CDC 1993c).

	Type of Water System							
	Community		Noncommunity		Individual		Total	
Type of deficiency	No.	(%)	No.	(%)	No.	(%)	No.	(%)
Untreated surface water	0	(0)	0	(0)	0	(0)	0	(0)
Untreated groundwater	1	(13)	7	(30)	2	(67)	10	(29)
Treatment	5	(63)	11	(48)	1	(33)	17	(50)
Distribution system	1	(13)	4	(17)	0	(0)	5	(15)
Unknown	1	(13)	1	(4)	0	(0)	2	(6)
Total	**9**	**(100)**	**23**	**(100)**	**3**	**(100)**	**34**	**(100)**

Infectious illnesses transmitted by recreational water use include folliculitis, otitis externa ("swimmer's ear"), diarrheal diseases, and such exotic infections as leptospirosis and primary amebic meningoencephalitis. Folliculitis and dermatitis caused by *Pseudomonas aeruginosa* are often reported among users of whirlpools and hot tubs.

Outbreaks of giardiasis have been traced to swimming pools (Porter, Ragazzoni, & Buchanon, 1988; CDC, 1988, 1990a, 1993a). Other disease outbreaks that have been associated with swimming include shigellosis (Makintubee, Mallonee, & Istre, 1987), viral disease (Lenaway, Brockman, Dolan, & Cruz-Uribe, 1989; Turner, Istre, Beauchamp, Baum, & Arnold, 1987), and cryptosporidiosis (CDC, 1990b, 1994b).

Increased rates of diarrheal illness among swimmers at beaches meeting EPA standards (Cabelli, Dufour, Levin, McCabe, & Haberman, 1979) prompted the EPA to issue tighter standards (Cabelli, 1983; Dufour, 1984). It is now recognized that providing temporary toilets to summer crowds is the single measure most likely to prevent outbreaks at beaches and other summer swimming areas (CDC, 1990a).

FOOD-BORNE INFECTIOUS DISEASE

Like water-borne disease, the great majority of acute illnesses transmitted by food are never reported; hence, the magnitude of this problem can only be estimated. From 1983 through 1987, 2,397 outbreaks of food-borne disease were reported in the United States, comprising 91,678 cases (CDC, 1990c). This is an annual average of 479 outbreaks and 18,335 cases, numbers consistent with the 300–600 outbreaks, involving 10,000–20,000 people, which are usually reported each year (Black, Cox, & Horwitz, 1978). It is estimated, however, that as many as six million cases, with 9,000 deaths, may occur annually in the United States (Office of Disease Prevention and Health Promotion, 1991).

Food Contamination

Any of several factors may be implicated in an episode of food-borne illness (Bryan, 1975, 1991; Levine, Labuza, & Morley, 1985). These include:

Improper Holding Temperatures. Inadequate refrigeration is responsible for the majority of bacterial food-borne disease. Whether bacteria are introduced during food production or food handling, they require time, warmth, and moisture to multiply sufficiently for the food to become infective. Holding food at temperatures below 40° F will prevent the multiplication of most bacteria.

Inadequate Cooking. This factor is responsible for many episodes of bacterial food-borne illness and most cases of food-borne parasitic disease. Food contaminated during its production and processing—such as *Salmonella*–contaminated meat—may be rendered safe by cooking it sufficiently to bring all parts of the meat to a temperature above 160° F. Similarly, encysted larvae of parasites such as tapeworms and *Trichinella* may be destroyed by adequate cooking.

Contaminated Equipment. Food grinders, meat slicers, cutting boards, and other utensils may be used to prepare contaminated food (e.g., raw meat) and subsequently employed, without proper cleaning, to prepare other foods, resulting in contamination.

Infected Food Handlers. Staphylococcus and *Salmonella* bacteria and hepatitis A virus, among others, are organisms that may be carried asymptomatically by food handlers. Proper personal hygiene, including hand washing, and heat-processing foods after handling are examples of effective protective measures.

Food From Unsafe Sources. Foods implicated in chemical outbreaks, such as toxic fish or mushrooms, are not contaminated by handling, nor can they generally be rendered safe in preparation. In these cases, the food itself is unsafe.

Organisms Responsible for Food-Borne Disease

The causes of the majority of food-borne outbreaks, like most water-borne outbreaks, are never identified. Of the approximately 40% for which an etiology is determined, about two-thirds are bacterial, 20%–25% are chemical, and the remainder are viral or parasitic in origin. In the past, the greatest number have been caused by one of three types of bacteria: *Salmonella* species, *Staphylococcus aureus*, and *Clostridium perfringens*. These bacteria have accounted for about 35% of the food-borne outbreaks for which a cause was identified. In more recent years, however, *Staphylococcus* has declined in importance, whereas the number of outbreaks and cases caused by *Shigella* species has increased. There are over 200 other known causes of food-borne illness (Bryan, 1975); only a few can be discussed here.

Bacteria. About 30% – 40% of bacterial food-borne outbreaks (approximately 25% of all food-borne outbreaks of known etiology) are caused by species of *Salmonella*. *Salmonella* food poisoning (like water-borne salmonellosis) is characterized by an incubation period of 18–24 hours and a clinical syndrome marked by fever, watery diarrhea that may contain blood or mucus, and vomiting. Symptoms usually subside within a few days, but a person can continue to infect others for weeks or even months.

Salmonella species commonly infect domestic animals raised for food production and current methods of processing and shipping foods in bulk make this organism a frequent contaminant of meat. At least 33% of poultry (and perhaps up to 80%), 15% of pork, and up to 10% of beef products are contaminated with *Salmonella* species. Eggs and animal products such as carmine dye also are often contaminated. The *Salmonella* bacterium is destroyed by cooking but may survive temperature less than 160° F. This creates problems for persons who like their roast beef rare and for commercial food preparers.

Salmonella may be passed on to other foods by contaminated utensils, surfaces, or personnel during the preparation of raw meat. Other sources of *Salmonella* in the environment include pets such as baby chicks and turtles. The incidence of reported cases of salmonellosis in the U.S. has been increasing steadily for the last 45 years (Figure 3.1).

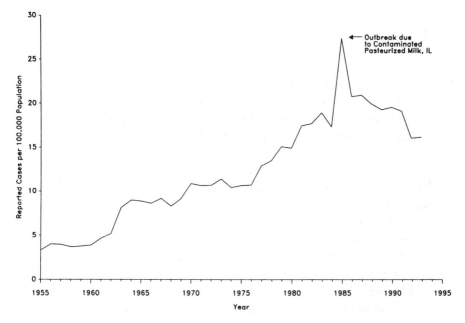

Figure 3.1 Reported cases of salmonellosis (excluding typhoid fever) in the United States, 1955–1993 (CDC, 1994a).

In 1985 *Salmonella typhimurium* caused the largest single food-borne outbreak ever reported in the United States. The vehicle was low-fat (2%) pasteurized milk produced by a dairy plant in Chicago. There were over 16,000 culture-confirmed cases; it is estimated that over 150,000 persons became ill. Of these, at least 2,777 were hospitalized and 14 died (CDC, 1990c).

Staphylococcus aureus is usually the cause of about one-quarter of all bacterial food-borne outbreaks, but in 1986 and 1987, the most recent years for which Centers for Disease Control surveillance data are available, this organism was responsible for only 8 (4%) of 202 such outbreaks (CDC, 1990b). Food-borne infection with this organism usually results in a gastrointestinal syndrome with vomiting, following an incubation period of two to four hours. The illness is self-limited, with symptoms usually subsiding in a few hours after onset.

Staphylococcus aureus is most commonly introduced into food by asymptomatic food handlers, who harbor the organism in their noses or throats. If the food is not adequately refrigerated, the bacteria will multiply and produce a toxin that is heat-stable, so it is not destroyed by cooking.

Clostridium perfringens was increasingly implicated as a cause of food-borne disease during the early 1980s when it was responsible for about 15% of all outbreaks. Between 1986 and 1987 it was implicated in only five outbreaks, however. This bacterium causes a lower intestinal syndrome of abdominal pain and diarrhea of sudden onset; there is often nausea but rarely vomiting or fever. The incubation period is usually 10–12 hours, but may be as short as 6 or as long as 24 hours. The illness usually resolves within a day.

The *Clostridium perfringens* bacterium is an anaerobic, spore-forming rod commonly found in raw meats and poultry. The spores often survive usual cooking temperatures and may then multiply to infective levels during slow cooling, slow rewarming after cooling, or both. Outbreaks almost always occur among those attending large catered or institutional meals.

From 1983 through 1987, *Shigella* species were responsible for 44 outbreaks of food-borne illness, accounting for 9,971 cases (CDC, 1990c). Shigellosis may present as dysentery, with fever and loose stools containing blood and mucus. In small children the acute phase is often accompanied by seizures. Alternatively, the disease may consist simply of watery diarrhea. Humans are the only significant reservoir of *Shigella.* Infection may occur after the ingestion of very small numbers (10–100) of bacteria. Food handlers are sometimes implicated, and flies may transfer the organism to susceptible foods (Benenson, 1990).

Clostridium botulinum causes botulism, a potentially fatal illness characterized by cranial nerve palsies followed by paralysis of the extremities and the muscles of respiration. From 1983 to 1987, 73 outbreaks of botulism were reported in the United States. Most outbreaks are small (one case is considered an outbreak); a total of 80–150 cases are reported each year.

The organism is anaerobic and spore-forming; the spores germinate and the bacteria produce toxin under conditions of low oxygen tension, such as in improperly canned food. The toxin is heat-labile, so it may be destroyed by cooking. Because of its severity, virtually all outbreaks of botulism are reported to public health authorities.

Listeria monocytogenes, usually carried by dairy products, has been responsible for some major food-borne epidemics; the largest occurred in Los Angeles in 1985. Of the 142 cases, 93 were in pregnant women. Ten neonates and 18 nonpregnant adults died, and there were 20 spontaneous abortions (Linnan et al., 1988).

Infection with *Vibrio vulnificus* is transmitted by ingestion of raw oysters—even those harvested in unpolluted waters. It has become increasingly common in the Gulf states since first reported in 1979 and has a case-fatality rate of over 20% (Levine et al., 1993)

Other bacteria reported with some frequency in food-borne outbreaks are: *Bacillus cereus* (CDC, 1994c); *Vibrio parahemolyticus*; and *Campylobacter* species. A total of 20 different species of bacteria were identified as the causes of at least one outbreak in the U.S. during the 5-year period 1977–1982 (CDC, 1985) and a similar number were implicated between 1983 and 1987 (CDC, 1990c). In January 1993, *E. Coli* serotype 0157:H7 was transmitted to several hundred people in four western states via hamburgers sold in a chain of fast-food restaurants, resulting in both bloody diarrhea and a serious childhood renal disease known as hemolytic-uremic syndrome (CDC, 1993c). Four children died in this outbreak, and similar instances of contamination and infection continue to occur in the United States.

Viruses

Although viral gastroenteritis may be transmitted by food, reports of such transmission are unusual. Between 1983 and 1987, 10 outbreaks of Norwalk virus infection and two of other viral gastroenteritides were reported, accounting for 1,722 cases. Hepatitis A is the only other viral illness commonly identified in food-borne outbreaks; 29 such outbreaks (1,067 cases) were reported during this period (CDC, 1990c). Hepatitis virus may be introduced into food by asymptomatic carriers who work as food handlers (CDC, 1993d).

Parasites

Trichinella spiralis is the most common food-borne parasite in the United States; it is transmitted through undercooked pork or occasionally through bear meat. The practice of feeding uncooked garbage to hogs generally has been abandoned in recent years and trichinosis has become less common. In the early 1950s, the incidence of trichinosis in the United States (where it is a reportable disease) was over 350 cases per year. Since then, the incidence has declined save for periodic outbreaks. Since 1981, fewer than 150 cases per year have been reported (CDC, 1994). The dietary habits of southeast Asian immigrants may place them at particular risk for trichinosis (Stehr-Green & Schantz, 1986).

Beef, pork, and fish tapeworms, transmitted through the undercooked flesh of the intermediate host, are occasionally acquired in the United States; *Giardia lamblia* (which is usually water-borne) and *Entameba histolytica* (which is usually transmitted person-to-person) sometimes may be transmitted through food. In the Far East, flukes such as *Clonorchis sinensis*, are transmitted through the consumption of raw crustaceans and occasionally may infect immigrants to the United States.

VECTOR-BORNE INFECTIOUS DISEASE

The term *vector* denotes a nonhuman carrier that can transmit disease organisms directly to humans. Vectors may be either biological or mechanical. In the former the pathologic microorganism must multiply or develop within the vector before it becomes infective. The time required to do so is the extrinsic incubation period of the disease. Mechanical vectors, on the other hand, simply transport microorganisms from one place to another; houseflies and cockroaches are examples.

As is true for most infectious disease, vector–borne illness is of much greater importance in the developing world than in industrialized countries. Malaria, transmitted by mosquitoes, is perhaps the most widespread and serious vector-borne disease. Other insect-borne diseases that are unknown in the United States, such as yellow fever, filariasis, and kala-azar, cause considerable suffering and death in much of the world. A summary of important vector-borne diseases is provided in Table 3.3.

Mosquitoes as Vectors

As shown in Table 3.3, mosquitoes transmit a variety of pathogenic organisms, including viruses, protozoa, and metazoa. The importance

Table 3.3   Some Insect Vectors and the Diseases They Transmit

Vector	Disease	Pathogen
	Mosquitoes	
Anopheles sp.	Malaria	*Plasmodium* sp.[a]
Culex sp.	Filariasis	*Wuchereria bancrofti* and *malayi*[b]
Culex sp.	Encephalitis	Arbovirus
Aedes aegypti	Yellow fever	Arbovirus
Aedes aegypti	Dengue	Arbovirus
	Biting flies	
Deer fly	Filariasis	*Loa loa*[b]
Black fly	River blindness	*Onchocerca volvulus*[b]
Tsetse fly	Sleeping sickness	*Trypanosoma gambiense* and *rhodesiense*[a]
Sand fly	Kala-azar	*Leishmania donovani*[a]
	Tropical ulcer	*L. tropica*[a]
	Cutaneous leishmaniasis	*L. mexicana*[a]
	Espundia	*L. Braziliense*[a]
	Other insects	
Gnats	Filariasis	*Mansonella ozzardi*[b]
Rat flea	Plague	*Yersinia pestis*[c]
	Murine typhus	*Rickettsia mooseri*[d]
Body louse	Epidemic typhus	*R. prowazekii*[d]
	Trench fever	*R. quintana*[d]
Mite	Rickettsialpox	*R. akari*[d]
Tick	Rocky mountain spotted fever	*R. rickettsi*[d]
Tick	Lyme disease	*Borrelia burgdorferi*[c]
Tick	Colorado tick fever	Arbovirus

[a] protozoa   [b] nematode   [c] bacteria   [d] rickettsia

of mosquitoes as vectors of disease, as well as their nuisance value, has led to widespread efforts to control them. Mosquito control requires a thorough knowledge of their life cycle and behavior, and the dynamics of the ecosystems they inhabit. All mosquitoes breed in stagnant water and produce aquatic larvae, but the preferred type of water (fresh water pond, salt marsh, etc.) varies between different species. The range of mosquito species is also variable; some species have a range of up to 20 miles, whereas the effective range of *Aedes aegypti* is limited to about one block (Savage, 1980).

In an area where control operations are to be initiated, surveillance is conducted to gain information regarding changes in the numbers and varieties of mosquitoes present. Many different types of traps can be used to collect adults; larvae are dipped manually from pools of stagnant water. In malarious areas, adult mosquitoes may be dissected and their stomachs and salivary glands examined microscopically to determine the rate of carriage of malaria parasites. There are three fundamental types of mosquito control—environmental, chemical, and biological. Their use in combination is termed integrated pest management.

Environmental control involves eliminating mosquito breeding sites and using screens and bed nets. These techniques are the oldest and were the chief tools in the celebrated campaigns of Major William Gorgas to eliminate yellow fever from Havana and the Panama Canal Zone in the early 1900s.

Environmental control measures also include eliminating human-made breeding sites, such as collections of water in tin cans, flower pots, discarded tires, and other refuse; and the use of proper irrigation practices. Modifying water flow and filling natural breeding sites in wetlands has been tried, but, in many cases, has not improved water flow enough to reduce mosquito populations in natural ecosystems.

Chemical control involves applying different chemicals to eradicate populations of mosquitoes in various developmental stages. Since World War II, a great number of insecticides, both larvacides and adulticides, have become available. These generally are classified as follows: stomach poisons, which must be ingested; contact poisons, which penetrate the insect's cuticle; or fumigants, which enter the insect's respiratory system (Pratt, Littig, & Barnes, 1960). They may also be classified as residual (environmentally persistent substances such as DDT) or nonresidual (quickly degraded compounds such as pyrethrins).

Insecticides have been used widely throughout the world in programs for the control of malaria and other vector-borne illnesses and a large share of whatever success these programs have attained has been attributed to these chemicals. In recent years, however, two major problems have emerged. The first is the problem of insect resistance to these chemicals. Over 200 species of insects have developed resistance to one or more insecticides, and compounds such as

DDT, which were once the mainstay of most mosquito-control programs in tropical areas, have now become almost useless in many places (Beck & Davies, 1981).

The second problem is increasing recognition of the dangers to the health of humans, agriculture, and natural ecosystems that are posed by the insecticides themselves. Acute poisoning incidents have always been a well-known threat, but the possible long-term consequences of insecticide exposure have only recently become a matter for concern. DDT, for instance, is known to be concentrated through the food chain, stored in fat, and secreted in human milk (Woodard, Ferguson, & Wilson, 1976; Bouwman, Becker, Cooppan, & Reinecke, 1992). It is known to cause weakening of the shells of eggs laid by exposed birds, but its effects in humans are still a matter of debate. Considerations such as these have led to the elimination of the use of DDT in the United States and the heavy regulation of other insecticides. DDT is still legal in a number of countries, and is illegally used in others (Dinham, 1993).

Ultralow volume application techniques—in which small amounts of insecticide are spread over a wide area by airplane—have come into use as a method for reducing the dangers of human exposure. The combination of chemicals with local environmental modification has also been successful. For example, bed nets impregnated with synthetic pyrethrins, such as permethrin, have shown promise in the tropics.

Biological control uses a variety of biological agents and methods to control various insect pests. These include microorganisms and sterilized males. So far the most successful biological control method has been the stocking of permanent bodies of water with small fish *(Gambusia* species) that feed on mosquito larvae. The control of mosquito populations with bacteria such as *Bacillus thuringiensis israeliensis* has been introduced recently and shows great promise (Laird, 1985; Entwistle, Cory, Balley, & Higgs, 1993). These biological methods are clearly preferable to filling productive wetlands and contaminating the environments with chemicals that pose risks to the health of humans as well as to other organisms.

Integrated pest management is used successfully in controlling a number of pests in agriculture and public health—including mosquito control. This approach combines environmental, chemical, and biological control strategies, using each when it is the most effective and giving priority to strategies with low potential for destruction or contamination of ecosystems. Success in rural areas of developing countries requires full community participation to identify and reduce breeding populations and to avoid indiscriminate use of chemicals that speed the development of insect resistance. In many developing countries—tropical Africa, for instance—no control method can be completely effective as mosquito habitat is extensive and economic resources are insufficient to support control efforts.

Diseases Transmitted by Mosquitoes

Malaria. Malaria is the most prevalent of the several diseases transmitted by mosquitoes (see Table 3.2). It is caused by a protozoan parasite that reproduces within the host's red blood cells and is characterized by periodic chills and fever. Adult hosts in endemic areas may have a high degree of acquired immunity and be relatively asymptomatic for long periods of time. Four species of the *Plasmodium* genus are responsible for human malaria: *P. vivax*, the most common, causes tertian malaria (a 3–day fever cycle); *P. malariae* causes quartan malaria (a 4–day fever cycle); *P. falciparum* causes malignant tertian malaria, the most serious form of the disease; and *P. ovale* causes ovale tertian malaria, a relatively mild illness.

Malaria is endemic throughout most of the nonindustrialized world. In 1955 the 8th World Health Assembly established a goal of global malaria eradication. Until about 1975 it did appear that programs of mosquito control and treatment of cases were bringing this disease under control. More recently, however, it has become evident that the prevalence of malaria is increasing. In Africa alone it is now estimated that malaria infects over 200 million people and contributes to the death of over one million (mostly infants and children) annually (Chin, 1986). Although Africa has the greatest prevalence of malaria, the greatest increases in incidence are occurring in Asia and Latin America. On these continents, people without resistance or immunity to the malaria parasites are migrating to regions of endemic malaria in search of work in mining and timber industries.

Until the early 1950s malaria was endemic in the southeastern United States. The urbanization of this region, coupled with chemical and environmental modification, resulted in the elimination of the disease, however. Cases continue to be imported into the United States. A peak number of 4,247 imported cases was recorded in 1970, during the Vietnam War; in 1991, 1,046 cases were imported (CDC, 1994d). Despite the presence of anopheline mosquitoes, transmission of malaria occurs only rarely in the United States (Brook, Genese, Bloland, Zucker, & Spitalny, 1994). This is apparently because a critical density of anopheline mosquitoes and infected persons is required to sustain transmission; the relatively few imported cases do not constitute a sufficient parasite reservoir.

Yellow Fever. This disease is caused by an arbovirus and is found today in South America and Africa. The virus attacks the liver, kidneys, and brain, and the illness is marked by jaundice and hemorrhage. Epidemics of yellow fever in the United States occurred as far north as New York in the 18th century. It was not until the early 1900s—following the pioneering work of Walter Reed and Carlos Findlay—that the mosquito vector was identified and the disease was eliminated from New Orleans (Williams, 1959).

Yellow fever occurs in two cycles: urban and jungle (or sylvatic). Jungle yellow fever is maintained in a mosquito–monkey cycle and is transmitted by several species of mosquito that breed and dwell in the jungle canopy. If a human is bitten by one of these vectors—as sometimes happens in clearing jungle land for farming or road building—the infected person may contract the disease and return to the city to initiate the urban, human-*Aedes aegypti* cycle.

Other Arboviruses. Many different arboviruses cause disease in humans but few of these are found in the United States. Most are transmitted by mosquitoes; some are spread by ticks. Arbovirus infections are marked by fever, headache, and myalgia and some produce hemorrhage and central nervous system damage.

Several types of arboviral encephalitis are transmitted in the United States. These include eastern equine, western equine, and St. Louis encephalitis. None are common, although outbreaks occasionally occur.

Dengue is an illness characterized by muscle aches and fever. It is fairly common in the Caribbean and elsewhere in the tropics. In 1980 the first U.S. cases since 1945 were reported in Texas (CDC, 1980), suggesting this disease might become more common in this country; but this has not occurred.

Flies as Vectors of Disease

As with mosquitoes, a knowledge of fly ecology is important to the control of these insects. The breeding patterns and flight ranges of different species vary widely. Fly traps and other devices are available as aids in surveillance.

Control of domestic flies is attained best through proper disposal of wastes. The use of screens is also important. Insecticides can be added to a variety of baits and strips, but flies are often resistant to many of these chemicals (Savage, 1980).

Sylvatic biting flies, which serve as biological vectors of many diseases, are difficult to control. For instance, blackflies *(Simulium* species), which transmit river blindness (onchocerciasis), breed only in fast-flowing water. Attempts to control this insect have involved aerial spreading of larvacides in hard-to-reach rapids in west Africa.

As shown in Table 3.3, a number of diseases are transmitted by biting flies. In the United States these insects are not significant carriers of disease, but they occasionally serve as mechanical vectors of tularemia—which is more frequently transmitted by ticks—or anthrax (American Academy of Pediatrics, 1991). However, the former is uncommon (generally fewer than 300 cases/yr) and the latter is essentially nonexistent in this country (CDC, 1994).

Biting flies such as blackflies and horseflies are thus mainly nuisances in the U.S., but are important vectors of parasitic disease in tropical countries. In some areas these exotic diseases are of great importance: Onchocerciasis is a major cause of blindness in parts of western Africa; sleeping sickness, which affects both humans and cattle, makes substantial tracts of otherwise arable land in Africa virtually uninhabitable.

Diseases also are transmitted by domestic flies. Houseflies breed in excrement, garbage, and other waste and have been implicated as mechanical vectors in the spread of typhoid fever, bacterial diarrheas, amebiasis, trachoma, and other diseases (Benenson, 1990). Their importance as vectors in the spread of infectious disease is largely unknown, however. Any of several species of fly may be responsible for myiasis, a condition in which eggs are deposited in a wound and fly larvae subsequently invade the surrounding tissue.

Other Insect Vectors

A variety of other biting insects serve as biological vectors for many illnesses, including those caused by parasites, bacteria, viruses, and rickettsiae (Table 3.3). In the United States, two of these are important: Lyme disease, transmitted primarily by the bite of ticks of the genus *Ixodes,* and Rocky Mountain spotted fever (RMSF), transmitted by ticks of the genus *Dermacentor.* The causative organism of Lyme disease is a spirochete bacterium, *Borrelia burgdorferi*; that of RMSF, a rickettsia, *Rickettsia rickettsii.*

Lyme disease was first described in 1975 and has now surpassed RMSF as the most common tick-borne disease in the United States. Human infection with another tick-borne ricketsia, *Ehrlichia canis,* was first reported in 1986; the number of reported cases have increased in each subsequent year (CDC, 1990d).

Plague, well-known for the devastation it caused in Europe in the Middle Ages, occurs occasionally (5-10 cases/yr) in the western United States, where rodents such as prairie dogs serve as reservoirs for the bacterium *Yersinia pestis.* Human cases occur chiefly in persons engaged in outdoor work, recreation, or animal handling.

Filariasis is an infection caused by several species of roundworm and is found in Africa, Asia, and the Pacific; as shown in Table 3.3, it has several vectors. It is characterized by subcutaneous nodules, recurring fevers, and with some species of parasite, lymphedema of the lower extremities and scrotum.

Other diseases for which insects serve as specific vectors are either rare (murine typhus and Colorado tick fever, for instance) or nonexistent in the United States. Some biting insects such as head lice and bedbugs are nuisances, but do not transmit disease.

Common household insects such as cockroaches have been shown to carry pathogenic organisms and are thought to serve as mechanical vectors of diarrheal and other diseases. Their actual role in disease transmission, however, remains largely undefined.

Rodent Vectors

Domestic rats and mice are highly adaptable creatures; they live in and around the various structures built by humans in both urban and rural areas. Surveillance is conducted chiefly by experienced inspectors searching for droppings, runways, and other signs of rodent presence.

Control efforts are based on both environmental and chemical methods. The former are preferred; they involve making dwellings and food as inaccessible as possible to rodents. Buildings can be "rat-proofed" by sealing holes around plumbing and under doors and by implementing sanitation programs. Leaks in sewers permit rats to move into buildings and should be repaired; refuse should be removed and properly stored prior to disposal.

Several rodenticides are used in rat control. During the last 15 years strains of rats resistant to some of these poisons—particularly anticoagulants such as warfarin—have emerged (Savage, 1980).

Rats serve as reservoirs of plague and murine typhus, diseases that are transmitted by the rat flea. They also are reservoirs of trichinosis. The house mouse is a reservoir for rickettsialpox, a rare illness that is transmitted by a mite that parasitizes the mouse.

Rats and mice are thought to serve as mechanical vectors of salmonellosis; they carry the bacteria in their intestines and may contaminate human food with their droppings. Rats also serve as mechanical vectors and reservoirs for leptospirosis, as do many other domestic and wild animals. Leptospirosis, a flu-like illness that sometimes causes hemorrhage and jaundice, is caused by a bacterium, *Leptospira icterohemorrhagiae*. Humans usually contract the disease when swimming or working in water contaminated with animal urine; the bacteria enter through open cuts or sores (Benenson, 1990).

Rats are biological vectors for rat-bite fever, a rare but occasionally fatal febrile illness caused by the bacteria *Streptobaccilus moniliformis* or *Spirillum minus*. Rat bites themselves are much more common than most of the infectious diseases carried by rats, particularly in inner-city neighborhoods. Children are often the victims. In the developing countries, one of the greatest problems posed by rats is their consumption of stored foodstuffs.

A recent epidemic in the southwestern United States has emphasized the importance of rodents as disease vectors and the role of environmental factors in vector-borne disease. In the spring of 1993, over 40 cases (including 26 fatalities) of a severe respiratory illness were linked to a hantavirus transmitted by deer mice (Hughes, Peters, Cohen, & Mahy, 1993; Nichol et al., 1993). This virus, along with other recently identified hantaviruses (CDC, 1994e), was apparently been endemic in a number of areas of the United States for an undetermined period. It became responsible for a disease epidemic because its vector underwent a "population explosion," linked to an abundance of pinon nuts and grasshoppers which, in turn, were linked to heavy rains and snows during the previous spring (Stone, 1993).

SOIL-BORNE PARASITIC DISEASE

Soil-borne parasites are among the most common infectious diseases in the world. It is estimated that one-quarter of the world's population (about 1 billion people) is infected with the large roundworm, *Ascaris lumbricoides* (Crompton, 1988), and about 700 million persons are infected with hookworm (Katz et al., 1989).

In the United States these infections are limited chiefly to the rural southeastern states. Although infections are not as widespread as in years past, prevalence is high in some communities. These parasites are transmitted when human feces are deposited on the ground and the eggs or larvae in the feces undergo a period of development in the soil. Humans are infected by ingesting the eggs, or when larvae invade the skin. Infections are therefore associated with rural poverty and its attendant conditions of poor sanitation and education.

Proper disposal of human feces is central to the control of these parasites. Construction of privies may be helpful. Periodic mass treatment of children in communities where ascariasis is prevalent provides at least temporary control. Wearing shoes protects against infection by hookworm and *Strongyloides* species. However, soil-borne nematodes are likely to remain common where rural poverty is present and soil and climatic conditions are favorable. Control of the parasites ultimately will depend on improved economic conditions for the poor.

Ascaris

Roundworm (*Ascaris lumbricoides*) ova are ingested by the host and hatch in the small intestine. A human host may harbor hundreds of worms; complications of infection include intestinal obstruction or perforation, obstruction of the common bile or pancreatic ducts, and appendicitis. In addition, a heavy infection may cause nutritional deficiencies in the host.

Hookworm

Ancylostoma duodenale was once very common in the southeastern United States and was responsible for widespread serious morbidity. The work of the Rockefeller Sanitary Commission from 1910 to 1920, which focused on educating the public about sanitation, was responsible for a great reduction in its prevalence (Mott & Roemer, 1948), and it has continued to decline since.

Hookworm ova hatch in the soil and the larvae enter the host's body by penetrating the skin—usually through bare feet. They migrate to the small intestine, where the adults attach themselves to the intestinal mucosa and actively suck blood. A heavy infection ("hookworm disease") can cause severe anemia, hypoproteinemia, edema, and congestive heart failure.

Whipworm

These parasites (*Trichuris trichiura)* enter the host's body when the ova are ingested. The larvae pass directly to the large intestine, where they mature and often cause diarrhea. A heavy infection can result in rectal prolapse.

Strongyloides

The ova of *Strongyloides* species hatch in the intestine of the host, and larvae are passed in the stool. The larvae may enter a free-living cycle in the soil or may invade the body of a new host through the skin and migrate to the small intestine. Larvae in the host's intestine may penetrate directly through the intestinal mucosa to establish a new migratory cycle, a process known as internal autoinfection. *Strongyloides* species are particularly dangerous to the malnourished or immunocompromised host: massive internal autoinfection takes place, larvae migrate aberrantly throughout the body (the "hyperinfection syndrome"), and shock and death may follow.

Animal Nematodes

The larvae of dog or cat hookworms may penetrate the skin of humans, but their migration is limited to the skin. A highly pruritic rash, known as cutaneous larva migrans or "creeping eruption," results. This condition is encountered not uncommonly in bathers on beaches where dogs run loose.

If the ova of dog or cat ascarids (*Toxocara canis* and *Toxocara cati*) are ingested by a human, the larvae migrate aberrantly and enter the liver, the eye, or even the brain—a disease known as visceral larva migrans. The condition is most common in the children of dog owners (Schantz, Weiss, Pollard, & White, 1980).

SUMMARY

On a worldwide basis, environmental infectious disease is the most important health problem, causing more morbidity and mortality than any other. In the U.S., environmental infectious disease has been partially controlled and no longer has the power to command public attention to the extent that chemical and radiation hazards do, nor to the extent that infections spread person-to-person do. Nonetheless, environmental infectious disease still causes significant morbidity and mortality in this and other developed countries, and the price of keeping it relatively well-controlled is eternal vigilance.

REFERENCES

American Academy of Pediatrics. (1991). *Report of the Committee on Infectious Diseases* (2nd ed.) Elk Grove Village, IL: Author.

Beck, J. W., & Davies, J. E. (1981). *Medical parasitology* (3rd ed.). St. Louis: C. V. Mosby.

Benenson, A. M. (Ed.). (1990). *Control of communicable diseases in man.* Washington, DC: American Public Health Association.

Black, R. E., Cox, R. C., & Horwitz, M. A. (1978). Outbreaks of foodborne disease in the United States, 1975. *Journal of Infectious Disease, 137,* 213-218.

Bouwman, M., Becker, P. J., Cooppan, R. M., & Reinecke, A. J., (1992). Transfer of DDT used in malaria control in malaria control to infants via breast milk. *Bulletin of the World Health Organization, 70,* 241-250.

Brook, J. H., Genese, C. A., Bloland, P. B., Zucker, J. R., & Spitalny, K. C. (1994). Malaria probably locally acquired in New Jersey. *New England Journal of Medicine, 331*, 22-23.

Bryan, F. A. (1975). *Disease transmitted by foods* (DHHS Publication No. CDC 75-8237). Atlanta, GA: Centers for Disease Control.

Bryan, F. A. (1991). Factors that contribute to outbreaks of food-borne disease. *Journal of Food Protection, 41*, 816-827.

Cabelli, V. J. (1983). *Health effects criteria for marine recreational waters* (EPA Publication No. 600/1-83-031). Research Triangle Park, NC: U.S. Environmental Protection Agency.

Cabelli, V. J., Dufour, A. P., Levin, M. A., McCabe, L. J., & Haberman, P. W. (1979). Relationship of microbial indicators to health effects at marine bathing beaches. *American Journal of Public Health, 69*, 690-696.

Centers for Disease Control. (1980). Dengue—United States. *Morbidity Mortality Weekly Report, 29*, 531-532.

Centers for Disease Control. (1985) *Foodborne disease outbreaks annual summary, 1982.* Atlanta, GA: Author.

Centers for Disease Control (1988). Water-related disease outbreaks, 1985. *Morbidity Mortality Weekly Report, 37* (No. SS-2), 15-24.

Centers for Disease Control. (1990a). Waterborne disease outbreaks. *Morbidity Mortality Weekly Report, 39* (No. SS-1), 1-13.

Centers for Disease Control (1990b). Swimming-associated cryptosporidiosis. *Morbidity Mortality Weekly Report, 39*, 343-345.

Centers for Disease Control. (1990c). Foodborne disease outbreaks, 5-year summary, 1983-1987. *Morbidity Mortality Weekly Report, 39* (No. SS-1), 15-57.

Centers for Disease Control. (1990d). Rocky Mountain spotted fever and human ehrlichiosis—United States, 1989. *Morbidity Mortality Weekly Report, 39*, 282-284.

Centers for Disease Control and Prevention. (1993b). Update: Cholera—Western Hemisphere, 1992. *Morbidity Mortality Weekly Report, 42*, 89-91.

Centers for Disease Control and Prevention. (1993d). Hepatitis A—Missouri, Wisconsin, and Alaska. *Morbidity Mortality Weekly Report, 42*, 526-529.

Centers for Disease Control and Prevention. (1993a). Surveillance for waterborne disease outbreaks—United States, 1991–1992. In CDC Surveillance Summaries, *Morbidity Mortality Weekly Report, 42* (SS-57) 1-22.

Centers for Disease Control and Prevention. (1993c). Surveillance for waterborne disease outbreaks—United States, 1991-1992. *Morbidity Mortality Weekly Report, 42* (No. SS-5), 1-22.

Centers for Disease Control and Prevention (1994a). Summary of notifiable diseases, United States, 1992. *Morbidity Mortality Weekly Report, 8.*

Centers for Disease Control and Prevention. (1994b). *Cryptosporidium* infections associated with swimming pools—Dane County, Wisconsin, 1993. *Morbidity Mortality Weekly Report, 43,* 561-563.

Centers for Disease Control and Prevention. (1993c). Update: Multistate outbreak of *Escherchia coli* 0157:H7 infections from hamburgers— Western United States, 1992-1993. *Morbidity Mortality Weekly Report, 42,* 258-63.

Centers for Disease Control and Prevention. (1994c). *Bacillus cereus* food poisoning associated with fried rice at two child day care centers— Virginia, 1993. *Morbidity Mortality Weekly Report, 43,* 177-178.

Centers for Disease Control and Prevention. (1994d). Malaria surveillance annual summary, 1991. Atlanta, GA.

Centers for Disease Control and Prevention. (1994e) Newly identified hantavirus—Florida, 1994. *Morbidity Mortality Weekly Report, 43,* 99-105.

Chin W. (1986). Malaria. In J. Last (ed.), *Maxcy-Rosenau Public Health and Preventive Medicine* (pp. 361-370). Norwalk, CT: Appleton-Century-Crofts.

Craun, G. F. (1979). Water-borne giardiasis in the United States. *American Journal of Public Health, 69,* 817-819.

Crompton, D. W. T. (1988). The prevalence of ascariasis. *Parasitology Today, 4,* 162-169.

Dinham, B. (1993). *The pesticide hazard: a global health and environmental audit.* London: Zed Books.

Dufour, A. P. (1984). *Health effects criteria for fresh recreational waters* (EPA Publication No. 600/1-84-004). Resesarch Triangle Park, NC: U. S. Environmental Protection Agency.

Entwistle, P. F., Cory, J. S., Balley, M. J., & Higgs, S. (eds.). (1993). *Bacillus thuringiensis, an environmental biopostiade: Theory and practice.* New York: Wiley.

Haley, C. E. W., Gunn, R. A., Hughes, J. M., Lippy, E. C., & Craun, G. F. (1980). Outbreaks of water-borne disease in the United States. *Journal of Infectious disease, 141,* 794-797.

Hayes, E. B., Matte, T. D., O'Brien, R., McKinley, T. W., Logsdon, G. S., Rose, J. B., Ungar, B. L., Word, D. M., Pinsky, P. F., & Cummings, M. L. (1989). Large community outbreak of *cryptosporidiosis* due to contamination of a filtered public water supply. *New England Journal of Medicine, 320,* 1372-1376.

Hopkins, D. R. & Ruiz-Tiben, E. (1990). Dracunculiasis eradication: Target 1995. *American Journal of Tropical Medicine Hygiene, 43,* 296-300.

Hughes, J. M., Peters, C. J., Cohen, M. L., & Mahy, B. W. (1993). Hantavirus pulmonary syndrome: An emerging infectious disease. *Science, 262*, 850–851.

Jakubowski, W. (1988) Purple burps and the filtration of drinking water supplies (Editorial). *American Journal of Public Health, 78*, 123-125.

Kaplan, J. E., Gary, G. W., Baron, R. C., Singh, N., Schonberger, L. B., Feldman, R., & Greenberg, H. B. (1982). Epidemiology of Norwalk gastroenteritis and the role of Norwalk virus in outbreaks of acute non-bacterial gastroenteritis. *Annals of Internal Medicine, 96*, 756-761.

Katz, M., Despommier, D. D., & Gwadz, R. (1989). *Parasitic Diseases* (2nd ed.). New York: Springer-Verlag.

Kent, G. P., Greenspan, J. R., Herndon, J. L., Mofenson, L. M., Harris, J. A., Eng, T. R., & Waskin, H. A. (1988). Epidemic giardiasis caused by a contaminated public water supply. *American Journal of Public Health, 78*, 139-143.

Laird, M. (1985). New answers to malaria problems through vector control? *Experentia. 41*, 446-456.

Lenaway, D. D., Brockman, R., Dolan, G. J., & Cruz-Uribe, F. (1989). An outbreak of an enterovirus-like illness at a community wading pool. *American Journal of Public Health, 78*, 889-890.

Levine, A. S., Labuza, T. P., & Morley, J. W. (1985). Food technology: A primer for physicians. *New England Journal of Medicine, 312*, 628-634.

Levine, W. C., Griffin, P. M., and the Gulf Coast *Vibrio* Working Group. (1993). *Vibrio* infections on the gulf coast: The results of a first year of regional surveillance. *Journal of Infectious Disease, 167*, 470-483.

Linnan, M. J., Mascola, L., Lou, X. D., Goulet, V., May, S., Salminen, C., Hird, D., Yonekura, M. L. Hayes, P., Weaver, R., Audurier, A., Plikaytis, B. D., Fannin, S., Kleks, A., Broome, C. V. (1988). Epidemic listeriosis associated with Mexican-style cheese. *New England Journal of Medicine, 319*, 823-828.

Makentubee, S., Mallonee, J., & Istre, G. R. (1987). Shigellosis outbreak associated with swimming. *American Journal of Public Health, 77*, 166-168.

Mott, F. D. & Roemer, M. I., (1948). *Rural health and medical care.* New York, McGraw-Hill.

Nicol, S. T., Spiropoulou, C. F., Morzunov, S., Rollin, P. E., Ksiazek, T. G., Feldmann, H., Sanchez, A., Childs, J., Zaki, S., & Peters, C. J. (1993). Genetic identification of a hantavirus associated with an outbreak of acute respiratory illness. *Science, 262*, 914-917.

Navin, T. R., Juranek, D. D., Ford, M., Minedew, D. J., Lippy, E. C., & Pollard, R. A. (1985). Case-control study of waterborne giardiasis in Reno, Nevada. *American Journal of Epidemiology, 122*, 269-275.

Office of Disease Prevention and Health Promotion, U. S. Public Health Service. (1991, January). Food Safety: Preventing foodborne disease. *Prevention Reports*, Department of Health and Human Services.

Pavia, A. T., Campbell, J. F., Blake, P. A., Smith, J. D., McKinley, T. W., & Martin, D. L. (1987)). Cholera from raw oysters shipped interstate. *Journal of American Medical Association, 285*, 2374.

Porter, J. D., Ragazzoni, H. P., & Buchanon, J. D. (1988). Giardia transmission in a swimming pool. *American Journal of Public Health, 78*, 659-662.

Pratt, H. D., Littig, K. W., & Barnes, R. C. (1960). *Survey and control of mosquitoes of public health importance* (USDHEW Publication No. VC-36). Atlanta, GA: U.S. Department of Health and Human Services.

Rosenberg, M. L., Koplan, J. P., Wachsmuth, I. K., Wells, J. G., Gangarosa, E. J., Guerrant, R. L., & Sack, D. A. (1977). Epidemic diarrhea at Crater Lake from enterotoxigenic *Escherichia coli. Annals of Internal Medicine, 86*, 714-718.

Savage, E. P. (1980). Disease vectors. In P. W. Purdom (Ed.), *Environmental Health*. New York: Academic Press.

Schantz, P. M., Weiss, P. E., Pollard, Z. F., & White, M. C. (1980). Risk factors for toxicaral ocular larva migrans: A case-control study. *American Journal of Public Health, 70*, 1273-1277.

Snow, J. (1855). *On the mode of communication of cholera* (2nd ed.) London: Churchill. Quoted in J. S. Mausner & A. K. Bahn (1974). *Epidemiology: An introductory text*. Philadelphia: W. B. Saunders.

Stehr-Green, J. K., & Schantz, P. M. (1986). Trichinosis in Southeast Asian refugees in the United States. *American Journal of Public Health, 76*, 1283-1289.

Stone, R. (1993). The mouse–pinon nut connection. *Science, 262*, 833.

Swerdlow, D. L. Woodruff, B. A., & Brady, R. C., Griffin, P. M., Tippen, S., Ddonnell, H. D., Jr., Geldreich, E., Payne, B. J., Meyer, A. Jr., Wells, J. G., Green, K. D., Bright, M., Beans, N. H., & Blake, P. A., (1992). A Waterborne outbreak in Missouri of *Escherichia coli* 0157: H7 associated with bloody diarrhea and death. *Annals of Internal Medicine, 117*, 812-819.

Turner, M., Istre, G., R., Beauchamp, H., Baum, M., & Arnold, S. (1987). Community outbreak of adenovirus type 7a infections associated with a swimming pool. *Southern Medical Journal, 60*, 712-715.

Williams, G. (1959). *Virus hunters*. New York: Alfred A. Knopf.

Woodard, B. T., Ferguson, B. B., & Wilson, D. J. (1976). DDT levels in milk of rural indigent blacks. *American Journal of Diseases of Children, 130*, 400-403.

SUGGESTED READINGS

American Academy of Pediatrics Committee on Infectious Diseases. (1994). *1994 Red book: Report of the committee on infectious diseases* (23rd ed.). Elk Grove Village, IL: Author.

Benenson, A. M. (Ed.). (1990). *Control of communicable diseases in man* (15th ed.). Washington, DC: American Public Health Association.

Feigin, R. D., & Cherry, J. D. (1992). *Pediatric infectious diseases* (3rd ed.). Philadellphia W. B. Saunders.

Last, J. M., & Wallace, R. B. (Eds.). (1992). *Maxcy-Rosenau-Last Public health and preventive medicine.* Norwalk, CT: Appleton & Lange.

Mandell, G. L., Douglas, R. G., & Bennett, J. E. (1990). *Principles and practice of infectious diseases* (3rd ed.). New York: Hurchill Livingstone.

Mitchell, R. (Ed.). (1993). *Environmental microbiology.* New York: Wiley.

Strickland, G. T. (1991). *Hunder's tropical medicine.* Philadelphia: W. B. saunders.

Warren, K. S., & Mahmond, A. A. F. (Eds.). (1990). Tropical and geographical medicine (7th ed.). New York: McGraw-Hill.

Chapter 4

Toxic Chemicals, Fibers, and Dusts

A. James Ruttenber and Renate D. Kimbrough

Members of the public and workers come in contact with a staggering number of chemicals. Fortunately, most do not enter the bodies of persons who are potentially exposed and even fewer exposures lead to doses that cause disease. But the list of chemicals shown to have produced disease through environmental exposures is quite long, and research on potential toxic effects has not kept pace with the introduction of new chemical products. The chemical industry generates new compounds and new production methods at a rate that outpaces the ability of health and regulatory agencies to carefully monitor their safety.

Classifying chemicals based on molecular structure, physical characteristics, sources, end uses, and toxic properties helps make sense out of the confusing array of compounds (Table 4.1). The first classification scheme uses a combination of chemical and physical properties, toxic effects, and uses. The second arranges chemicals by mechanisms of toxicity. Both groupings are useful, though the former is more helpful for remembering specific chemicals because many of them produce a variety of toxic effects by many different mechanisms. The chemicals covered in this chapter are commonly involved in environmental health problems and represent the types of exposures and toxic effects encountered in the practice of environmental health. There are many good texts and computer databases that cover

Table 4.1   Classification of Toxic Chemicals, Fibers, and Dusts

I.   Classification by Chemical and Physical Properties
    A.   Metals and Metallic Compounds
    B.   Dusts and Fibers
    C.   Gases
       Irritants
       Asphyxiants
    D.   Organic Chemicals
       Pesticides
       Herbicides
       Halogenated Polyaromatic Compounds
       Volatile Organic Compounds
    E.   Toxins

II. Classification by Mechanism of Toxicity
    A.   Carcinogens
    B.   Neurotoxins
    C.   Mutagens
    D.   Allergens
    E.   Teratogens
    F.   Reproductive Toxicants
    G.   Metabolic Toxicants

the identification, measurement, and toxicology of environmental chemicals. These are listed in the reference section for this chapter and in the Introduction. Familiarity with reference sources on the toxicology of chemicals is essential to the practice of environmental health and saves having to memorize a large body of facts.

METALS AND METALLIC COMPOUNDS

Lead

Lead is probably the most discussed and analyzed of all the environmental chemicals and has been studied over many centuries. Because it is a component of many industrial products, it exposes humans through a variety of routes. Sources of lead include paint, leaded gasoline, batteries, and drinking water from distribution systems that have lead pipes, fixtures, or solder.

The United States and a few other nations have removed lead as an "antiknock" agent in most preparations of gasoline and have experienced substantial declines in concentrations of lead in air and soil as well as declines in the average blood lead concentrations in members of the public. Similar reductions have been noted for exposures to lead-based paints following governmental regulations, educational programs, and remediation. However, most of the world's population is still exposed through these two routes because, except in North America and some European countries, lead is not carefully regulated.

Lead forms salts with many elements and complex compounds with organic molecules (e.g., the gasoline additive, tetraethyl lead). These compounds can be ingested, inhaled, or absorbed through the skin. Depending on the chemical properties of lead compounds, between 5% and 50% of ingested lead is absorbed by the gastrointestinal tract of an adult (Centers for Disease Control and Prevention [CDC], 1991). Gastrointestinal absorption by children is greater than for adults, exceeding 50% for some lead compounds in drinking water.

Inhalation can result in uptakes in blood of 50%–70% of lead in inspired air, depending on particle size and solubility. Inorganic lead does not pass through the skin, but organic lead does. About 90% of the lead that reaches the bloodstream is deposited in the skeleton. The remainder is stored in soft tissues and blood, or is excreted.

Lead is toxic to the kidney and the nervous system—particularly to the nervous system of the fetus and young child. By complexing with the sulfhydryl groups, lead interferes with the function of enzymes, thereby damaging many different organs and physiologic processes. Damage to enzymes involved with heme synthesis ultimately causes anemia with microcytic, hypochromic cells.

In the nervous system, lead is directly toxic to Schwann cells, causing segmental demyelination of peripheral nerves, and leading to decreased conduction velocity in motor nerves. Peripheral neuropathy is the most common neurologic manifestation of lead toxicity in adults. Lead is also directly toxic to neurons and alters neurotransmitter function. Encephalopathy appears more frequently in children with high exposures, apparently because lead compounds pass through the blood–brain barrier more easily in children than in adults.

Exposure to environmental lead has been associated with hyperactivity, fine motor dysfunction, and learning disorders in children. Recent reports have associated lowering of intelligence quotient (IQ) scores and other measures of intelligence with blood lead levels near or lower than current public health guidelines in the United States (Baghurst et al., 1992; Needleman, Schell, Bellinger, Leviton & Allred, 1990).

A positive association between blood levels and elevated blood pressure has been reported (Hertz-Picciotto & Croft, 1993; Maheswaran, Gill, Beevers, 1993; Schwartz, 1991), and lead may also cause acute and chronic damage to the kidneys. Environmental and occupational exposures have been associated with adverse reproductive outcomes, including spontaneous abortion, decreased sperm counts, minor congenital anomalies, and stillbirths (Fischbein, 1992).

Lead toxicity appears to vary linearly with dose and the forementioned pathology is more severe with higher doses. In 1991 CDC revised its recommendations for lead toxicity and advised community-wide intervention if many children in a community have blood lead concentrations ≥ 10 µg/dL. The CDC also recommended investigation of the home environments of individual children with blood lead concentrations ≥ 15 µg/dL (CDC, 1991).

Since the late 1970s, when lead was phased out of gasoline in the United States, average blood lead levels dropped substantially (Pirkle et al., 1994). Of U. S. children 1 to 5 years of age between 1988–1991, 8.9% (approximately 1.7 million) had blood lead concentrations equal to or greater than 10 µg/dL; the risk for exposure at this level was higher for poor, minority, and urban children (Brody et al., 1994). Lead-based paint remains the chief source of lead poisoning in the United States, even though concentrations in residential paint were strictly regulated starting in 1978 (CDC, 1991).

Mercury

Whereas lead is usually toxic as a salt or in complexes with organic molecules, mercury is toxic as a salt, as an organic compound, and in its elemental state. The pathology associated with each of these forms is quite different.

At room temperature, elemental or metallic mercury is a liquid and is slightly volatile. It is used in the electrolytic production of chlorine gas (the chloralkali process) and in metal extraction. Elemental mercury is poorly absorbed by the gastrointestinal tract, but is well absorbed (approximately 80%) in the lungs if it is in the vapor phase.

Mercury forms salts with many anions and these are used in a number of industries and are ingredients in a variety of products, including fungicides and medicines. Mercury salts are moderately absorbed (7%–15%) by the gastrointestinal tract and can be inhaled if particles are small enough.

Mercury also forms organic compounds. Methylmercury used to be a popular fungicide for treating seeds before planting but has been replaced by phenylmercury—a less toxic compound.

In nature, methylmercury is formed when mercury salts are metabolized by bacteria in aquatic ecosystems. Approximately 90% of ingested methylmercury is absorbed in the gastrointestinal tract and is then distributed throughout the body because of its high lipid solubility; other organic forms of mercury are less extensively absorbed and distributed.

Like lead, mercury exerts its toxic effects by binding with the sulfhydryl groups of proteins and with other organic compounds. Organic mercury compounds are distributed to many organs, but cause the most damage to the brain and kidneys. In the brain, toxicity from elemental mercury produces the clinical picture of encephalopathy and irritability that is dose dependent and subsides with removal from exposure. Workers in the felt hat industry in the early 20th century developed this syndrome (Neal & Jones, 1938) and have been described as "mad hatters."

Elemental mercury and mercury salts can damage the glomeruli and collecting tubules of the kidney, and chronic high doses can cause renal failure. Ingested mercury produces abdominal pain and inhaled elemental mercury (mercury vapor) induces severe pulmonary fibrosis.

Young children exposed to mercury salts can develop *acrodynia* (from the Greek roots that translate as *extremity* and *pain*). This disease is characterized by rash (it is sometimes called "pink disease" or erythroedema because of the characteristic red hands and feet), irritability, pruritus, hypertension, excess sweating, hypotonia, and photophobia (Chamberlain & Quillian, 1963). Reports of acrodynia have been rare since the 1960s, when mercury salts were removed from teething powder and drugs—the most common routes of exposure in the past.

One of the most striking examples of a human disease from an environmental exposure is the epidemic of Minamata disease caused by methylmercury. In 1950, a Japanese chemical plant in Minamata City began discharging mercury-containing liquid wastes to the near-by Minamata Bay. The plant used mercuric oxide as a catalyst in the production of acetaldehyde and vinyl chloride (Ellis, 1989). Bacteria in the bay sediment converted inorganic mercury to methylmercury, which, because of its lipid solubility, contaminated the marine food chain and, subsequently, humans who consumed seafood.

The first patients exhibited delirium, disturbed speech, and abnormal gait. Those poisoned were mostly fishermen and their families who lived along the sea near Minamata City. Before the first human cases were diagnosed, dead fish had been seen in the bay, and neighborhood cats developed an erratic pattern of behavior that became known as the "dancing disease"—the poisoned cats staggered, convulsed, and ran in circles (Smith & Smith, 1975).

Residents of Minamata who were exposed to methylmercury developed a variety of signs and symptoms, including numbness around their mouths and in their extremities, speech and hearing impairment, constriction of visual fields, ataxia and gait impairment, sensory disturbances, choreiform movements, and seizures (Tedeschi, 1982). Children born to exposed mothers developed abnormal motor function and severe central nervous system damage and were frequently diagnosed as having cerebral palsy.

In November 1956 seafood from Minamata Bay was identified as the source of the illness, but it took the Japanese government until 1958 to warn the public against eating seafood from the bay. Cases of Minamata disease continued to appear through the early 1970s, and over 2,500 seacoast residents have been diagnosed as having Minamata disease (Tamashiro, Arakaki, Akagi, Futatsuka, & Roht, 1985).

Another outbreak of Minamata disease occurred in Niigata between 1964 and 1965, where an acetaldehyde plant released mercury that contaminated fish and shellfish in the Agano River.

Outbreaks of methylmercury poisoning have also occurred after consumption of seed grain treated with fungicidal preparations of methylmercury in Iraq, Guatemala, Ghana, and Pakistan (Elhassani, 1983).

Recently, environmental exposures to mercury have been documented in homes painted with latex paint that contained phenylmercuric acetate as a fungicide and bactericide (Agocs et al., 1990). In 1990, this additive was banned in the United States. Mercury exposures have also been documented in the Amazon region, where gold miners use metallic mercury to extract gold. Since the mid-1980s, many miners have been exposed to dangerous concentrations of mercury vapor when they heated the gold-mercury amalgam in order to evaporate mercury. Wastes from gold processing have also contaminated aquatic ecosystems with elemental mercury which has subsequently been converted to methylmercury—posing health risks to those who consume aquatic species.

FIBERS AND DUSTS

Asbestos

Fibers are defined as particles that are at least three times as long as they are wide. Asbestos is a fibrous material composed of different types of hydrated magnesium silicates. Coiled asbestos fibers are called serpentine asbestos; chrysotile (white) asbestos is in this group. Straight fibers are in the amphibole group, which comprises crocidolite (blue) asbestos, amosite (brown) asbestos, as well as other fibers. Asbestos fibers visible to the naked eye are actually bundles of much finer fibrils with diameters as small as a few angstroms. These small fibers can be best seen with an electron microscope.

Valued for its insulating and fire-resistant properties, asbestos has been used in many products. These include insulation for steam pipes and boilers, ceiling materials, brake linings for motor vehicles, asbestos-cement pipe, roofing, and textiles. Because it is a naturally occurring mineral, there are areas throughout the world with high asbestos concentrations in soil and air.

Inhaled small asbestos particles are first deposited in respiratory bronchioles and alveoli and are then translocated to interstitial tissue or to the lymphatics. Along the way they may be phagocytized by alveolar or interstitial macrophages, which release reactive oxygen molecules that injure the alveoli and stimulate fibrosis. This process can lead to asbestosis if there is prolonged exposure to high concentrations of respirable fibers. Asbestos fibers can work their way into the pleural lining and, through processes similar to those in the lung, produce fibrous scars called *pleural plaques*. Asbestos fibers can also be ingested and deposited at different sites in the gastrointestinal tract, or can perforate the bowel mucosa and deposit in the peritoneum, where they induce fibrosis. Fibers can also be transported in the blood stream to the kidneys, where they deposit in the glomeruli.

There is evidence that a variety of chemical and physical processes are involved in asbestos-induced bronchogenic carcinoma in the lung, and mesothelioma in the pleura and peritoneum (McClellan et al., 1992). Asbestos has caused lung disease and mesothelioma in thousands of workers in many different industries, including shipyards, building insulation and construction trades, plumbing and pipe fitting, brake manufacturing and repair, and railroads. Increases in the risk for cancers of the gastrointestinal tract, larynx, kidney, and ovary have also been reported (Rom, 1992), but epidemiologic evidence for these sites is less convincing than for lung cancer and mesothelioma. The multiplicative interaction of risks for lung cancer from asbestos and smoking has been well established (Hammond, Selikoff, & Seidman, 1979).

Although the first case of asbestosis was recognized in 1906 and asbestos was linked to lung cancer in the 1950s (Rom, 1992), the use of asbestos in industrial products was not regulated until the 1960s. It was not until the 1980s that public health agencies began efforts to have asbestos removed from all products and from buildings.

Other Fibers and Dusts

Naturally occurring fibers other than asbestos have been implicated as carcinogens and pulmonary irritants. Residents of Turkish villages show increased rates of lung cancer and pulmonary fibrosis that are apparently caused by exposure to erionite fibers occurring naturally in the soils of the region (Baris et al., 1978, 1987). Erionite is similar to asbestos and may cause pulmonary damage through mechanisms like those proposed for asbestos.

Man-made fibers have also been implicated in pulmonary disease. They can be grouped as continuous glass filaments, insulation wool composed of glass, rock, or slag, refractory ceramic fibers, and glass microfibers (World Health Organization, 1988; McClellan et al., 1992; Bunn, Bender, Hesterberg, Chase, & Konzen, 1993). These fibers have been used extensively as insulating materials, and as replacements for asbestos. In general, human and animal studies have not shown a relation between exposure to fibrous glass (fiberglass) and pulmonary disease, but animal studies suggest that refractory ceramic fibers induce both interstitial fibrosis and lung cancer (Bunn et al., 1993).

The potential for respiratory disease from both natural and man-made fibers is related to a number of factors: concentration in air, duration of exposure, fiber diameter and length, and fiber composition and durability. Although man-made fibers are similar to asbestos with regard to many of these features, it has not been established whether one or more of the groups of man-made fibers causes pulmonary disease in humans.

Mineral dusts composed of small particles of such materials as silica and coal also induce progressive and permanent pulmonary fibrosis—termed silicosis and anthracosis, respectively. They have caused disease in workers in hard rock and coal mining, in steel mills and foundries (where sand is used in molds), in abrasive cleaning operations such as sandblasting, and in ceramics industries. The mechanism for pulmonary pathology is similar to that of asbestosis— immune responses mediated by macrophages release damaging chemicals and trigger cellular responses that produce fibrosis in pulmonary tissue.

Dusts composed of organic compounds (bioaerosols) cause asthma and hypersensitivity pneumonitis. They are produced by plants in natural ecosystems, in agriculture and industries that process plant and animal products, and by microorganisms that contaminate all kinds of environmental media, including organic matter and the ventilation systems in buildings.

IRRITANT AND ASPHYXIANT GASES

The irritant gases (Figure 4.1) are best represented by the common air pollutants ozone (O_3), oxides of nitrogen (nitrous [or nitrogen] oxide

[N$_2$O], nitrogen monoxide [NO], nitrogen dioxide [NO$_2$]), and oxides of sulfur (primarily sulfur dioxide, SO$_2$). The sources and toxic effects of these air pollutants are described in Chapter 6. Irritant gases can produce a spectrum of damage in the lung—from mild irritation to fibrosis—depending on the magnitude and duration of exposure.

Asphyxiant gases (Figure 4.1) displace oxygen in the lower airways and can lead to asphyxiation and death. Methane (CH$_4$) is a colorless, odorless, inflammable gas. When it emanates from decaying natural vegetation, it is called marsh gas. It is the main component of natural gas and is commonly produced by decaying organic matter in garbage dumps and landfills and by manure. Because methane is lighter than air, it is only a problem in enclosed places, such as in the Third World, where living quarters may be connected to manure storage areas.

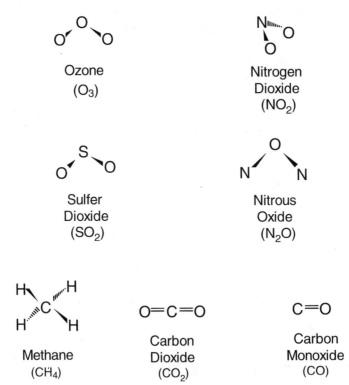

Figure 4.1 Chemical and structural formulas for common irritant and asphyxiant gases.

Carbon dioxide (CO_2, Figure 4.1) is colorless and odorless but, when inhaled, it leaves a sour taste in the mouth. It is produced naturally by respiration in plants and animals, by microbial decomposition of organic matter, and during the combustion of plant and fossil fuels. It is used in the chemical industry and is a waste product of industry as well.

Carbon dioxide is an asphyxiant and produces narcosis as well as asphyxiation. In 1986 about 1,700 people were killed when a cloud of CO_2 erupted from the sediments of Lake Nyos in Cameroon (Freeth, 1992; Kling et al., 1987). The source of the eruption was a chamber of molten rock deep under the water. The gas percolated into the lower part of the lake and was trapped by a layer of cold water. An unknown "trigger"—perhaps strong wind, falling rocks, heavy rainfall, or a sudden surge of gas—disrupted the cold water layer, releasing the trapped gas. Because CO_2 is heavier than air, it flowed through low-lying areas and asphyxiated villagers as they slept.

Carbon Monoxide

Carbon monoxide (CO, Figure 4.1) is a byproduct of combustion, particularly from automobiles and heaters that burn oil, gas, or charcoal. This colorless, odorless gas combines with hemoglobin to form carboxyhemoglobin, thereby acting as a chemical asphyxiant. Carbon monoxide from combustion of fuels can build up inside poorly ventilated buildings and is a common cause of death from indoor air pollution (Cobb & Etzel, 1991). Automobiles increase CO levels in urban air (Chapter 6) and are also a major cause of carbon monoxide poisoning in enclosed spaces.

ORGANIC CHEMICALS

Of the chemicals contaminating the environment, the organic compounds are certainly prominent. Carbon atoms provide their primary structure, whereas a wide variety of other atoms determine their chemical characteristics and toxicity. The simplest organic chemicals are hydrocarbons—compounds composed of chains (aliphatic hydrocarbons) or rings (aromatic hydrocarbons) of carbon atoms with attached atoms of hydrogen. Though organic chemists use plenty of terms to classify these compounds based on their composition and structure, environmental scientists find it more convenient to organize them by a combination of their molecular structure, physical characteristics, and uses in agriculture and industry.

Pesticides

Pesticides eradicate or control organisms that damage crops, buildings, and ornamental vegetation. This general term encompasses a variety of more specific categories, including desiccants, fungicides, herbicides, insecticides, insect growth regulators, miticides, nematicides, plant growth regulators, rodenticides, and soil fumigants. Generally, the pesticides that pose the greatest risk to human health are the organic chemicals used as insecticides, herbicides, fumigants, and rodenticides.

Organophosphorus compounds (Figure 4.2) are organic compounds that contain phosphate groups. Parathion is an organophosphate that is acutely toxic to humans and has caused many fatal poisonings by intentional and inadvertent direct ingestion and by contamination of food (Diggory et al., 1977). For these reasons its use has been severely restricted in the United States, but it is produced and used without such restrictions in many other countries (Dinham, 1993). Malathion, a less-toxic organophosphate, has been used in attempts to prevent the spread of the Mediterranean fruit fly in California. It has also been used in Pakistan to control DDT-resistant mosquitoes. There are hundreds of other organophosphorus compounds marketed worldwide, and the acute human toxicity of different compounds varies considerably.

In the United States organophosphates are responsible for more toxic exposures than any other group of pesticide (Litovitz et al., 1993). Most severe poisonings follow acute episodes of high exposure—usually by accidental ingestion of solutions in unmarked or poorly marked containers. Children are particularly at risk for such exposure.

Organophosphates are well absorbed by the skin, conjunctiva, gastrointestinal tract, and the lungs. These compounds irreversibly inhibit the enzyme acetylcholinesterase, producing an acute syndrome characterized by diarrhea, salivation, airway obstruction, rest-

Organophosphates

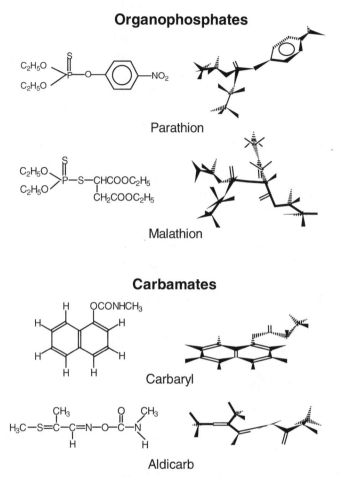

Parathion

Malathion

Carbamates

Carbaryl

Aldicarb

Figure 4.2   Chemical and structural formulas for selected organophosphate and carbamate pesticides.

lessness, anxiety, miosis, and muscle fasciculations. High doses can cause convulsions, coma, and death by respiratory failure. Acute organophosphate poisoning by some compounds can be followed by syndromes of intermediate and delayed neurotoxicity (Senanayake & Karalliedde, 1987).

Carbamate pesticides (Figure 4.2) are derivatives of carbamic acid that reversibly inhibit the enzyme acetylcholinesterase. Carbaryl (Sevin®)—the pesticide produced at the Union Carbide plant in Bhopal, India—and aldicarb (Temik®) are popular carbamate pesticides. Of the insecticides currently on the market, aldicarb has one of the lowest LD_{50}s in animals. It has concentrated in toxic levels in some shallow aquifers and has occasionally poisoned humans who consumed agricultural products such as watermelons that were contaminated through improper application of this insecticide (Green, Heurmann, & Wehr, 1987). Compared with organophosphates, the effects of carbamates are similar but, because enzyme inhibition is reversible, they are usually less severe and of shorter duration. However, fatal poisonings from carbamates have been reported.

Organochlorine pesticides are chlorinated organic compounds with structures of varied complexity (Figure 4.3). DDT (dichlorodiphenyltrichloroethane) was an extremely popular insecticide from the 1950s to the 1970s. Because it accumulates in food chains and is toxic to birds, it has been banned in the United States and many other countries. However, DDT continues to be used by Third World countries to eradicate mosquitoes in the control of malaria.

DDT is an example of a pesticide that has been banned because of its toxicity to natural ecosystems—not because of its human toxicity. However, it has been shown to be a carcinogen, a teratogen, and a mutagen in laboratory studies of animals. DDT also produces tremors and acute central nervous system toxicity in humans (Anger & Johnson, 1985). Although a recent study suggested a relation between DDT and breast cancer in humans (Wolff, Toniolo, Lee, Rivera, & Dubin, 1993), another found no such relation (Krieger et al., 1994). Moreover, most studies of humans with low-to-moderate tissue concentrations of DDT have shown no risk for disease.

Chlorinated cyclodienes are organochlorine compounds with complex ring structures; they include aldrin, chlordane, dieldrin, eldrin, heptachlor, and toxaphene (Figure 4.3). At high doses, members of this family of insecticides produce acute neurotoxicity in humans, including tremors and seizures.

Chlordane has been used extensively in the eradication of termites and other domestic insects. In the laboratory it causes liver toxicity and cancer in mice and immune system changes in their pups. In humans, chlordane produces stupor and seizures and ingestion of only a few grams can be fatal. This compound is extremely persistent in the environment and concentrates in food chains. If incorrectly applied in the soil around buildings and in basements, chlordane can

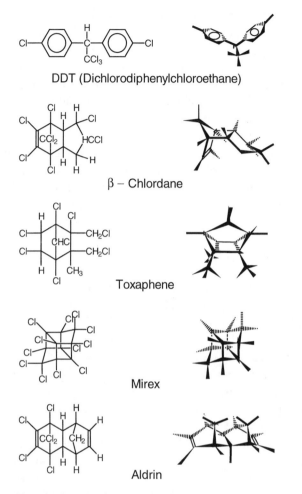

DDT (Dichlorodiphenylchloroethane)

β – Chlordane

Toxaphene

Mirex

Aldrin

Figure 4.3   Chemical and structural formulas for selected organochlorine pesticides.

contaminate the air inside buildings and expose humans to toxic concentrations. Because of this problem, chlordane was voluntarily taken off the U.S. market in 1988 and later banned by the EPA. Companies based in the United States still market it abroad (Dinham, 1993).

Toxaphene is a mixture of many different chlorinated hydrocarbons that are particularly toxic to fish. The popularity of this compound in the United States declined after it was shown to be an animal carcinogen in laboratory tests. It is, however, used throughout the world.

Mirex is a chlorinated hydrocarbon that has been applied to control fire ants in the southeastern United States. In terms of acute toxicity, it is less potent than DDT. However, it is persistent in ecosystems, concentrates in food chains, and has produced liver disease and tumors in animals in laboratory tests. In the environment mirex may degrade to chlordecone (Kepone®), an organochlorine pesticide that has a similar complex ring structure. Mirex was banned by the U.S. Environmental Protection Agency (EPA) in 1977. In the 1970s Kepone® caused severe neurologic disease and reduced the concentration and motility of sperm in heavily exposed workers at a poorly run Virginia production facility (Taylor, Selhorst, Houff, & Martinez, 1978). Kepone® is no longer produced in the United States.

Phenoxyaliphatic Acids

Herbicides have been used extensively in agriculture and in the Vietnam War. The phenoxyaliphatic acids (Figure 4.4) include 2,4-D (2,4-dichlorophenoxyacetic acid) and 2,4,5-T (2,4,5-trichlorophenoxyacetic acid). These two compounds have received attention because both are contaminated by polychlorinated dibenzo-p-dioxins; 2,4,5-T is contaminated by 2,3,7,8-tetrachlorodibenzo-p-dioxin (TCDD), the most toxic of the dioxins. Agent Orange, which was used extensively as a defoliant in the Vietnam War (Orians & Pfeiffer, 1970), is a mixture of 2,4-D and 2,4,5-T.

Both 2,4-D and 2,4,5-T inhibit oxidative phosphorylation, cause a mild heat exhaustion syndrome, and are toxic to muscle and possibly to peripheral nerves (Ellenhorn & Barceloux, 1988). Hepatotoxicity has been noted for 2,4-D in a number of species, and it may be a carcinogen (International Agency for Research on Cancer [IARC], 1977; Lilienfeld & Gallo, 1989). In mice, 2,4,5-T is a teratogen; there is conflicting evidence for the carcinogenicity of this compound.

A few epidemiologic studies of industrial and agricultural exposures to phenoxyaliphatic acids indicate increased risks for soft tissue sarcomas and non-Hodgkin's lymphoma, and there is weaker evidence for the relation between these compounds and Hodgkin's disease—another type of malignant lymphoma (Hoar et al., 1986; Hoar

Phenoxyaliphatic Acids

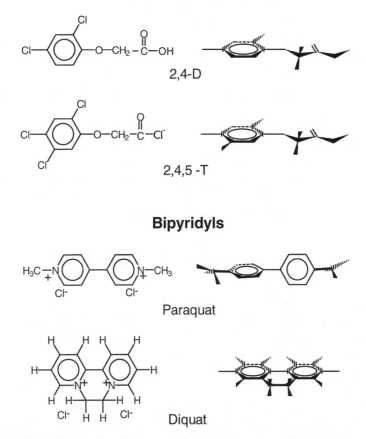

2,4-D

2,4,5 -T

Bipyridyls

Paraquat

Diquat

Figure 4.4   Chemical and structural formulas for selected herbicides.

Zahm et al., 1990; Stellman & Stellman, 1992). There is still debate over these findings, and in many studies it is not clear whether disease risk is associated with either 2,4-D, 2,4,5-T, or TCDD alone, or one compound in combination with one or two of the others. In the United States, use of 2,4-D has been restricted to pastures, rangeland, and rice crops, and suspended for food crops and for vegetation in aquatic and recreational areas. In 1990, 2,4-D was withdrawn from the market in Sweden in light of evidence for its carcinogenicity (Hardell, 1994).

Bipyridyls

Bipyridyl herbicides (Figure 4.4) include paraquat along with the less popular diquat. Paraquat is extremely toxic and is heavily regulated in the United States. Some Latin American countries and the United States still allow paraquat to be sprayed on marijuana fields, and paraquat is used in agriculture in many countries.

Both paraquat and diquat are poorly absorbed by the skin and gastrointestinal tract. In spite of paraquat's low gastrointestinal absorption, the oral route is the most common one for poisoning. Ingestion can be intentional; it also occurs by mistake when paraquat is stored in beverage containers. Paraquat causes severe fibrosis and necrosis in the lung, but this damage is not seen with diquat. Both compounds can cause significant damage to the epithelium of the gastrointestinal tract and to other tissues.

Polychlorinated Biphenyls and Dibenzofurans

Polychlorinated biphenyls (PCBs, Figure 4.5) include 209 chloro-biphenyl congeners—each with a different arrangement of chlorine atoms about the biphenyl rings. PCBs have been used widely in the past in electrical transformers and capacitors, wood sealants, plasticizers, and carbonless copying paper. They are fat soluble, and many congeners are very stable. Because of these chemical characteristics, PCBs concentrate in sediments and aquatic food chains.

The United States banned PCBs from industry in 1971, and their use has been banned or restricted by many other countries. They are still found in old transformers, capacitors, and other products. Today a major route of exposure to humans is through consuming fish from aquatic ecosystems contaminated by industries that used PCBs in the past.

Polychlorinated dibenzofurans are unwanted contaminants of a number of industrial chemicals and are produced in waste incineration, the chlorine bleaching of paper pulp, and the industrial production of the fungicide pentachlorophenol. Dibenzofurans are contaminants of some PCB mixtures and are commonly found with another unwanted group of by-products, the polychlorinated dibenzo-p-dioxins.

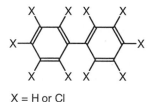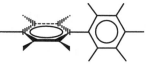

X = H or Cl

Polychlorinated Biphenyls (PCBs)

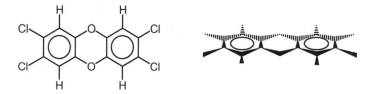

2,3,7,8-Tetrachlorodibenzo-p-dioxin (TCDD)

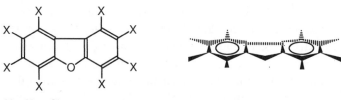

X = H or Cl

Polychlorinated Dibenzofurans

Figure 4.5   Chemical and structural formulas for selected halogenated polyaromatic hydrocarbons.

PCBs are absorbed in the lungs, through the skin and by the gastrointestinal tract. They accumulate in fatty tissue and are excreted in human milk. Most humans carry trace amounts of PCBs in their tissues. Toxic effects attributed to PCBs include acute eye irritation, nausea, respiratory difficulty, chloracne, toxic hepatitis, and sensory peripheral neuropathy. It is unclear whether PCBs caused these effects or whether they were caused by the chlorinated dibenzofurans which have contaminated some of the PCB mixtures to which humans were exposed.

Outbreaks of poisoning occurred in Japan in 1968 (*Yusho disease*) and in Taiwan in 1978 (*Yucheng disease*). In both instances, rice oil was accidentally contaminated by a mixture of PCBs and other toxic compounds that leaked from heating units in rice oil production facilities. Many who consumed the contaminated rice oil in Japan and Taiwan developed chloracne. Adults in one or both outbreaks exhibited a number of other abnormal findings including nausea, vomiting, appetite loss, weakness, swelling of the limbs, abnormal liver function, and dark, discolored skin (Kimbrough, 1987). In both outbreaks, children exposed in utero showed hyperpigmentation, and some Taiwanese children were born with erupted teeth and later exhibited impaired tooth development (Rogan et al., 1988). A follow-up of persons exposed in Japan showed an increase in mortality from liver cancer for men but not for women (Kuratsune, Nakamura, Ikeda, & Hirohata, 1987). Infants born to women exposed in the Taiwan incident had a high mortality rate (Hsu et al., 1985) and showed evidence of mild behavioral and activity disorders (Chen et al., 1994).

In the Japanese outbreak, researchers first identified PCBs in the rice oil and thought they caused the illness. Further investigation showed that the rice oil contained many other chemicals in relatively high concentrations, including polychlorinated dibenzofurans, polychlorinated quarterphenyls, and polychlorinated dibenzo-p-dioxins. Polychlorinated dibenzofurans appear to be the most toxic of the mixture, and were most likely responsible for the noted toxic effects. This conclusion is supported by evidence from workers with high exposures to PCBs exclusively, who have not shown the ill effects observed in the Japanese and Taiwanese outbreaks.

In capacitor plants with relatively high air levels of PCBs, workers have experienced skin and eye irritation, nausea, and respiratory difficulties. In some plants where PCBs were used, chloracne was also reported. It is not clear whether the chloracne was caused by PCBs or by chlorinated dibenzofurans, which may have been present as contaminants. In other factories with similar exposures to PCBs chloracne was not observed.

Highly chlorinated commercial mixtures of PCBs have caused liver tumors in rodents. Like DDT, polychlorinated biphenyls have been shown to be tumor promoters and to have estrogenic effects in animals (IARC, 1991; Safe, 1987; Silberhorn, Glauert, & Robertson, 1990).

Chlorinated Dibenzo-p-dioxins

Polychlorinated dibenzo-p-dioxins (commonly termed dioxins, Figure 4.5) comprise a group of stable, environmentally persistent chemicals that are byproducts in the manufacture of other chlorinated compounds such as chlorinated phenols and their derivatives, hexachlorobenzene, and all products that are produced using these compounds as starting materials. Dioxins are also formed during the chlorine bleaching of pulp and paper and by combustion in forest fires, incinerators, automobile engines, and cigarettes.

The most toxic and most studied of the dioxins is 2,3,7,8-tetrachlorodibenzo-p-dioxin (commonly abbreviated TCDD). TCDD is very toxic in a number of laboratory animal species. In mice, rats, and guinea pigs, it has increased mortality, decreased weight gain, and altered concentrations of a number of enzymes; TCDD has also increased the incidence of gross and microscopic pathologic changes, including hepatocellular carcinomas and squamous cell carcinomas at a number of sites (Kociba et al., 1978). Laboratory studies have also linked TCDD to developmental and reproductive abnormalities, immune suppression, and disruption of regulatory hormones (EPA, 1994). In a recently published study, TCDD was shown to produce endometriosis in Rhesus monkeys 10 years after termination of chronic exposure (Rier, Martin, Bowman, Dmowski, & Becker, 1993). Additional studies will have to be conducted before the importance of this finding can be assessed.

The onset of acute effects from short-term exposures to dioxins are usully delayed for 2 weeks or more after first exposure. Chloracne, liver enlargement, and neuromuscular disease have been diagnosed in humans exposed to TCDD.

Groups of humans have been exposed in occupational settings or following accidental or purposeful environmental releases; TCDD and other dioxins are also found in low concentrations (in the ng/kg range) in members of the general public (Orban, Stanley, Schwemberger, & Remmers, 1994). In the Vietnam War, both

Americans and Vietnamese were exposed to Agent Orange, which contained TCDD as a contaminant. Many Vietnam veterans have claimed their health has been affected by exposure to Agent Orange, and reports from Vietnam also raise the question of human health risks. Even though a number of epidemiologic studies of Vietnam veterans have been conducted (Stellman & Stellman, 1992), it has been hard to establish causal relations between exposure and disease. The main problem has been the absence of data and methods for determining the exposure status of subjects in epidemiologic studies.

Vietnamese researchers have found evidence of adverse pregnancy outcomes and cancer in members of the general public who were exposed to these herbicides (Constable & Hatch, 1985; Sterling & Arundel, 1986). These studies are difficult to interpret for reasons similar to those for the studies of U. S. veterans. Furthermore, many are unpublished and few are available to the international scientific community for review.

An explosion at a chemical plant that was manufacturing 2,4,5-trichlorophenol released large quantities of TCDD to the atmosphere around Seveso Italy in 1976. As many as 37,000 residents were exposed to varying concentrations of TCDD. About 300 of this group—most of them children—developed chloracne and other skin lesions within months after exposure. Some who lived in the highly exposed areas developed polyneuropathy and other abnormal neurologic conditions as well as hepatomegaly (Pocchiari, Silano & Zampieri, 1979). An epidemiologic study of the community exposed in Seveso is still underway, and recent analyses suggest increases in the incidence of a number of different cancers (Bertazzi et al., 1989, 1993). Such data will always be difficult to interpret, however, as exposures were not well characterized and the number of subjects in the high exposure areas is small.

Studies of workers exposed to TCDD in the manufacture of 2,4,5-T have also shown increased mortality for all cancers combined, soft tissue sarcoma, and respiratory tract cancers (Zober, Messerer, & Huber, 1990; Fingerhut et al., 1991; Manz et al., 1991; Kogevinas et al., 1993). Because it has been difficult in epidemiologic studies to separate the effects from combined exposure to TCDD, the phenoxy herbicides, and contaminants of these products, it may be prudent, according to Axelson (1993) to regard the entire complex of exposures as risky.

Volatile Organic Compounds

Volatile organic compounds (VOCs, Figure 4.6) is a term used to describe a diverse group of simple organic compounds, including solvents and halogenated hydrocarbons. These compounds are stable and commonly contaminate aquifers, soil, and the atmosphere. When assessing contamination from chemical sources, environmental scientists often quantify these compounds as a group rather than measuring each separately.

Solvents (a classification based on function rather than chemical structure) are liquid at room temperature; most are volatile and many are used for purposes other than removing grease and dirt. Formaldehyde is used extensively in industry as a solvent, in the synthesis of chemicals, and in building materials. Urea-formaldehyde foam insulation, particle board, and carpet adhesives all contain formaldehyde and emit this chemical to indoor air, particularly when

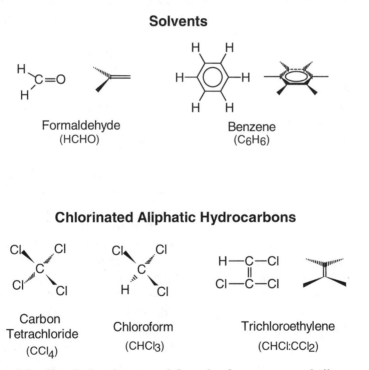

Solvents

Formaldehyde
(HCHO)

Benzene
(C6H6)

Chlorinated Aliphatic Hydrocarbons

Carbon
Tetrachloride
(CCl4)

Chloroform
(CHCl3)

Trichloroethylene
(CHCl:CCl2)

Figure 4.6 Chemical and structural formulas for common volatile organic compounds.

materials are new. Wood and tobacco smoke also contain this compound. Formaldehyde irritates mucous membranes and causes allergic dermatitis and asthma. This compound has also been shown to produce nasal cancer in animals, and there is limited evidence that it is also a human carcinogen (Landrigan, 1992).

Benzene is an industrial solvent and a starting compound in many chemical syntheses. It is a natural contaminant of motor fuels and is used in the petrochemical and rubber industries. Like other solvents, benzene is acutely toxic to the central nervous system. It produces a syndrome of acute toxicity characterized by euphoria, headache, and drowsiness. Stupor, coma, and convulsions may follow high exposures. Benzene blocks mitosis of cells in bone marrow and causes aplastic anemia; it is also a mutagen and has been shown to cause myelogenous leukemia in humans.

Chlorinated aliphatic hydrocarbons (Figure 4.6) are halogenated hydrocarbons composed of various arrangements of chlorine, carbon, hydrogen, and oxygen. Carbon tetrachloride (CCl_4) is used to manufacture many chemicals, including halogenated hydrocarbon refrigerants. It is a common pollutant of aquifers, rivers, and lakes. Chloroform (CCl_3) is another chlorinated hydrocarbon used as a solvent and a chemical feedstock in industry; it has also been used as an anesthetic. Chloroform is produced in trace amounts when organic compounds in water are treated with chlorine for drinking water purification. Both carbon tetrachloride and chloroform produce acute and chronic damage to the liver and kidneys and are considered potential human carcinogens.

Trichloroethylene (TCE) is an industrial solvent and degreasing agent. It was once used to extract caffeine from coffee and as a human anesthetic (it is still used in animal surgery). Acute exposure to high doses of TCE can produce potentially fatal cardiac arrhythmias. TCE also causes acute renal tubular necrosis and transient necrosis of liver cells. Although some laboratory experiments have shown TCE to produce liver and lung cancers in mice, there is still debate over whether TCE should be classified as a human carcinogen.

TCE is particularly mobile in soil and water, and improper handling and disposal has resulted in extensive contamination of many aquifers. Airports, military bases, nuclear weapons production plants, and the computer microchip industry have been the major contributors to such environmental contamination. Tetrachloroethylene (perchloroethylene or PCE), a solvent commonly used in dry cleaning and degreasing, may also contaminate soil and water. Because it is more volatile than TCE, it is less likely to contaminate ground and surface water. In one study (Kyyronen, Taskinen, Lindbohm, Hemminki, & Heinonen, 1989), tetrachloroethylene was associated with spontaneous abortion in women who worked in the dry–cleaning industry.

TOXINS

The term *toxin,* though often used to describe any toxic agent, is more correctly applied to biologically active, naturally occurring organic compounds that are usually composed of proteins. Humans are exposed to toxins in food, water, the atmosphere, through dermal contact, and by the bites of animals and insects. Bacterial toxins are well-known, and their effects include cell swelling, platelet adhesion, vasodilation, hypotension, paralysis, and cell death (Marrack & Kappler, 1990). Toxins operate through a variety of mechanisms —some have enzymatic activity, some increase levels of cyclic adenosine monophosphate in target cells, and some elicit immune responses.

Most bacterial food poisonings occur through gastrointestinal infections from the bacteria in food, as discussed in Chapter 3. Some species of bacteria, such as *Vibrio cholerae* (the bacterium that causes cholera), release toxins into food and do not actually infect humans.

Fish are common sources of acute, toxin-associated food-borne outbreaks. Twenty to 40 ciguatera and scombroid poisoning outbreaks per year are reported in the United States (CDC, 1990). Ciguatoxin is produced by *Gambierdiscus toxicus* and other marine dinoflagellates, which are found in association with sessile algae and detritus in coral reef ecosystems (Auerbach & Halstead, 1989). As this toxin is passed through the food chain, it concentrates in successive organisms and reaches highest concentrations in the fish (amberjack, snapper, grouper, and barracuda) that feed in this ecosystem. Ciguatoxin poisoning results in a variety of gastrointestinal and neurologic symptoms.

Scombroid fish poisoning follows the consumption of inadequately refrigerated fish of the suborder Scombroidei (albacore, blue- and yellow-fin tuna, and mackerel) and other dark-fleshed species. Scombrotoxism is characterized by flushing, headache, and allergic symptoms that are similar to those produced by histamine, which has been measured in high concentrations in fish implicated in such poisonings. Presumably, histamine is produced in the bacterial decomposition of amino acids in fish muscle. Although some have argued that histamine may not be the sole agent, high concentrations have been measured in urine from subjects in a recent outbreak (Morrow, Margolies, Rowland & Roberts, 1991), strongly implicating this toxin as the causative agent.

Other dinoflagellate species produce neurotoxins that contaminate filter-feeding clams, oysters, mussels, and crabs. Paralytic shellfish poisoning, which can progress from mild paresthesias to respiratory arrest, is most frequently caused by saxitoxin (Yentson, 1984), but has been linked to other dinoflagellate toxins. Neurotoxic shellfish poisoning is a milder condition caused by less-toxic toxins such as those produced by the dinoflagellate *Ptychodiscus breve*, which causes "red tides" under physical, biological, and chemical conditions that favor its growth.

Alkaloids are nitrogen-containing toxins present in from 10% to 25% of all plant species (Geehr & Kunkel, 1989; Winter, 1990). Although alkaloids poison animals more frequently than humans, they are common in edible plants and are toxic to humans at high doses. Tropane alkaloids are cholinesterase inhibitors and are present in a number of fruits and vegetables of the Solanaceae family, including chili pepper, potatoes, apples, eggplants, belladonna, and Jimson weed. Pyrrolizidine alkaloids are hepatotoxic and carcinogenic; they are produced by many different plant species, some of which are used as herbal teas or folk medicines. Outbreaks of liver disease have been linked to consumption of grain that was contaminated when weeds containing these alkaloids were harvested along with the grain (Mohabbat et al., 1976; Tandon et al., 1976).

Some toxic amino acids are produced by plants that are used as food, as evidenced by the group of amino acids found in seeds of the genus of *Lathyrus,* which cause the chronic neurological disease lathyrism. This disease is still prevalent in India and other countries where the seed is eaten when other foods are in short supply. Neurotoxic and carcinogenic amino acids have also been identified in seeds of the Cycad, which are used to make flour in Guam and other areas of the western Pacific region (Spencer, Kisby, & Ludolph, 1991).

Other plant toxins include glucosinolates, which are produced by the crucifer family (cabbage, kale, and brussels sprouts) and interfere with thyroid function (Winter, 1990); glycosides with a variety of toxic effects including cardiotoxicity (the digitalis-producing foxglove, for example) and the generation of hydrogen cyanide; and oxalates (concentrated in spinach and rhubarb leaŸes) which form kidney stones and produce acute gastrointestinal and neurologic syndromes.

A number of plant toxins are carcinogens. Safrole, which produces liver cancer in rats, is found in the sassafras plant and in oils of camphor and nutmeg. Caffeic acid, the naturally occurring carcinogen that poses the greatest risk to humans through dietary exposure, is found in lettuce, coffee, apples, potatoes, and carrots (Gold, Slone, Stern, Manley, & Ames, 1992).

Mycotoxins, low molecular weight compounds produced by many different species of molds, are toxic to humans and other animals primarily as contaminants of food chains. Aflatoxins comprise a group of toxins produced by some strains of *Aspergillus* species that contaminate peanuts and animal feed. Aflatoxins B_1 and its metabolite M_1 (found in milk of cows that consumed feed contaminated by aflatoxin B_1) are animal carcinogens and aflatoxin B_1 is a potent hepatotoxin that has been linked to the high incidence of liver cancer in Africa and Asia (Bressac, Kew, Wands & Ozturk, 1991). There is also evidence that hepatitis B infection, alone or in conjunction with aflatoxin B_1, causes liver cancer in these areas (Hsia et al., 1992; Wogan, 1992). A number of other mycotoxins cause a variety of diseases by many different mechanisms (Hsieh & Gruenwedel, 1990).

Mushrooms contain a variety of toxins that can poison humans and other animals that eat them. Mushroom toxins produce a variety of effects, including gastrointestinal discomfort, hallucinations, and severe liver and kidney damage. Mushroom toxins are usually grouped according to the type of symptoms they produce and to their chemical properties (Concón, 1988; Geehr & Kunkel, 1989; Hsieh & Gruenwedel, 1990). These toxins include cyclopeptides (produced by species of *Amanita* and *Galerina),* which are extremely toxic to liver cells and cause fatal poisonings; monomethylhydrazine, a metabolite of the toxin gyromitrin (produced by species of *Gyromitra,* the false morels), which causes hemolysis and is toxic to the liver and kidneys; muscarine and muscimol, parasympathomimetic alkaloids produced by a variety of species, including *Amanita muscaria*; the psychoactive compounds ibotenic acid (in *Amanita muscaria* and *A. pantheria*), and the hallucinogens psilocybin and psilocin (produced by *Psilocybe* and *Paneolus species*).

SUMMARY

Toxic chemicals are widespread in the environment and therefore have the potential for causing significant damage to human health. In contrast to the ubiquity and toxicity of these substances, few adverse health effects have been clearly demonstrated with epidemiologic techniques. Damage to human health has primarily been shown in workers and in a few well-known episodes such as the Minamata Bay incident. In many other instances it has been possible to document exposure, but more difficult to demonstrate intake, dose, or health effects conclusively. As discussed in Chapter 10, however, the absence of epidemiologic evidence is not adequate to exclude health risks—particularly in studies of small populations.

Though we have compiled an impressive body of literature on the toxicity of a wide variety of chemicals, we know little about the health risks from chronic exposures to low concentrations of chemicals, or from exposures to mixtures of chemicals. Because toxicity testing will not keep pace with the introduction of new chemicals into the environment, practitioners of environmental health will have to continue to rely on health surveillance and environmental monitoring programs in order to protect the public.

REFERENCES

Agocs, M. M., Etzel, R. A., Parrish, R. G., Paschal, D. C., Campagna, P. R., Cohen, D. S., Kilbourn, E. M., & Hesse, J. L. (1990). Mercury exposure from interior latex paint. *New England Journal of Medicine, 323*, 1096-1101.

Anger, K. W., & Johnson, B. L. (1985). Chemicals affecting behavior. In J. L. O' Donoghue (Ed.), *Neurotoxicity of industrial and commercial chemicals*, Vol. I. (pp. 51-148). Boca Raton, FL: CRC Press.

Auerbach, P. S., & Halstead, B. W. (1989). Hazardous aquatic life. In P. S. Auerbach & E. C. Geehr (Eds.), *Management of wilderness and environmental emergencies* (pp. 932-1028). St. Louis: C. V. Mosby.

Axelson, O. (1993). Seveso: Disentangling the dioxin enigma? *Epidemiology, 4*, 389-392.

Baghurst, P. A., McMichael, A. J., Wigg, N. R., Vimpani, G. V., Robertson, E. F., Roberts, R. J., & Tong, S. L. (1992). Environmental exposure to lead and children's intelligence at the age of seven years: the Port Pirie cohort study. *New England Journal of Medicine, 327*, 1279-1284.

Baris, Y. I., Sahin, A. A., Ozismi, M., Kerse, I., Ozen, E., Kolacan, B., Altinors, M., & Goktepeli, A. (1978). An outbreak of pleural mesothelioma and chronic fibrosing pleurisy in the village of Karain/Urgup in Anatolia. *Thorax, 33,* 181-192.

Baris, I., Simonato, L., Artvinli, M., Pooley, F., Saracci, R., Skidmore, J., & Wagner, C. (1987). Epidemiological and environmental evidence of the health effects of exposure to eronite fibers: A four-year study in the Cappadocian region of Turkey. *International Journal of Cancer, 39,* 10-17.

Bertazzi, P. A., Zocchetti, C., Pesatori, A. C., Guercilena, S., Sanarico, M.,& Radice, L. (1989). Ten-year mortality study of the population involved in the Seveso incident in 1976. *American Journal of Epidemiology, 129*, 1187-1200.

Bertazzi, P. A., Pesatori, A. C., Consonni, D., Tironi, A., Landi, M. T., & Zocchetti, C. (1993). Cancer incidence in a population accidentally exposed to 2,3,7,8-tetrachlorodibenzo-para-dioxin. *Epidemiology, 4,* 398-406.

Bressac, B., Kew, M., Wands, J., & Ozturk, M. (1991). Selective G to T mutations of p53 gene in hepatocellular carcinoma from southern Africa. *Nature, 350,* 429-431.

Brody, D. J., Pirkle, J. L., Kramer, R. A., Flegal, K., Matte, T. D., Gunter, E. W., & Paschal, D. C. (1994). Blood levels in the US population: Phase 1 of the Third National Health and Nutrition Examination Survey (NHANES III, 1988-1991). *JAMA, 272,* 277-283.

Bunn, W. B., Bender, J. R., Hesterberg, T. W., Chase, G. R., & Konzen, J. L. (1993). Recent studies of man-made vitreous fibers: Chronic animal inhalation studies. *Journal of Occupational Medicine, 35,* 101-113.

Centers for Disease Control and Prevention. (1990). Foodborne disease outbreaks, 5-year summary, 1983-1987. *Morbidity Mortality Weekly Report, 39* (No. SS-1), 15-57.

Centers for Disease Control and Prevention. (1991). *Preventing lead poisoning in young children.* Atlanta, GA: U.S. Department of Health and Human Services.

Chamberlain, J. L., & Quillian, W. W. (1963). Acrodynia: A long-term study of 62 cases. *Clinical Pediatrics, 2,* 439-443.

Chen, Y-C J., Yu, M-L M., Rogan, W. J., Gladen, B. C., Hsu, C-C. (1994). A 6-year follow-up of behavior and activity disorders in the Taiwan Yu-cheng children. *American Journal of Public Health, 84,* 415-421.

Cobb, N., & Etzel, R. A. (1991). Unintentional carbon monoxide-related deaths in the United States, 1979 through 1988. *JAMA, 266,* 659-63.

Concon, J. (1988). *Food toxicology, part A: principles and concepts.* New York: Marcel Dekker.

Constable, J. D., & Hatch, M. C. (1985). Reproductive effects of herbicide exposure in Vietnam: Recent studies by the Vietnamese and others. *Teratogenesis, Carcinogenesis, and Mutagenesis , 5,* 231-250.

Diggory, H. J. P., Landrigan, P. J., Latimer, K. P., Ellington, A. C., Kimbrough, R. D., Liddle, J. A., Cline, R. E., & Smrek, A. L. (1977). Fatal parathion poisoning caused by contamination of flour in interna-tional commerce. *American Journal of Epidemiology, 106,* 145-153.

Dinham, B. (1993). *The pesticide hazard.* London: Zed Books.

Elhassani, S. B. (1983). The many faces of methylmercury poisoning. *Journal of Toxicology. Clinical Toxicology, 19,* 875-906.

Ellenhorn, M., & Barceloux, D. (Eds.). (1988). *Medical toxicology: Diagnosis and treatment of human poisoning.* New York: Elsevier.

Ellis, D. (1989). *Environments at risk.* Berlin: Springer-Verlag.

Fingerhut, M. A., Halpern, W. E., Marlow, D. A., Piacitelli, L. A., Honchar, P. A., Sweeney, M. H., Greife, A. L., Dill, P. A., Steenland, K., & Suruda, A. J. (1991). Cancer mortality in workers exposed to 2,3,7,8-tetrachlorodibenzo-*p*-dioxin. *New England Journal of Medicine, 324,* 212-218.

Fischbein, A. (1992). Occupational and environmental lead exposure. In W. Rom (Ed.), *Environmental and occupational medicine* (pp. 735-758). Boston: Little, Brown.

Freeth, S. (1992, August 15). The deadly cloud hanging over Cameroon. *New Scientist,* 23-27.

Geehr, E. C., & Kunkel, D. B. (1989). Poisonous Mushrooms. In P. S. Auerbach & E. C. Geehr (Eds.), *Management of wilderness and envi-ronmental emergencies* (pp. 932-1028). St. Louis: C. V. Mosby.

Gold, L. S., Slone, T. H., Stern, B. R., Manley, N. B., & Ames, B. N. (1992). Rodent carcinogens: Setting priorities. *Science, 258,* 261-265.

Green, M. A., Heurmann, M. A., & Wehr, M. (1987). An outbreak of water-melon-borne pesticide toxicity. *American Journal of Public Health, 77,* 1431-1434.

Hammond, E. C., Selikoff, I. J., & Seidman, H. (1979). Asbestos exposure, cigarette smoking and death rates. *Annals of the New York Academy of Sciences, 321,* 473-490.

Hardell, L. (1994). Chlorophenols, phenoxyacetic acids, and dioxins. In C. Zenz, O. B. Dickerson, & E. P. Horvath (Eds.). *Occupational medicine* (3rd ed.). St. Louis: Mosby.

Hertz-Picciotto, I., & Croft, J. (1993). Review of the relation between blood lead and blood pressure. *Epidemiologic Reviews, 15*, 353-373.

Hoar, S. K., Blair, A., Holmes, F. F., Boysen, C. D., Robel, R. J., Hoover, R., & Fraumeni, J. F. (1986). Agricultural herbicide use and risk of lym-. phoma and soft-tissue sarcoma. *JAMA, 256*, 1141-1147.

Hoar Zahm, S., Weisenburger, D. D., Babbitt, P. A., Saal, R. C., Vaught, J. B., Cantor, K. P., & Blair, A. (1990). A case-control study of non-Hodgkin's lymphoma and the herbicide 2,4-dichloro phenoxyacetic acid (2,4-D) in Eastern Nebraska. *Epidemiology, 1*, 349-356.

Hsieh, D. P. H., & Gruenwedel, S. H. O. (1990). Microbial toxins. In C. K. Winter, J. N. Seiber, & C. F. Nuckton. *Chemicals in the human food chain.* New York: Van Nostrand Reinhold.

Hsia, C. C., Kleiner, D. E., Axiotis, C. A., Di Bisceglie, A., Nomura, A. M. Y., Stemmermann, G. N., & Tabor, E. (1992). Mutations of the p53 gene in hepatocellular carcinoma: Roles of hepatitis B virus and aflatoxin contamination in the diet. *Journal of the National Cancer Institute, 84*, 1638-1641.

Hsu, S-T, Ma, C-I, Hsu, S. K-H, Wu, S-S, Hsu, N-H, Yeh, C-C, & Wu, S-B. (1985). Discovery and epidemiology of PCB poisoning in Taiwan: A four-year follow–up. *Environmental Health Perspectives, 59*, 5-10.

International Agency for Research on Cancer. (1977). Chlorinated dibenzodioxins. *IARC Monographs on the Evaluation of Carcinogenic Risks of Chemicals to Man.* Lyon, France.

International Agency for Research on Cancer. (1991). Occupational exposures in insecticide application, and some pesticides. *IARC Monographs on the Evaluation of Carcinogenic Risks of Chemicals to Man, 53.* Lyon, France.

Kimbrough, R. D. (1987). Human health effects of polychlorinated biphenyls (PCBs) and polybrominated biphenyls (PBBs). *Annual Review of Pharmacology and Toxicology, 27*, 87-111.

Kling, G. W., Clark, M. A., Compton, H. R., Devine, J. D., Evans, W. C., Humphrey, A. M., Koenigsberg, E. J., Lockweed, J. P., Tuttle, M. L., & Wagner, G. N. (1987). The 1986 Lake Nyos gas disaster in Cameroon, West Africa. *Science, 236*, 169-174.

Kociba, R. J., Keyes, D. G., Beyer, J. E., Carreon, R. M., Wade, C. E., Dittenber, D. A., Kalnins, R. P., Frauson, L. E., Park, C. N., Barnard, S. D., Hummel, R. A., & Humiston, C. G. (1978). Results of a two-year chronic toxicity and oncogenicity study of 2,3,7,8-tetrachlorodibenzo-p-dioxin in rats. *Toxicology and Applied Pharmacology, 46*, 279-303.

Kogevinas, M., Saracci, R., Winkelmann, R., Johnson, E. S., Bertazzi, P. A., Bueno de Mesquita, B. H., Kauppinen, T., Littorin, M., Lynge, E., Neuberger, M., & Pearce, N. (1993). Cancer incidence and mortality in women occupationally exposed to chlorphenoxy herbicides, chlorophenols, and dioxins. *Cancer Causes and Control, 4,* 547-553.

Krieger, N., Wolff, M. S., Hiatt, R. A., Rivera, M., Vogelman, J., & Orentreich, N. (1994). Breast cancer and serum organochlorines: A prospective study among white, black, and asian women. *Journal of the National Cancer Institute, 86,* 589-599.

Kuratsune, M., Nakamura, Y., Ikeda, M., & Hirohata, T. (1987). Analysis of deaths seen among patients with Yusho. *Chemosphere, 10,* 2085-2088.

Kyyronen, P., Taskinen, H., Lindbohm, J., Hemminki, K., & Heinonen, O. P. (1989). Spontaneous abortions and congenital malformations among women exposed to tetrachloroethylene in dry cleaning. *Journal of Epidemiology and Community Health, 43,* 346-351.

Landrigan, P. J. (1992). Formaldehyde. In W. Rom (Ed.), *Environmental and occupational medicine* (2nd ed.), (pp. 269-291). Boston: Little, Brown.

Landrigan, P. J., & Nicholson, W. J. (1992). Benzene. In W. Rom (Ed.), *Environmental and occupational medicine* (2nd ed., pp. 861-865). Boston: Little, Brown .

Lilienfeld, D., & Gallo, M. (1989). 2,4-D, 2,4,5-T, and 2,3,7,8-TCDD: An overview. *Epidemiologic Reviews, 11,* 28-58.

Litovitz, T., Holm, K. C., Clancy, C., Schmitz, B. F., Clark, L. R., Oderda, G. M. (1993). 1992 Annual report of the American Association of Poison Control Centers Toxic Exposure Surveillance System. *American Journal of Emergency Medicine, 11,* 494-555.

Marrack, P., & Kappler, J. (1990). The staphylococcal enterotoxins and their relatives. *Science, 248,* 705-711.

Maheswaran, R., Gill, J. S., & Beevers, D. G. (1993). Blood pressure and industrial lead exposure. *American Journal of Epidemiology, 137,* 645-653.

Manz, A., Berger, J., Dwyer, J. H., Flesch-Janys, D., Nagel, S., & Waltsgott, H. (1991). Cancer mortality among workers in chemical plant contaminated with dioxin. *Lancet, 338,* 959-964.

McClellan, R. O., Miller, F. J., Hesterberg, T. W., Warheit, D. B., Bunn, W. B., Kane, A. B., Lippmann, M., Mast, R. W., McConnell, E. E., & Reinhardt, C. F. (1992). Approaches to evaluating the toxicity and carcinogenicity of man-made fibers: Summary of a workshop held November 11-13, 1991, Durham, North Carolina. *Regulatory Toxicology and Pharmacology, 16,* 321-364.

Mohabbat, O., Srivastava, R. M., Younos, M. S., Sediq, G. G., Merzad, A. A., & Aram, G. N. (1976). An outbreak of hepatic veno-occlusive disease in North Western Afghanistan. *Lancet, 2* (7980), 269-271.

Morrow, J. D., Margolies, G. R., Rowland, J., & Roberts, L. J. (1991). Evidence that histamine is the causative toxin of scombroid-fish poisoning. *New England Journal of Medicine, 324,* 716-720.

Neal, P., & Jones, R. R. (1937). Chronic mercurialism in the hatters' fur-cutting industry. *JAMA, 110,* 337-343.

Needleman, H. L., Schell, A., Bellinger, D., Leviton, A., & Allred, E. N. (1990). The long-term effects of exposure to low doses of lead in childhood: an 11-year follow-up report. *New England Journal of Medicine, 322,* 83-88.

Orban, J. E., Stanley, J. S., Schwemberger, J. G., & Remmers, J. C. (1994). Dioxins and dibenzofurans in adipose tissue of the general U.S. population and selected subpopulations. *American Journal of Public Health, 84,* 439–445.

Orians, G. H., & Pfeiffer, E. W. (1970). Ecological effects of the war in Vietnam. *Science, 168,* 544-554.

Pirkle, J. L., Brody, D. J., Gunter, E. W., Kramer, R. A., Paschal, D. C., Flegal, K. M., & Matte, T. D. (1994). The decline in blood lead levels in the United States: The National Health and Nutrition Examination Surveys. *JAMA, 272,* 284-291.

Pocchiari, R., Silano, V., & Zampieri, A. (1979). Human health effects from accidental release of tetrachlorodibenzo-p-dioxin (TCDD) at Seveso, Italy. *Annals of New York Academy of Sciences, 320,* 311-320.

Rier, S. E., Martin, D. C., Bowman, R. E., Dmowski, W. P., & Becker, J. L. (1993). Endometriosis in Rhesus monkeys *(Macaca mulatta)* following chronic exposure to 2,3,7,8-tetrachlorodibenzo-p-dioxin. *Fundamental and Applied Toxicology, 12,* 433-441.

Rogan, W. J., Gladen, B. C., Hung, K-L., Koong, S-L., Shih, L-Y., Taylor, J. S., Wu, Y-C., Yang, D., Ragan, N. B., & Hsu, C-C. (1988). Congenital poisoning by polychlorinated biphenyls and their contaminants in Taiwan. *Science, 241,* 334-336.

Rom, W. (1992). Asbestos-related diseases. In W. Rom (Ed.), *Environmental and occupational medicine* (2nd ed., pp. 269-291). Boston: Little, Brown.

Safe, S. (Ed.). (1987). *Environmental toxin series 1. Polychlorinated biphenyls (PCBs): Mammalian and environmental toxicology.* New York: Springer-Verlag.

Schwartz, J. (1991). Lead, blood pressure, and cardiovascular disease in men and women. *Environmental Health Perspectives, 91,* 71-75.

Senanayake, N., & Karalliedde, L. (1987). Neurotoxic effects of organophosphorus insecticides: An intermediate syndrome. *New England Journal of Medicine, 316,* 761-763.

Silberhorn, E. M., Glauert, H. P., & Robertson, L. W. (1990). Carcinogenicity of polyhalogenated biphenyls: PCBs and PBBs. *Critical Reviews in Toxicology, 20,* 440-496.

Smith, W. E., & Smith, A. (1975). *Minamata*. New York: Holt, Reinhart and Winston.

Spencer, P. S., Kisby, G. E., & Ludolph, A. C. (1991). Slow toxins, biologic markers, and long-latency neurodegenerative disease in the western Pacific region. *Neurology, 41*(Suppl. 2), 62-66.

Stellman, J. M., & Stellman, S. D. (1992). Health effects of phenoxy herbicides and Agent Orange. In W. Rom (Ed.), *Environmental and occupational medicine* (2nd ed., pp. 1041-1049). Boston: Little, Brown.

Sterling, T. D., & Arundel, A. (1986). Review of recent Vietnamese studies on the carcinogenic and teratogenic effects of phenoxy herbicide exposure. *International Journal of Health Services, 16*, 265-278.

Tandon, B. M., Tandon, R. K., Tandon, H. D., Narndranathan, M., & Joshi, Y. K. (1976). An epidemic of veno-occlusive disease of liver in Central India. *Lancet, 2*(7980), 271-272.

Tamashiro, H., Arakaki, M., Akagi, H., Futatsuka, M., & Roht, L. (1985). Mortality and survival for Minamata disease. *International Journal of Epidemiology, 14*, 582-588.

Tedeschi, L. G. (1982). The Minamata disease. *American Journal of Forensic Medicine and Pathology, 3*, 335-338.

Taylor, J. R., Selhorst, J. B., Houff, S.A., & Martinez, A. J. (1978). Chlordecone intoxication in man. 1. Clinical observations. *Neurology, 28*, 626-635.

U.S. Environmental Protection Agency (1994). *Health assessment document for 2,3,7,8-tetrachlorodibenzo-p-dioxin* (TCDD) and related compounds (EPA/600/BP-92/001a, b, c). Washington, DC: Author.

Winter, C. K. (1990). Toxins of plant origin. In C. K. Winter, J. N. Seiber, & C. F. Nuckton (Eds.), *Chemicals in the human food chain*. New York: Van Nostrand Reinhold.

Wogan, G. N. (1992). Aflatoxins as risk factors for hepatocellular carcinoma in humans. *Cancer Research, 52*(Suppl.), 2114s-2118s.

Wolff, M., Toniolo, P., Lee, E., Rivera, M., & Dubin, N. (1993). Blood levels of organochlorine residues and risk of breast cancer. *Journal of the National Cancer Institute, 85*, 648-652.

World Health Organization. (1988). Environmental health criteria. Manmade mineral fibres. *International Program on Chemical Safety:Vol. 77*. Geneva: Author.

Yentson, C. M. (1984). Paralytic shellfish poisoning. An emerging perspective. In Ragelis, E. P. (Ed.), *Seafood toxins*. Washington, DC: American Chemical Society.

Zober, A., Messerer, P., Huber, P. (1990). Thirty-four-year mortality follow-up of BASF employees exposed to 2,3,7,8-TCDD after the 1953 accident. *International Archives of Occupational and Environmental Health, 62*, 139-157.

SUGGESTED READINGS

Amdur, M. O., Doull, J., & Klaassen, C. D. (Eds.). (1991). *Casarett and Doull's Toxicology: The basic science of poisons* (4th ed.). New York: Pergamon.

Cockerham, L., & Shane, B. (Eds.). (1994). *Basic environmental toxicology.* Boca Raton, FL: CRC Press.

Committee on Pesticides in the Diets of Infants and Children. (1993). *Pesticides in the diets of infants and children.* Washington, DC: National Academy Press.

Dinham, B. (1993). *The pesticide hazard.* London: Zed Books.

Ellenhorn, M. J., & Barceloux, D. G. (1988). *Medical toxicology: Diagnosis and treatment of human poisoning.* New York: Elsevier.

Kimbrough, R. D., Mahaffey, K. R., Grandjean, P., Sandoe, S-H., & Rutstein, D. D. (1989). *Clinical effects of environmental chemicals.* New York: Hemisphere.

Lewis, R. J. (1992). *Sax's dangerous properties of industrial materials* (8th ed., Vols.1-3). New York: Van Nostrand Reinhold.

Lippmann, M. (1992). *Environmental toxicants: Human exposures and their health effects.* New York: Van Nostrand Reinhold.

Rom, W. (Ed.). (1992). *Environmental and occupational medicine* (2nd ed.). Boston: Little, Brown.

Rumack, B. H., & Spoerke, D. G. (1994). *Handbook of mushroom poisoning* (2nd ed.). Boca Raton, FL: CRC Press.

Scialli, A. (1991). *A clinical guide to reproductive and developmental toxicology.* Boca Raton, FL: CRC Press.

Winter, C. K., Seiber, J. N., Nuckton, C. F. (Eds.). (1990). *Chemicals in the human food chain.* New York: Van Nostrand Reinhold.

Chapter 5

Ionizing and Nonionizing Radiation

A. James Ruttenber and Herman T. Blumenthal

In our daily lives, we are exposed to many types of radiation, some natural and some artificially produced. Physicists describe radiation as photons that have properties of both particles and waves. The different types of radiation can be conveniently ordered along the *electromagnetic spectrum,* which arranges them according to wavelength, frequency, and energy (Figure 5.1). This is possible because the product of frequency and wavelength is constant and equal to the speed of light (3×10^8 m/sec), and because wavelength is inversely proportional to the energy of a photon, which can be calculated by multiplying frequency by Planck's constant (4.14×10^{-15} electron volt/sec).

At the low-energy, low-frequency, and long-wavelength end of the electromagnetic spectrum are the nonionizing types of radiation such as the extremely low-frequency radiation emitted by electric power lines as well as radio waves, microwaves, infrared radiation, and visible light. Ultraviolet (UV) light spans the gap between nonionizing and ionizing radiation because ultraviolet radiation of short wave lengths has enough energy (more than 10 electron volt) to remove an orbital electron and create an ion.

In the ionizing region of the electromagnetic spectrum are X-rays, gamma rays, and cosmic rays. Alpha particles, beta particles, and neutrons also have enough energy to induce ionization. We will use the electromagnetic spectrum as a "road map" throughout this

The Electromagnetic Spectrum

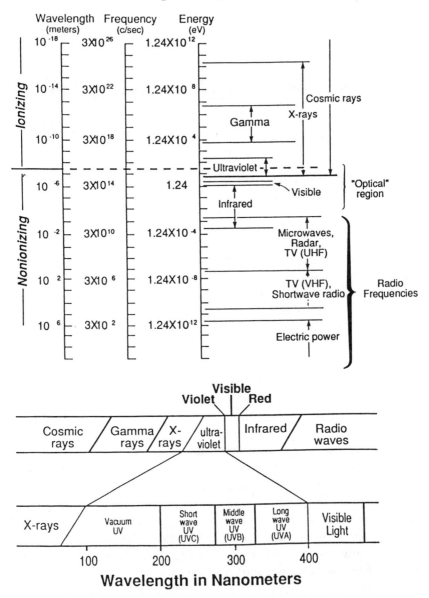

Figure 5.1   The electromagnetic spectrum (from Glaser [1992], with permission). Note: c/sec = cycle/second; eV = electron volt.

chapter. It will help put the different types of radiation in perspective and clearly delineate the boundary between nonionizing and ionizing radiation.

NONIONIZING RADIATION

Compared with ionizing radiation, which has wavelengths less than 100 nanometers (nm) and frequencies greater than 3×10^9 megahertz (1 hertz [Hz] = 1 cycle/sec; 1 megahertz [MHz] = 10^6 Hz), radiation of longer wavelengths does not have enough energy to remove electrons from atoms and produce ions. Except for visible light, nonionizing radiation usually goes undetected by human sensory systems—unless its intensity is high enough to produce heat.

Extremely Low-Frequency Electric and Magnetic Fields

An electrical field and its corresponding magnetic field are produced any time an electric current flows between two points. Fields produced by currents with frequencies between 1 and 3,000 Hz are called *extremely low-frequency electromagnetic fields* (EMFs). They are strongest around high–voltage transmission lines, lower voltage distributor lines, radar and communications systems that involve low-frequency modulation, appliances such as electric blankets, electric shavers, microwave ovens, television screens, and the flyback transformers in video-display terminals.

Because electrical activity is involved in a number of normal physiological functions, low-frequency electric and magnetic fields can produce a variety of effects in living systems. For instance, nerve cells communicate with one another by electrical impulses, electrocardiograms and electroencephalograms record electrical wave patterns in the heart and brain, and pulsed electromagnetic fields are used to enhance the healing of wounds and bone fractures (Becker, 1990).

Some types of electromagnetic exposure, such as radar at short distances, produce enough thermal energy to induce burns and cataracts. The thermal energy produced in tissues by most environmental exposures to EMFs is generally acknowledged to be less than the heat released by the metabolic processes in the exposed organism, and the amount of energy is too small to break chemical bonds or to form ions. Therefore, EMFs probably impact biological systems by interfering with bioelectric processes at the molecular level.

EMFs affect the flow of ions and other molecules across cell membranes, alter the responses of cells to hormones, including corticosteroids, testosterone, and melatonin. They also influence concentrations of neurotransmitters and growth factors, and impact other biochemical processes. Altering these processes can, in turn, impact the function of the immune system and patterns of cellular communication that may help control neoplasia. Cell membranes and their receptor molecules appear to be more sensitive to low frequency magnetic fields than to electric fields.

Recently, the epidemiologic evidence for a relation between EMFs and cancer has increased, and scores of scientific papers have been published on this issue (Hendee & Boteler, 1994; Savitz, 1993). The epidemiologic evidence is strongest for the relation between childhood leukemia and certain configurations of electrical power lines outside the homes of children. Residential EMFs have also been related to brain cancers in children, and to all childhood cancers combined. Studies of the relation between cancer in adults and residential EMFs show fewer positive findings than the studies of children, but those exploring the association between occupational EMF exposure and cancer, when viewed together, are more suggestive of a relationship than the studies of residential exposures (Bates, 1991; Loomis, Savitz, & Ananth, 1994; Savitz & Calle, 1987).

The epidemiologic findings have stimulated interest in the possible mechanisms responsible for this effect, as this is important for establishing a causal relation between exposure and disease (Chapter 10). There is no evidence that EMFs directly damage deoxyribose nucleic acid (DNA); there is evidence, however, that they produce changes in DNA synthesis and ribose nucleic acid (RNA) transcription and alter patterns of melatonin secretion by the pineal gland (Blask, 1989; Wilson, Chess, & Anderson, 1986). Because melatonin has been shown to control cell proliferation and suppress tumor growth, EMFs may promote cancer by upsetting the melatonin-regulated control of preneoplastic cells; they may also promote tumor growth by other mechanisms that have yet to be identified.

There are reports of developmental abnormalities in animals exposed in the laboratory to EMFs, but the findings are inconsistent (Chernoff, Rogers, & Kavet, 1992; Ubeda, Leal, Trillo, Jimenez, & Delgado, 1983). Data from human studies of congenital malformations (Nordstrom, Birke, & Gustavsson, 1983) and fetal loss (Wertheimer & Leeper, 1986, 1989) have been questioned with regard to methodologic flaws (Shore, 1992). Though the evidence that EMFs pose risk as a teratogen or as a disrupter of growth and development is less compelling than it is for cancer, more studies are needed before this risk can be ruled out.

Other studies on the effects of EMFs have shown small effects on human heart rate, evoked cerebral potential and reaction time, and changes in hormone concentrations in rats (Hendee & Boteler, 1994). Research on neurologic and behavioral effects of EMFs has produced contradictory results, with some studies of rats suggesting reduced rates of response to stimuli and behavioral changes following in-utero exposure (McGivern, Sokol, & Adey, 1990; Salzinger, Freimark, McCullough, Phillips, & Birenbaum, 1990).

In the 1980s, there was speculation that radiation from video display terminals (VDTs) posed a health risk. Although VDTs produce extremely small exposures to X-rays, they also generate EMFs from their flyback transformers. In contrast to preliminary studies that suggested congenital malformations and spontaneous abortions were related to work in front of VDTs, recent studies with better designs have found no increased risk (Schnorr et al., 1991).

Because sources of low-frequency electromagnetic radiation produce a variety of combinations of electric and magnetic field strengths, it is more difficult to define the dose resulting from an exposure than in the case of ionizing radiation. However, measurement devices for both types of fields have been improved in recent years and will hopefully provide better exposure estimates in studies of human exposure.

Most toxic substances exhibit a direct relation between the size of dose and the magnitude of the physiologic response. Studies of EMFs have not shown such a relationship—they are biologically active at certain combinations of field strength and frequency, and the rate of change in one or both of these fields may also be related to their biological effects.

Although many countries have established exposure limits for EMFs and radiofrequency radiation, the U. S. government is still considering proposals for such regulations (Sliney & Cuellar, 1992). In lieu of federal government regulations, some states have established exposure limits, and the American Conference of Governmental Industrial Hygienists (1994) has developed guidelines for occupational exposures. In cases where the health risks from an exposure are difficult to assess, and where scientific evidence supports a theoretical risk, it is important to consider the social costs of minimizing exposure. If exposure can be effectively minimized without great cost, then it makes sense to implement the reduction. Recently, some electric power utilities and local governments have begun to take this approach of "prudent avoidance," (Morgan, Nair, & Florig, 1989) and are now burying new power lines in urban areas or routing aboveground lines to avoid residential areas rather than deal with the uncertainty over their possible health risks.

Static Magnetic Fields

In contrast to electric and magnetic fields associated with transmitting electric power with alternating currents, static magnetic fields do not have wave-like properties. The most ubiquitous exposure to humans is from the magnetic field of the earth, which can fluctuate widely due to solar storms and weather patterns in the troposphere. The earth's static magnetic field also influences the flux of ionizing cosmic radiation. There have been few studies of the biologic effects of the earth's magnetic field, though one suggested a possible link with anencephalus, which was hypothesized to be mediated by cosmic radiation rather than the magnetic field itself (Archer, 1979).

Humans are also exposed to static magnetic fields in the workplace by electrolysis cells used to generate chlorine gas and extract aluminum from its ore, as well as from electric welding apparatus and induction furnaces. A new source of exposure is magnetic resonance imaging (MRI), which can expose patients to extremely high field strengths. Studies of the health effects of static magnetic fields are sparse, and have generally not revealed health risks. There is some evidence for biologic effects in laboratory studies (Kanal, Shellock,

& Talagala, 1990), but studies of workers in the aluminum industry have produced conflicting results (Milham, 1979; Rockette & Arena, 1983; Mur et al., 1987).

Ultrasound, Radiofrequencies, and Microwaves

As diagrammed in Figure 5.1, radiofrequencies comprise electromagnetic radiation with frequencies between zero and 300×10^{12} Hz (300 gigahertz [GHz]). Radiofrequency radiation includes 60 Hz electric power transmission as well as microwaves. Other types of radiofrequency radiation include electromagnetic radiation used in ultrasound (radiation at frequencies from 0.02 to about 30 mHz), radio and television transmission, radar, and microwaves (300 MHz to 300 GHz) (Figure 5.1).

Compared with other regions of the electromagnetic spectrum, little is known about the health effects of frequencies between 60 Hz and a few hundred megahertz. It is clear, however, that many organisms can detect these fields, and birds, fish, and turtles use them for navigation. Environmental exposures to humans in this region of the electromagnetic spectrum include living or working near television and radio broadcast towers. There have been some studies that examined the association between radiofrequency radiation and human disease, but the results are not definitive.

Microwaves are produced by radar, microwave ovens, and medical diathermy equipment (which is used in heat-therapy for joint and muscle pain). Energy from microwaves and from shorter wavelengths in the radiofrequency range causes biologic damage through the heat it produces. Burns, corneal opacities, and cataracts are produced by these radiations. The extent to which heat is produced is a function of the intensity (power) of the radiation.

Ultrasound is mechanically produced acoustic radiation, as opposed to the other forms of nonionizing radiation, which are electromagnetic. Humans are most frequently exposed to ultrasound during medical procedures, particularly for the evaluation of fetal growth and development. Most studies of in utero ultrasound exposure have identified no health risks (Lyons, Dyke, Toms, & Cheang, 1988; Stark, Orleans, Haverkamp, & Murphy, 1984).

Infrared and Visible Radiation

Infrared radiation, with wavelengths between 0.7 and 1,000 µm, generates heat, which may cause burns to the skin or retina, corneal opacities, or cataracts. Workers such as glassblowers are at risk for this type of exposure. Visible light, with wavelengths between 400 and 760 nanometers (nm), is produced by optical sources such as spotlights, projectors, and floodlights. Visible light can damage the retina and degrade color and night vision, and may produce temporary or permanent damage to the eye. Lasers, which emit intense beams of light that range between the infrared and ultraviolet bands, are the most worrisome sources of visible light, and can severely damage the cornea, lens, and retina.

Ultraviolet Radiation

The sun is the major source of UV exposure to humans, and this exposure increases with altitude. Ultraviolet light of all wavelengths is also produced by a number of industrial processes and manufactured items, including electric lights, welding arcs, germicidal lamps and tanning lamps.

UV-A (315–400 nm) induces some tanning, but minimal erythema. It damages the cornea and retina, and may induce skin cancer. UV-A is not absorbed by oxygen and ozone in the stratosphere, but is absorbed by oxygen and a number of air pollutants in the troposphere. Photochemical smog (Chapter 6) requires the energy of UV-A to fuel complex photochemical reactions at the earth's surface.

UV-B (280-315 nm) is a potent stimulator of skin pigmentation and the main cause of sunburn and skin cancer. This band of wavelengths also damages protein molecules in the lens of the eye and excessive exposure can produce cataracts (AMA Council on Scientific Affairs, 1989). UV-C (100-280 nm) is the most biologically damaging type of ultraviolet radiation and is used to kill bacteria in laboratories, hospitals, and industry.

The oxygen in the earth's stratosphere absorbs most UV-C from the sun and is thereby converted to ozone. Ozone, in turn, absorbs UV-B and releases more oxygen, which is then available to absorb more UV-C. These photochemical reactions are responsible for the filtering effect of the stratospheric ozone layer. Chlorofluorocarbons and other halogenated compounds quickly destroy ozone (Chapter 6); releases from industries and consumer products worldwide have been slowly removing this filtering system for both UV-B and UV-C. Scientists are worried about the increased risks for skin cancer that are predicted by increases of UV-B , and about the potential damage to plant productivity from UV-C.

Ultraviolet radiation directly damages human skin by fragmenting the elastic fibers of the dermis, resulting in wrinkles resembling those of aging skin, and by damaging DNA, which may lead to cancer. Basal cell carcinoma is by far the most common skin cancer attributable to UV radiation. Most basal cell cancers enlarge slowly at the site of origin and do not metastasize. UV also induces squamous cell carcinomas and these may spread to regional lymph nodes. Both types of skin cancer can be easily cured by local excision if diagnosed early enough.

Malignant melanomas have also been associated with exposure to sunlight—particularly during childhood. The presence of hereditary nevi also increases the risk for malignant melanoma—particularly for those exposed to UV radiation during childhood. The cells of melanomas spread not only to regional lymph nodes—they commonly enter the bloodstream and can spread to virtually every organ in the body. Excision is an effective treatment only if a melanoma is detected soon after arising.

It appears that from the 1960s to the 1980s the incidence of malignant melanomas and squamous cell skin cancers has more than tripled (Glass & Hoover, 1989). The recent epidemic is probably due to modern lifestyles that include many outdoor activities. Because there is evidence that the greatest risk for UV radiation induction of both squamous cell carcinomas and malignant melanomas is from exposure during childhood, these increases may be due to an increase in outdoor activities of children.

Because malignant melanomas are frequently fatal and because other skin cancers require costly but preventable health-care intervention, public health measures are needed to counteract the risks from modern lifestyles and reduced protection by the stratospheric ozone layer. Most sunscreen lotions absorb UV-B, and some are now being formulated to filter UV-A, thereby reducing another possible cause of skin cancer. Because indoor sun lamps also emit UV-A and UV-B, designing bulbs that minimize UV-B may also reduce the risk for skin cancer (Walter et al., 1990). Wearing sunglasses that absorb UV-B is also a recommended prevention measure—particularly for children living in regions receiving intense UV radiation.

IONIZING RADIATION

Atomic Structure

The ionizing radiation with the greatest public health significance comes from inside the atom, which is composed of a nucleus with positively charged protons and neutrons with no charge, surrounded by one or more orbits of negatively charged electrons. Protons and neutrons, in turn, are composed of various arrangements of quarks and leptons, which are considered to be the fundamental nuclear particles. The atom contains mostly empty space, however. If the nucleus of an atom was 1 cm in diameter, then the closest electron would be 1 km away. Atoms appear solid because of the forces that hold the particles together.

The number of protons in an atom determines its chemical properties. Atoms of the same element always have the same number of protons, but the number of neutrons may vary. Isotopes are atoms with the same number of protons, but with different numbers of neutrons. Each isotope has a unique combination of protons and neutrons, which together account for its atomic mass. The ratio between the number of protons and neutrons determines the stability of an isotope—too many or too few neutrons per proton creates instability.

Unstable or radioactive isotopes undergo atomic decay, releasing energy and particles as they are transmuted into other isotopes of the same element or into isotopes of other elements. The process of nuclear decay ends with the formation of a stable isotope. The time involved in the decay of one isotope to another is measured as the *half-life* of the isotope—the time it takes for a group of atoms of the same isotope to be reduced by 50% through atomic decay. Isotopes have half-lives measured in seconds, days, and years.

Depending on the number of protons and neutrons in the nucleus, the process of nuclear decay involves the release of one or more of the following types of matter and energy: *alpha particles,* which are helium nuclei with two protons and two neutrons, *beta particles*—electrons that originate from the nucleus, and *neutrons* and *gamma rays*—photons with properties of waves and particles. *X-rays* are photons released when electrons outside the nucleus release energy.

Alpha particles are comparatively large and have a strong positive electrical charge. They release their energy over short distances and therefore produce dense patterns of ionization. Because of this, they are said to have a high *linear energy transfer (LET)*. Alpha particles can penetrate only a few centimeters of air and just a few cell layers in human tissue.

Beta particles release energy over greater distances and can penetrate a few meters in air, as well as the epidermal layer of skin. Gamma and X-rays travel even greater distances and can penetrate the body easily. Because these three types of radiation release energy over long distances, they have a low LET. Like gamma and X-rays, neutrons travel great distances and can penetrate the body. Because they are more energetic than the other particles, they have a high LET.

Units of Measurement for Ionizing Radiation

The need to have units and standards for exposure was realized soon after the harmful biological effects of radiation became evident. One of the first physical units of X-ray exposure was the smallest amount that would fog a photographic plate. To account for biological damage, dose units were based on exposures that produced observable acute effects. The earliest maximum standard for exposure to radiation workers was a cumulative 1–month exposure equal to 10% of an acute exposure that produced erythema.

Modern radiation standards are based on physical units (Table 5.1; Kathren & Petersen, 1989). The first units of physical measurement were related to the properties of radium-226 and expressed with "conventional" units that are still popular in the United States. In 1948 the General Conference of Weights and Measures—an international body chartered to develop a unified system of measures based on the metric system—began the revision of radiation units. It adopted an international system of units, called the *Systeme Internationale*

Table 5.1 Terms and Units for Ionizing Radiation

Unit	SI	Conventional
Activity	Becquerel (Bq) (1 dis/sec)	Curie (Ci) $(3.7 \times 10^{10}$ dis/sec)
Environmental concentration	Activity per area, volume, or mass	Activity per area, volume, or mass
Absorbed dose	Gray (Gy) (1 Gy = 1 J/kg)	Rad (1 rad = 10^{-2} J/kg)
Equivalent dose	$H_T = \sum_R W_R \times D_{T,R}$ In sievert (Sv) (1 Sv = 100 rem)	$H_T = \sum_R W_R \times D_{T,R}$ In rem (1 rem = 0.01 Sv)
Effective dose	$E = \sum_T W_T \times H_T$ In sievert (Sv)	$E = \sum_T W_T \times H_T$ In rem

Notes:

dis $=$ disintegration

H_T $=$ equivalent dose in tissue or organ T

W_R $=$ radiation weighting factor that accounts for the biological effects of a specified type and energy of radiation. It reflects the relative biological effectiveness of the radiation.

$D_{T,R}$ $=$ absorbed dose

W_T $=$ weighting factor for tissue or organ T, which includes the probability of attributable fatal cancer; weighted probability of attributable non-fatal cancer; weighted probability of severe hereditary effects; and relative length of life lost.

E $=$ effective dose

(*SI*), which has become the international standard for reporting. The SI units for activity, exposure, and dose are listed in Table 5.1, along with factors for converting conventional units to SI units. Because many health physicists have not become used to the SI units, it is customary in the United States to report findings with both, usually with the conventional units in parentheses.

The *activity* of an isotope is the number of atoms undergoing nuclear decay or transformation per unit time—in other words, the rate of decay of radioactive material. The curie is a unit of activity and is defined as 37 billion (3.7×10^{10}) atomic disintegrations per second—the approximate decay rate of one gram of radium. The *becquerel,* the SI unit of activity, is defined as one disintegration per second. Environmental concentrations of radioactivity are commonly measured as activity per unit mass or volume of an environmental medium.

Exposure to ionizing radiation has a unique definition in health physics, where it is defined as the ability of X- or gamma radiation to produce ions in air, and is quantified with a conventional unit called the roentgen or with the SI units of coulomb per kilogram. This definition of exposure is of little relevance in determining health risks from ionizing radiation. As is the case for toxic chemicals, the environmental concentration of a radionuclide—expressed as activity per unit mass or volume of environmental medium (Chapter 1)—is the measure of exposure most useful for determining health risks.

Ionizing radiation exposes the body from the outside with photons, neutrons, and beta particles (*external exposure*), or from the inside via inhaled or ingested radioactive material (*internal exposure*). External and internal doses, which are more relevant for determining health risks (Chapter 1), can be computed for a uniform exposure to the entire body, or for specific organs or tissues. Such doses are called *whole body doses, organ doses*, and *tissue doses*, respectively. Whole body doses are more commonly received from external exposures than from internal ones. Internal doses are usually computed for individual organs because most radionuclides concentrate in specific organs rather than distribute uniformly throughout the body.

External doses are computed with formulae or computer programs that incorporate measures of the energy of the photon or particle, the distance from the source to the organism, and other factors that can modify the deposition of energy. Internal doses are computed with formulae that convert intake or activity per unit organ weight to organ dose by applying different conversion factors that account for deposition of specific radionuclides in specific organs. Computer models such as the ones described in Chapters 1 and 2 can be used to compute both intake and dose when data are not available for intake and activity in specific organs (Till & Meyer, 1983; Moskowitz, Pardi, DePhillips, & Meinhold, 1992).

The *absorbed dose* (Table 5.1), measured in units called the rad and the gray (Gy) (in SI units, 1 Gy = 100 rad), is the measure of the deposited energy per unit mass of tissue. The absorbed dose does not, however, account for the unique abilities of the different types of radiation to damage biologic tissue to different degrees. Such adjustment is needed because high-LET radiation produces dense patterns of ionization and is more damaging per unit absorbed dose than low LET radiation, which disperses energy over greater distances.

The *equivalent dose* International Commission on Radiological Protection [ICRP] (a new term that replaces the dose equivalent, which is computed in a similar way) is the measurement that reflects these differences in biologic effects for the purpose of radiation protection (ICRP, 1991). The *rem* and *sievert* (Sv) are the units for this measurement (1 Sv = 100 rem). An equivalent dose is the absorbed dose adjusted by a radiation weighting factor (W_R), which is based on the *relative biological effectiveness* (*RBE*) of one radiation compared with another to induce cancer at low doses. The RBE is similar to the quality factor used to compute the dose equivalent (Kathren & Petersen, 1989), and is related to the LET of the radiation. For low LET radiation from X-rays, gamma rays, and beta particles, the W_R is one, and a rad equals a rem. For high LET radiation, the W_R is greater than 1. For alpha particles, it is 20, and for neutrons, the W_R ranges from 5 to 20, depending on the energy of the neutron (ICRP, 1991).

To account for the differences in doses from annual exposures resulting in the internal deposition of radionuclides with different physical and biological half-lives (Chapter 2), the doses to organs are estimated for specific time periods—usually for 50 years. Such estimates are made with a unit termed the *committed dose equivalent,* and are designed to protect workers who are chronically exposed to radionuclides that remain in their bodies for long periods of time.

For radon gas (radon-222), which provides radiation exposure mainly through its radioactive decay products that have short half-lives, a different unit is needed. This is because the relative concentrations of these decay products can vary from place to place, and there is a need to have a term that combines their energies. The *working level (WL)* is any combination of the short-lived progeny of radon that, in 1 liter of air, will result in 1.3×10^5 million electron volts (MeV) of alpha energy. Because a measure of cumulative exposure is needed for radiation protection purposes, the product of time and exposure in WL is used. By convention, the *working level month*

(WLM) is the product of the exposure in WL and the duration in hours, divided by 170 (the approximate number of hours in 1 working month, as this measure was developed to protect uranium miners). It is possible to compute an absorbed dose for an organ or tissue from exposure radon progeny, but this approach is used mainly for research purposes.

Radiation Protection Standards

In the 1930s, "tolerance doses" for radiation workers were set at 1–2 mGy (0.1–0.2 rad per day) by various professional and scientific organizations, based on observations of the health of medical workers (Shapiro, 1990). In 1956 the Biological Effects of Atomic Radiations (BEAR) Committee of the U.S. National Academy of Sciences and the British Medical Research Committee both recommended that a radiation worker younger than 30 be limited to a cumulative whole body dose of 0.5 Sv (50 rem) up to age 30, and to 0.5 Sv (50 rem) between ages 30 and 50, or to 0.05 Sv (5 rem) per year for this period.

Also in 1956, the U.S. National Council on Radiation Protection and Measurements (NCRP)—an advisory group chartered by Congress and funded by contributions from government, scientific groups, and industry—recommended that the public be limited to 10% of the occupational dose. This recommendation was also made by the ICRP—an international advisory funded by various international health and scientific organizations.

In 1977 the ICRP revised its safety standards and concluded that radiation workers should not be permitted to take more dangerous risks than those in other occupations. It determined that a risk for death of 1 in 10,000 per year is acceptable for radiation workers (ICRP, 1977, 1979). In its revised safety standards, the ICRP also recommended a system to adjust for differences in the risk for cancers between doses received by different organs of the body. For instance, the risk for cancer from a dose to the entire body of 0.01 gray (1 rad) of gamma radiation is much greater than the same dose to the lung. The ICRP proposed weighting factors to adjust for these differences: 0.25 for gonads; 0.15, breast; 0.12, red bone marrow; 0.12, lung; 0.03, thyroid; 0.03, bone surfaces; and 0.30 for all other organs (ICRP, 1991). A dose computed with these factors—which mainly adjust the risk for fatal cancer—was termed the *effective dose equivalent* (EDE). Such an approach provides a way to combine doses from internal and external exposures for radiation protection purposes only. Using the EDE for epidemiologic studies is not appropriate, as they have already been adjusted for estimated cancer risk.

In 1977 the ICRP recommended that a worker receive an annual EDE of less than 0.05 Sv (5 rem), though they made an exception for those workers who entered the workforce at older ages. The new recommendations allowed a higher annual dose—up to 0.125 Sv (12.5 rem) EDE—as long as a worker's lifetime cumulative radiation dose did not exceed an average of 5 rem per year EDE for every year of age above 18. At this time, the ICRP also made recommendations for annual limits of intake for internal exposures to radionuclides and recommended that maximum doses to the general public be kept at 10% of the worker doses.

The current U.S. radiation protection standards are, in general, based on the 1977 ICRP recommendations. The U.S. Nuclear Regulatory Commission (USNRC) and Department of Energy (DOE) each have a limit of 50 mSv (5 rem) total effective dose equivalent (or TEDE, the sum of the EDE from external radiation and the committed effective dose equivalent from internal exposure) per year, and do not adjust for the age of a worker. The DOE also requires special approval for a worker to exceed 20 mSv (2 rem) TEDE in any 1 year, and has an administrative rule that the lifetime TEDE for a worker should not exceed 1 rem per year of age. These agencies have additional regulations for unique exposures and target tissues, such as doses to the fetus and for the prevention of noncancer effects; they also regulate internal exposure to radionuclides with *annual limits on intake* (intakes that result in a specified committed effective dose equivalent) and *derived air concentrations* (air concentrations that, under usual working conditions, will result in the annual limit on intake) (Hallenbeck, 1994).

The current regulations for doses to the general public vary according to source and circumstances of exposure (Hallenbeck, 1994; Shleien, 1992). For nuclear power plants regulated by the USNRC, the limit is 1 mSv (0.1 rem) TEDE per year, although a dose of 5 mSv (0.5 rem) may be permitted with prior authorization. For the production of nuclear fuel and the operation of nuclear power plants, the U.S. Environmental Protection Agency (EPA) limits the annual dose equivalent from all radionuclides except radon and its decay products to 0.25 mSv (0.025 rem) to whole body or to any organ other than the thyroid, and 0.75 mSv (0.075 rem) to the thyroid. The EPA and DOE also regulate radionuclides in drinking water with a variety of different concentration limits.

Recently, the recommended dose limits have been critically reviewed by the ICRP and the NCRP. To reduce risks for cancer from occupational exposures, the ICRP (1991) recommended an effective dose (the ICRP simplified the term EDE to effective dose; see Table 5.1) limit of 20 mSv/yr (2 rem/yr) averaged over 5 years and not to exceed 5 mSv (5 rem) in any single year. The ICRP also recommended that once pregnancy has been declared by a worker, the equivalent dose to the abdominal surface be limited to 2 mSv (0.2 rem). For the general public, the recommended limits for cancer protection are 1.0 mSv/yr (0.1 rem/yr) effective dose, averaged over 5 years (ICRP, 1991). Limits for noncancer effects to the skin and lens of the eye have also been recommended by the ICRP for workers and members of the public; these limits are much higher than those for cancer protection.

To reduce cancer risks for workers, the NCRP (1993) recommends an annual TEDE limit of 50 mSv (5 rem) and a cumulative TEDE limit equal to the product of 10 mSv (1 rem) and a worker's age in years. For the general public, the NCRP recommends a cancer protection limit of 1 mSv (0.100 rem) per year for continuous or frequent exposures and 5 mSv (0.5 rem) for infrequent exposures. Like the ICRP, the NCRP recommends limits for noncancer effects that are much higher than those for cancer.

It is not yet clear to what extent the new international and national recommendations will be adopted by the USNRC, DOE, and other federal and state agencies that regulate radiation exposure in the United States. It is evident, however, that certain regulations are currently less protective than the newly recommended levels.

The current U. S. occupational exposure limit for radon and its progeny is 4.0 WLM per year. Based on current estimates, this level of exposure puts miners at much greater risk than other radiation workers. A number of governmental and labor groups have argued for lowering this standard (Moure, 1981), but to date the standard has remained unchanged since it was set in the 1970s.

Monitoring Exposures to Ionizing Radiation

Occupational Exposures. All countries that have nuclear industries require some system of personal monitoring and record keeping. External radiation exposure is monitored with film badges or thermoluminescent detectors (TLDs), which are worn on the trunk between the waist and shoulders and on other areas if they are subjected to exposure rates higher than those for the trunk. Both devices record cumulative exposures to gamma rays, beta particles, and neutrons in combination, or separately if special filters and analytical procedures are used. The exposure readings from film badges or TLDs can be converted to equivalent or effective doses for any desired exposure period.

A number of other monitoring devices for external exposures are used in the nuclear industry for area monitoring to determine exposures in different work areas, or for assessing acute exposures. For industries that expose workers to radionuclides that could provide internal doses via inhalation, ingestion, or dermal absorption, special monitoring procedures are required. Such internal exposures can be evaluated with analyses of urine or feces, or by in vivo counting procedures such as whole body or and lung counting. For in vivo counting, special detectors are arranged to intercept radiation from the entire body or from specific organs.

Environmental Exposures. In the United States, nuclear facilities are required to estimate annual doses to the public and show that they are lower than regulatory limits. The same techniques that are used to evaluate exposures and doses to workers are used to assess exposures to the public. For external exposures, TLD detectors can be used to record cumulative doses. For most internal exposures, however, in vivo counting procedures are inappropriate, as they are not sensitive enough to detect the small levels of radioactivity deposited internally. The most commonly used technique for assessing public exposure is the modeling of exposure and dose based on release rates and measured concentrations in environmental samples.

Health Effects From Exposure to Ionizing Radiation

History. Some of the early atomic scientists and their assistants suffered damage from their exposures during experiments. Marie Curie had several radiation burns on her hands and she died of leukemia. Her daughter, the atomic scientist Irene Joliot-Curie, also died of leukemia. In experimenting with the fluoroscope, Thomas Edison developed skin burns within days of exposure, and one of his assistants died of bone cancer.

These events were not known to the general public in the late nineteenth and early twentieth centuries, and many believed that radioactivity had beneficial effects. Radioactive substances were added to both cosmetics and medicines during this period (Macklis, 1990; Macklis, Bellerive & Humm, 1990), and spas where one could bathe in and drink naturally radioactive water were popular all over the world.

During the early years of X-ray use, so little was known about the energy output of the machines that harmful effects from overexposure were experienced not only by patients, but also by technicians and radiologists as well. Fluoroscopic examinations were particularly dangerous because longer and more intense exposures were used in this procedure.

A much publicized event of the 1920s finally alerted the public to the dangers of radioactivity. As many as 4,000 women in the United States were employed to paint luminescent watch dials with paint containing radium and its radioactive decay products. The painters shaped their brushes with their lips, thereby receiving large doses of gamma radiation to their jaws and nearby tissues. Some 4 million watches were produced with this technique. Many women developed massive jaw ulcerations, pathological fractures, loss of teeth, and bone cancer; there is also evidence that a number of other cancers may have been caused by exposures from this occupation (Martland, 1929; Rowland & Lucas, 1984).

Because of the long latency between exposure to ionizing radiation and the onset of cancer, many of the consequences of these exposures did not become known for decades. Retrospective studies continue to identify the dangers of early uses of radiation in medicine and industry.

From 1928 to the early 1960s, a suspension of radioactive thorium called thorotrast was injected into patients to improve the X-ray images of soft tissues (Telles, Thomas, Popper, Ishak, & Falk, 1979). Patients who underwent this procedure have been determined to be at increased risk for hepatic angiosarcoma, leukemia, and possibly other cancers (Looney, 1960; Falk, Telles, Ishak, Thomas, & Popper, 1979).

In the early years of medical applications of ionizing radiation, many children received X-ray therapy to the head, neck, and chest for disorders such as ringworm, tonsillitis, acne, scarlet fever, asthma, and erroneously diagnosed "enlargement" of the thymus. These procedures also resulted in increased rates of a number of different cancers (National Research Council, 1990).

The most information concerning the relation between doses from ionizing radiation and risks for cancer comes from studies of the survivors of the bombings of Hiroshima and Nagasaki in 1945. The first victims died of burns, injuries, and acute radiation sickness. Soon after the bombings, the survivors developed severe and often fatal infections from radiation-induced bone marrow suppression. Years later, increases in the frequencies of a number of different cancers were discovered (Stewart & Kneale, 1990; Shimizu, Schull, & Kato, 1990; Yamazaki & Schull, 1990).

The nuclear weapons industry also produced radiation-related disease. United States scientists who helped build the atomic bomb developed acute radiation sickness from accidents with fissionable material (Hubner & Fry, 1980). Uranium miners who worked the Colorado Plateau of the United States developed increased rates of lung cancer from exposure to the decay products of radon gas (Hornung & Meinhardt, 1987). Workers in the nuclear weapons industry have shown excesses of some cancers (Wilkinson, 1991), and further research is needed to determine the magnitude of these risks.

Recent revelations about the early years of nuclear weapons development in the Soviet Union and former East Germany indicate that uranium miners, nuclear workers, and residents around nuclear facilities, such as the one near Chelyabinsk, Russia, may have been exposed to much higher doses than their American counterparts (Akleyev & Lyubchansky, 1994; Cochran & Norris, 1991; Cochran, Norris, & Suokko, 1993; Kahn, 1993).

Atmospheric fallout from above-ground nuclear weapons tests has exposed virtually everyone on the planet. In areas that received high concentrations of fresh fallout, such as the Marshall Islands and the Utah counties downwind from the Nevada Test Site, epidemiologic studies have shown increases in cancers among exposed persons

(Hamilton, van Belle, & Logerfo, 1987; Stevens et al., 1990; Kerber et al., 1993).

Biological Effects of Radiation

Many of the adverse health effects of radiation were discovered through studies of persons exposed during medical procedures. Others were revealed through the long-term studies of survivors of the Hiroshima–Nagasaki bombings. Additional evidence comes from studies of animals exposed in the laboratory. The effects of radiation exposure fall into three categories: (1) cell killing from high doses that can result in acute radiation sickness and sterility if reproductive tissue is exposed, (2) genetic damage from exposure to the ovaries and testes, and (3) neoplastic transformation of somatic cells.

The biological effects are produced when photons or particles released from radioactive atoms ionize atoms or molecules within cells. Ions are formed by the direct interaction of a photon or particle with a molecule in DNA or cell membranes, or indirectly when they ionize other atoms or molecules and produce free radicals (molecules containing unpaired electrons). Free radicals then react with enzymes and DNA, thereby disrupting biochemical processes and producing changes that lead to cell death, neoplasia, or heritable genetic damage. They can also damage the DNA in cell nuclei, leading to neoplasia and cancer in somatic tissue, and genetic effects in reproductive tissue. Cells have DNA repair mechanisms that can correct such damage and immune surveillance can destroy transformed cells, but these defenses are not completely effective.

Cells differ in their sensitivity to radiation. Shortly after the birth of an organism, some of the cells in the nervous system, the heart, and the kidney lose the ability to divide. These cells are comparatively resistant to ionizing radiation. Others divide periodically throughout the lifespan of an organism and vary in their sensitivity to radiation. Bone marrow and lymphoid cells are particularly sensitive. At moderate levels of exposure they are killed and at low levels they exhibit abnormal numbers of chromosomes, chromosomes with structural defects, or both. Cells that divide on a regular or cyclic basis constitute a third category. These cells are relatively resistant to radiation unless they are exposed during cell division.

Radiation Sickness and Other Acute Effects

Acute radiation sickness is caused by whole body absorbed doses above 100 rad (1Gy) administered over a short time period. The intensity, site, and onset of effects vary with dose. At doses above 1 Gy (100 rad), damage to the bone marrow causes clinically important decreases in concentrations of granulocytes and platelets (Gale & Butturini, 1991). The LD_{50} for humans is between 2 and 3 Gy (200 and 300 rad) (Morris & Jones, 1989), and at doses above 5 Gy (500 rad), survival is improbable unless special supportive measures are employed. This is because bone marrow function is unlikely to spontaneously recover. At doses in excess of 8 Gy (800 rad), death may result from damage to tissues of the gastrointestinal tract, central nervous system, or skin.

The signs and symptoms of acute radiation sickness include nausea, vomiting, and internal bleeding; central nervous system function is affected by whole-body absorbed doses above 6 Gy (600 rad). Locally focused intense exposure to ionizing radiation produces severe burns, massive cell death, and ulcers that are difficult to heal, as experienced by the early radiation scientists and, more recently, by the plant operators and firefighters during the Chernobyl nuclear accident (Gale, 1987).

Medical management of victims involves treating local tissue damage, preventing death from infection or bleeding, and attempting to stimulate bone marrow recovery. Techniques for improving bone marrow recovery involve administration of molecularly cloned hematopoietic growth factors or replacing damaged marrow with a transplant (Gale & Butturini, 1991).

Damage from In Utero Exposures

Fetal tissues are particularly sensitive to radiation exposure because they are undergoing rapid cell division. The manifestations of this sensitivity have been noted in children of mothers who had X-rays of the pelvis to determine whether the pelvic girdle was adequate for vaginal delivery—a technique called X-ray pelvimetry. These children have been shown to be at increased risk for leukemia at whole-body absorbed doses above 5 mGy (0.5 rad) (Stewart, 1971; NRC, 1990).

In utero exposure in animals has produced gross structural malformations, growth retardation, sterility, and central nervous system abnormalities, and damage is related to the time during embryogenesis when the exposure occurs. Children exposed in utero during the bombings of Hiroshima and Nagasaki were at increased risk for microcephaly and mental retardation from fetal absorbed doses of 0.5-1.0 Gy (50-100 rad) or above—particularly when the exposure occurred between 8 and 15 weeks gestational age (NRC, 1990). An inverse relation between in utero radiation dose and both intelligence test scores and school performance was also noted for children exposed during this period (Yamazaki & Schull, 1990).

Genetic Damage

Early in the history of radiobiology, studies of plants and fruitflies showed that ionizing radiation produced mutations that could be inherited. There was great interest, therefore, in determining whether radiation-induced mutations were produced in exposed humans, and whether these mutations could be inherited by their offspring.

Inherited genetic effects can appear as visible chromosome abnormalities, proteins with altered conformations or charges, spontaneous abortions, or premature death (NRC, 1990). These effects can be studied in the offspring of an exposed parent, or in children of later generations.

Studies of genetic effects in the first and second generations of children born to survivors of the Hiroshima and Nagasaki bombings have not shown statistically significant elevations. However, when data for a number of genetic effects in the first-generation offspring are combined, they suggest a slight positive relation. Neel (1991) concluded that a gonadal dose between 1.7 and 2.2 Sv (170–220 rem) was the most likely estimate for the dose that would double the background rates for the combination of all effects studied (stillbirths, cumulative mortality, cancer with onset before the age of 20 years, sex-chromosome aneuploids, and mutations affecting protein structure or function) in the first-generation offspring. The Committee on the Biological Effects of Ionizing Radiation (BEIR V) concluded than the doubling dose for humans is not likely to be smaller than the dose (about 1 Sv [100 rem]) estimated from studies in mice (NRC, 1990).

Recently, genetic damage from ionizing radiation to parents has also been hypothesized to increase the risk for leukemia in their children (Gardner et al., 1990a, 1990b). There is evidence from a few other studies that preconception exposure to ionizing radiation or other carcinogens increases the risk for cancer in offspring. This hypothesis needs further testing before it can be critically assessed.

Cancer

Exposure to ionizing radiation also results in cancer, as has been demonstrated in a large number of studies of persons exposed to radiation from a variety of sources. Figure 5.2 summarizes the fatal cancers associated with acute exposures to comparatively high doses from the bombing of Hiroshima and Nagasaki. Other types of cancer have been found to be in excess of background rates in studies of persons exposed during medical procedures and in the nuclear industry. Although we know a great deal about the carcinogenicity of radiation, we will learn much more as the cohorts of exposed persons age, and the causes of death are determined for all members.

There is still much debate over the quantitative estimates of risk for cancer per unit dose of ionizing radiation. Many sophisticated modeling techniques have been applied to data from the Hiroshima and Nagasaki survivors and to other exposed groups (NRC, 1990). Estimates of risk per unit dose vary, depending on the dose–response model and other assumptions about exposed groups. There is also much debate over extrapolating risks from high total doses to low ones, and from doses received acutely to those accrued over long periods of time—such as doses to the public from radionuclides released by nuclear facilities and from natural background radiation.

The estimates of risk made by BEIR IV (NRC, 1988) for internal exposures and BEIR V (NRC, 1990) for external exposures are probably the most widely used. For exposures to radon decay products, BEIR IV (NRC, 1988) estimates the lifetime risk for lung cancer mortality to be 3.5×10^{-4} per working level month. This estimate is based on studies of uranium miners exposed to cumulative doses much higher than those received by the general public. Therefore, the risks per unit dose may be lower for members of the public.

For external exposures, BEIR V (NRC, 1990) estimates that a single dose of 0.1 Sv (10 rem) to the total body results in an excess

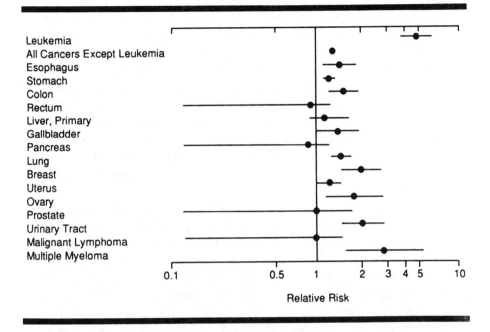

Figure 5.2   Relative risk and 90% confidence intervals for cancer mortality between 1950–1985 at a dose of 1 Gy (100 rad) shielded kerma [a measure of energy released by photons in matter; doses in kerma can be converted to absorbed doses for different organs with specific conversion factors (NRC, 1990), which average about 0.6]. From Shimizu, Schull, & Kato (1990) with permission.

mortality risk for all cancers of 7.7×10^{-3} in males, and 8.10×10^{-3} in females. BEIR V also concludes that continuous exposures delivering the same total dose over longer time periods have lower risks.

SOURCES OF HUMAN EXPOSURE

Background Radiation

Little attention was paid to natural background radioactivity prior to detecting radioactive fallout from atmospheric weapons testing. Background radiation from cosmic, terrestrial, and internal sources then became a point of reference from which to determine risks from fallout and the nuclear weapons and power industries. Although all ionizing radiation presents some risk, whether its source is natural or man-made, it has been difficult to quantify the proportion of cancers and genetic defects that might be attributed to natural sources of radiation and the magnitude of this risk is still a topic of debate.

Cosmic rays are highly penetrating and originate mostly in outer space, though some come from solar flares. As they move through the atmosphere, they expose organisms directly or indirectly by interacting with other elements and producing secondary radiations and new radionuclides, including carbon-14 and tritium (radioactive hydrogen-3), which become incorporated into the earth's environment and the tissues of living organisms.

The earth's crust contains radioactive materials that were formed at the birth of our universe. Materials with half-lives of 100 million years or more have survived to the present. Of these, potassium-40 and the radioactive decay chains of uranium-238 and thorium-232 (NCRP, 1987) are the most abundant. Potassium-40 is present in all plants and animals, including humans. All rocks and soils contain radioactive isotopes of uranium and thorium, which decay by releasing alpha and beta particles and gamma rays. Phosphate rock contains comparatively high concentrations of uranium-238 and its decay products. Decay products of uranium include radon gas, which escapes into the atmosphere and into water and exposes humans mainly through inhalation. Some radionuclides are also carried by rain into drinking water

Radon gas has a half-life of 3.8 days. Two of its short-lived decay products, polonium-218 and polonium-214, emit alpha particles which, if inhaled, can give substantial doses to the lung. The buildup of radon inside buildings has become an issue of concern in recent years. Radon seeps from soil into buildings through cracks in foundations and from spaces around water pipes. Radon dissolved in water can enter the air of buildings from faucets and showers. Uranium-rich building materials may also contribute to indoor radon levels.

Weathertight homes prevent the escape of radon gas to the outside atmosphere and therefore increase radon exposure to building occupants. Surveys of homes in Sweden, Finland, Britain, and the U.S. have revealed radon concentrations that are hundreds of times higher than outdoors.

Estimates of the health risks from indoor radon range from 5,000 - 40,000 fatal lung cancers each year (Council on Scientific Affairs, 1991; National Academy of Sciences, 1991). It is also estimated that about 12% of U. S. homes may have radon concentrations exceeding 4 picocuries (approximately 0.02 WL) per liter of air—the current level for which remedial action is recommended. The EPA has estimated that about 8 million people in the United States may have undesirably high levels of radon in their water supplies, and that water-borne radon may cause more cancer deaths than all other drinking water contaminants combined.

Medical Applications

By 1960 most physicians had abandoned X-ray therapy for benign conditions such as acne, eczema, psoriasis, and for reducing scar tissue. X-rays have continued to be used extensively in diagnostic and therapeutic procedures. Leukemia is now treated by total body irradiation to destroy bone marrow, followed by a bone marrow transplant from a compatible donor.

Improvements in the design of X-ray equipment, training of technicians, and routine inspections of equipment have reduced exposures from many procedures in diagnostic radiography, and doses from these have been reduced substantially over the years. Some new techniques, however, give patients higher doses than those from traditional radiographs. For instance, computed tomography (CT) is used extensively to locate and diagnose many different types of pathology. In this procedure hundreds of sharply focused X-ray beams rotate around the body and produce cross-sectional images.

An extensive expansion in the use of internally administered radionuclides has taken place over the past few decades, not only for the diagnosis and treatment of disease, but also for basic biological and medical research. Positron emission tomography (PET) scans involve the use of radioisotopes with short half-lives. This technique helps to locate and diagnose lesions of the brain as well as to study chemical and circulatory changes in the brain.

Radionuclides continue to be used in the treatment of cancer and polycythemia as well as in the diagnosis and treatment of hyperthyroidism and other disorders. Radioimmunoassays involving antibodies tagged with radionuclides are used extensively in medical diagnostic laboratories and many of the new procedures in the fields of molecular biology and genetics also involve the use of radionuclides. Techniques are now being developed to deliver radioactive antibodies to specific tissues for the destruction of cancer cells. Between 1960 and 1970 the use of radiopharmaceuticals increased about five times, and their use has grown faster since then.

The expanding use of radioactive substances involves exposures not only to patients but also to workers. Such procedures require the disposal of a rapidly expanding volume of radioactive waste. Slightly over 80% of all man-made radiation exposure to the general public is from medical applications.

Sterilization of Medical Products and Foods

Recently, gamma rays have been used by industry to sterilize medical products and food. The U.S. Food and Drug Administration has approved radiating fruits, grains, nuts, vegetables, chicken, and pork to prevent spoilage. Many other countries have developed irradiation facilities. Although it does not make foods radioactive, irradiation may produce carcinogenic peroxides and other toxic chemicals (Louria, 1990; Piccioni, 1988).

Because many foods have to be irradiated immediately after harvest, portable irradiation units may have to be used to treat crops in the field. The sources for gamma rays used in food irradiation are highly radioactive and pose health risks for workers who do not have adequate training. In addition, the public may be at risk for exposure through transportation accidents involving portable irradiation units.

Food irradiation has been promoted for use in Third World countries, where alternatives to refrigeration may be needed. Occupational and public health risks from the use of highly radioactive sources by untrained, unregulated, and poorly supervised personnel will be much greater than in countries that have had more experience with radiation.

The limited experience with irradiation of medical supplies in the United States has already resulted in accidents that have contaminated irradiation facilities and exposed workers unnecessarily. The clean up of minor leaks of cesium-137 sources in one U.S. facility has cost taxpayers over $30 million.

If food irradiation becomes widespread, traditional techniques for detecting spoilage and contamination with human pathogens may not be adequate. It is possible that efforts to reduce bacterial contamination of foods by irradiation may actually generate more severe health problems. It is not clear that the benefits from this technology will outweigh the risks.

Nuclear Power

Worldwide there are about 400 nuclear power plants in 26 countries. These reactors generated about 17% of the world's electricity in 1988 (U.S. DOE, 1991). In the United States there are 110 operating reactors that produced about 20% of the country's electricity in 1990 (Ahearne, 1995).

There are two important public health concerns regarding the normal operation of nuclear plants—effects on nearby populations and exposure of plant workers to radiation. Every year millions of curies of radioactive gases and liquids—predominantly isotopes of noble gases and tritium—are released from each reactor. Although these releases result in environmental concentrations that exceed background levels, the doses that members of the public receive from them are low compared with other sources of radiation—including natural ones.

Even though workers in the U. S. nuclear power industry usually receive annual doses well below the regulatory limits, they are higher than those for most jobs that involve radiation exposure. The annual collective dose (the product of the number of workers in the industry and their annual doses) for U. S. nuclear power plant workers is larger than the annual collective dose for any single industry (NCRP, 1989; NRC, 1992).

Accidents at nuclear power plants can expose workers and the public to high doses of radiation and contaminate ecosystems over large areas. Recent experience with major reactor accidents has also shown that clean up is incredibly expensive.

Nuclear power plants have lifespans of about 30 years because metal components become brittle after exposure to intense radiation fields. In the United States, federal regulations require that old nuclear power plants be dismantled and that radioactive materials be disposed of safely. The decommissioning may be immediate, or it may be delayed for a 30- to 50-year period of "safe storage" to allow a significant decrease in radioactivity. This process involves dismantling the reactor, removing all radioactive waste from the site, and restoring the site for public use—or at least to a condition that prevents human exposure and environmental migration of radionuclides.

Worldwide, 17 reactors—including five in the United States—are waiting for, or are undergoing decommissioning. Presently there are no disposal sites for the high–level radioactive wastes from these plants, though processes for selecting and evaluating sites are under way in the United States and other countries.

It appears that nuclear power will not grow to be a major source of electricity in the last years of the 20th century. In the United States orders for new nuclear power plants peaked in 1973, when 43 were ordered. By 1978 orders were down to two per year. Since then no new orders have been placed, and all orders placed between 1974 and 1978 have been canceled.

There are a number of reasons why plant construction has virtually ceased and public opposition to nuclear power continues. The Three Mile Island and the Chernobyl accidents, as well as frequent reports of minor accidents, have created a loss of confidence in the safety of nuclear plants. The disinterest on the part of investors—who have seen the cost of nuclear power rise exponentially in the past two decades—has also been a major roadblock to growth in the nuclear power industry.

These reservations might be overcome if a new generation of inherently safe reactors could be developed, and independent analyses showed nuclear power to be comparable to fossil fuel sources with regard to expense and environmental damage. Until extensive conservation measures have been implemented, however, it seems senseless to commit to a rebirth of this industry.

Nuclear Weapons Production

In the United States there are 17 major nuclear weapons facilities located in 12 different states. Large quantities of highly radioactive waste have accumulated over the years these facilities have been in operation (Office of Technology Assessment [OTA], 1991). There have also been repeated disclosures of mismanagement, safety violations, environmental contamination, accidents resulting in the spread of nuclear material, unsafe working conditions, and equipment failures. Scientists and the public have focused criticism on a number of facilities, including Hanford in Washington, Rocky Flats in Colorado, the Fernald Feed Materials Production Center in Ohio, the Savannah River site in South Carolina, the Oak Ridge Reservation in Tennessee, and the Idaho National Engineering Laboratory in Idaho (Ruttenber, 1995). In addition to exposures from the weapons industry, the public is at risk from accidents with involving the nuclear weapons themselves (Hubner & Fry, 1980).

With the apparent end of the cold war, the risk for environmental contamination and human exposure has been substantially reduced. Large volumes of highly radioactive waste still has to be processed and safely stored, and the facilities that have stopped production will have to be decommissioned. An explosion or fire during these operations could expose the public to hazardous levels of radiation, and workers will be placed at risk while decontaminating facilities containing unknown combinations of chemical and radioactive wastes (OTA, 1993).

Consequences of Nuclear War

The only instance of military use of atomic bombs on civilian populations is the bombing of Hiroshima and Nagasaki near the end of World War II. Together, the two bombs caused about 190,000 deaths. Half occurred in the first week after the blasts and were caused by trauma from collapsing buildings, the intense pressure from the blast itself, and from high doses of radiation (The Committee for the Compilation of Materials on Damage Caused by the Atomic Bombs in Hiroshima and Nagasaki, 1981).

In the years following World War II an enormous number of nuclear weapons, each many times more powerful than those dropped on Hiroshima and Nagasaki, have accumulated in stockpiles in the United States, Great Britain, the former Soviet Republics, France, China, and Israel. Other countries, such as India, Pakistan, and South Africa have developed smaller, but still potentially devastating weapons.

In the 1950s and 1960s elaborate civil defense programs were developed by the U.S. government, based on the supposition that with a week's warning, two-thirds of the U.S. population could survive in "fallout shelters" for up to a month, then emerge and rebuild their cities. Proponents of this program believed that nuclear war was survivable.

The idea of an effective civil defense program has now largely been abandoned by most scientists and physicians. In the 1980s the U.S. government attempted to modernize its plans for responding to nuclear war. The plans, developed by the Federal Emergency Management Agency (FEMA), were met with widespread public and professional criticism. This criticism did not derail the federal efforts to "survive" a nuclear war. Rather, the FEMA plans are now in place, but they have been kept out of public view and many of the plans are "classified."

Another consideration with regard to nuclear war is the extensive climate modification that could occur—commonly referred to as "nuclear winter" (Turco et al., 1983; Carrier, 1986). Using computer models, scientists have estimated the amount of soot and other debris that would be injected into the atmosphere and stratosphere. They argue that the solar radiation entering the atmosphere would be reduced to an extent that would alter the global climate and have profound effects on agriculture and natural ecosystems. Although there are many uncertainties in these models, the basic concept appears to be credible.

As the cold war winds down, the plans for decommissioning the weapons in the stockpiles of the United States and countries in the former Soviet Union have made nuclear war much less likely. It appears that the current threats are from the decommissioning of weapons facilities, the disposal of accumulated radioactive wastes, and from the detonation of weapons by "terrorist" operations.

Disposing of Nuclear Waste

The problem of how to store radioactive waste has been a matter of concern for over 30 years. From the early 1940s to the mid-1970s nuclear weapons and power industries placed production goals ahead of environmental and health concerns. Often, radioactive wastes were released to the environment during normal operations, and accumulated wastes were disposed of in ways that contaminated ecosystems. Nuclear power plants have generated large quantities of waste, but have produced much less environmental damage and fewer health risks to the public.

Nuclear waste is primarily classified according to how it is generated. *High-level* wastes comprise fission products from nuclear reactors, including those used in weapons production. Wastes from all other sources are termed *low-level* wastes. High-level wastes usually have high concentrations of radioactivity in relatively small volumes of material and low-level waste usually has low activity per unit volume. Radioactive wastes are not exclusively products of the nuclear industry—they also include by-products of all types of mining and mineral extraction, since raw ores contain variable quantities of radioactive elements.

The U.S. Low Level Waste Policy Act of 1980 subdivided low level wastes into three categories. Class A wastes contain low concentrations of radionuclides generated by medical and research institutions. Class B wastes have moderate concentrations of radionuclides with short half-lives and include filters from ventilation systems in nuclear power plants and radionuclides from uranium and plutonium production facilities. Class C wastes contain high concentrations of radionuclides and include some waste from nuclear power plants.

In the United States, low level waste makes up only 3% of the volume and 1% of the radioactivity of all radioactive wastes. In the first decades of the nuclear industry, low level waste was dumped into the ocean or disposed of by shallow land burial. By 1962, however, 95% of low level waste was stored in land burial sites; in 1970 ocean dumping was terminated.

The Nuclear Waste Policy Act of 1982 covers materials such as spent fuel rods from nuclear power plants, transuranic (elements with atomic numbers higher than uranium's) wastes, mill tailings (by-products of uranium mining and uranium processing), and the highly radioactive waste deriving from the separation of fission products during the reprocessing of spent nuclear fuel rods. The 1980 Low-Level Act required states, either individually or jointly, to find permanent low-level storage sites by 1986. To date, only seven states have developed agreements. It also appears that the U. S. Department of Energy will continue to have trouble with opening its transuranic waste storage site in New Mexico.

In order to permanently store high-level wastes, they must first be immobilized in glass—a process called vitrification. Glass blocks would be placed in underground chambers filled with rocks. This process may be imperfect, and scientists are worried about leaching of immobilized radioactive material (Burns, 1988).

In the United States there has been a series of setbacks in selecting and designing a site for the permanent storage of high-level waste. Currently, research is being conducted to determine the feasibility of storing high-level wastes at the DOE's Nevada Test Site. Scientists worry about adequate immobilization of wastes and members of the public who live near proposed sites object to possible health risks and reduced property values.

RADIATION DOSES FROM THE ENVIRONMENT

Recently the risks from environmental exposures to naturally occurring radon gas have been recognized. Prior to the middle 1980s the risks from radon and its decay products were not included in the estimates of background radiation, which were made for external exposures to radiation exclusively.

If doses from natural background radiation are computed as effective dose equivalents, then doses from external and internal sources can be combined for the purpose of comparing risks (NCRP, 1987). As illustrated in Table 5.2, the average person receives about 3 mSv (300 mrem) per year from natural background radiation—two-thirds from radon and one-third from a combination of cosmic radiation, gamma radiation emitted from radioactive elements in the earth's crust, and inhalation and ingestion of radionuclides in soil, water, air, and food. Exposures from medical diagnosis and treatment account for about 18% of the total dose from natural and artificial sources, and exposures from the nuclear weapons and power industries result in less than 1%. These estimates are based on normal operations from the nuclear industries and distribute doses over the entire population. They do not reflect the health risks to regional populations from an accident at a power plant or weapons facility; nor do they account for the economic impact of a large clean-up operation after such an accident.

Table 5.2   Average Annual Effective Dose Equivalent of Ionizing Radiations to a Member of the U.S. Population

Source	Dose equivalent[a]		Effective dose equivalent	
	mSv	mrem	mSv	percentage
Natural				
Radon[b]	24	2,400	2.0	55
Cosmic	0.27	27	0.27	8.0
Terrestrial	0.28	28	0.28	8.0
Internal	0.39	39	0.39	11
Total natural	—	—	3.0	82
Artificial				
Medical				
x-ray diagnosis	0.39	39	0.39	11
Nuclear medicine	0.14	14	0.14	4.0
Consumer products	0.10	10	0.10	3.0
Other				
Occupational	0.009	0.9	<0.01	<0.3
Nuclear fuel cycle	<0.01	<1.0	<0.01	<0.03
Fallout	<0.01	<1.0	<0.01	<0.03
Miscellaneous[c]	<0.01	<1.0	<0.01	<0.03
Total artificial	—	—	0.63	18
Total natural and artificial	—	—	3.6	100

[a]To soft tissues.

[b]Dose equivalent to bronchi from radon daughter products. The assumed weighting factor for the effective dose equivalent relative to whole-body exposure is 0.08.

[c]Department of Energy facilities, smelters, transportation, etc.

Source: National Academy of Sciences (1990), with permission.

REFERENCES

Ahearne, J. F. (1995). Does nuclear power have a future? In J. P. Young & R. S. Yalow (Eds.), *Radiation and public perception: Benefits and risks.* Washington, DC: American Chemical Society.

AMA Council on Scientific Affairs. (1989). Harmful effects of ultraviolet radiation. *JAMA, 262,* 380-384.

American Conference of Governmental Industrial Hygienists. (1994). *1994-1995 threshold limit values for chemical substances and physical agents and biological exposure indices*. Cincinnati: Author.

Akleyev, A. V., & Lyubchansky, E. R. (1994). Environmental and medical effects of nuclear weapon production in the Southern Urals. *The Science of the Total Environment, 142*, 1-8.

Archer, V. E. (1979). Anencephalus, drinking water, geomagnetism and cosmic radiation. *American Journal of Epidemiology, 109*, 88-97.

Bates, M. N. (1991). Extremely low frequency electromagnetic fields and cancer: The epidemiologic evidence. *Environmental Health Perspectives, 95*, 147-156.

Becker, R. O. (1990). *Cross currents: The promise of electromedicine, the perils of electropollution*. Los Angeles: Jeremy P. Tarcher.

Blask, D. E. (1989). The emerging role of the pineal gland and melatonin in oncogenesis. In B. W. Wilson, R. G. Stevens, & L. E. Anderson (Eds.), *Extremely low frequency electromagnetic fields: The question of cancer*. Columbus, OH: Battelle Press.

Burns, M. E. (Ed.). (1988). *Low-level radioactive waste regulation. Science, politics and fear*. Chelsea, MI: Lewis Publishers.

Carrier, G. F. (1986). Nuclear winter: The state of the science. In F. Soloman & R. Q. Marston (Eds.), *The medical implications of nuclear war*. Washington, DC: National Academy Press.

Chernoff, N., Rogers, J. M., & Kavet, R. A. (1992). A review of the literature on potential reproduct.

Cochran, T. B., & Norris, R. S. (1991). A first look at the Soviet bomb complex. *Bulletin of the Atomic Scientists. 47*, 25-31.

Cochran, T. B., Norris, R. S., & Suokko, K. L. (1993). Radioactive contamination at Chelyabinsk-65, Russia. *Annual Review of Energy and the Environment, 18*, 507-528.

The Committee for the Compilation of Materials on Damage Caused by the Atomic Bombs in Hiroshima and Nagasaki. (1981). *Hiroshima and Nagasaki: The physical, medical, and social effects of the atomic bombings*. New York: Basic Books.

Council on Scientific Affairs. (1991). Health effects of radon exposure. *Archives of Internal Medicine, 151*, 674-677.

Eisenbud, M. (1987). *Environmental radioactivity from natural, industrial, and military sources* (3rd ed.). New York: Academic Press.

Falk, H., Telles, N. C., Ishak, K. G., Thomas, L. B., & Popper, H. Epidemiology of thorotrast-induced hepatic angiosarcoma in the United States. *Environmental Research, 18*, 65-73.

Gale, R. P. (1987). Immediate medical consequence of nuclear accidents: Lessons from Chernobyl. *JAMA, 258*, 625-628.

Gale, R. P., & Butturini, A. (1991). Medical response to nuclear and radiation accidents. *Occupational Medicine: State of the Art Reviews, 6,* 581-596.

Gardner, M. J., Snee, M. P., Hall, A. J., Powell, C. A., Downes, S., & Terrell, J. D. (1990a). Results of case-control study of leukaemia and lymphoma in West Cumbria. *British Medical Journal, 300,* 423-29.

Gardner, M. J., Hall, A. J., Snee, M. P., Downes, S., Powell, C. A., & Terrell, J. D. (1990b). Methods and basic data of case-control study of leukaemia and lymphoma among young people near Sellafield nuclear plant in West Cumbria. *British Medical Journal, 300,* 429-34.

Glaser, Z. (1992). Non-ionizing radiation control. In K. L. Miller & W. A. Weidner (Eds.), *Handbook of management of radiation protection programs.* Boca Raton, FL: CRC Press.

Glass, A. G., & Hoover, R. (1989). The emerging epidemic of melanoma and squamous cell skin cancer. *JAMA, 262,* 2097-2100.

Hallenbeck, W. H. (1994). *Radiation protection.* Boca Raton, FL: Lewis.

Hamilton, T. E., van Belle, G., & Logerfo, J. P. (1987). Thyroid neoplasia in Marshall Islanders exposed to nuclear fallout. *JAMA, 258,* 629-636.

Hendee, W. R., & Boteler, J. C. (1994). The question of health effects from exposure to electromagnetic fields. *Health Physics, 66,* 127-136.

Hornung, R. W., & Meinhardt, T. J. (1987). Quantitative risk assessment of lung cancer in U. S. uranium miners. *Health Physics, 52,* 417-430.

Hubner, K. F., & Fry, S. A. (1980). *The medical basis for radiation accident preparedness.* New York: Elsevier/North-Holland.

International Commission on Radiological Protection. (1977). *Recommendations of the International Commission of Radiological Protection,* ICRP Publication 26. New York: Pergamon.

International Commission on Radiological Protection. (1979). *Limits for intakes of radionuclides by workers,* ICRP Publication 30. New York: Pergamon.

International Commission on Radiological Protection. (1991). *1990 recommendations of the International Commission on Radiological Protection,* ICRP Publication 60. New York: Pergamon.

Kahn, P. (1993). A grisly archive of key cancer data. *Science, 259,* 448-451.

Kanal, E., Shellock, F., & Talagala, L. (1990). Safety considerations in MR imaging. *Radiology, 176,* 593-606.

Kathren, R. L., & Petersen, G. R. (1989). Units and terminology of radiation measurement: A primer for the epidemiologist. *American Journal of Epidemiology, 130,* 1076-1087.

Kerber, R. A., Till, J. E., Simon, S. L., Lyon, J. L., Thomas, D. C., Preston-Martin, S., Rallison, M. L., Lloyd, R. D., & Stevens, W. (1993). A cohort study of thyroid disease in relation to fallout from nuclear weapons testing. *JAMA, 270,* 2076-2082.

Loomis, D. P., Savitz, D. A., & Ananth, C. V. (1994). Breast cancer mortality among female electrical workers in the United States. *Journal of the National Cancer Institute, 86*, 921-925.

Looney, W. B. (1960). An investigation of the late clinical findings following thorotrast (thorium dioxide) administration. *American Journal of Roentgenology, Radium Therapy and Nuclear Medicine, 83*, 163-185.

Louria D.B. (1990) Zapping the food supply. *Bulletin of the Atomic Scientists, 46*, 34-36.

Lyons, E. A., Dyke, C., Toms, M., & Cheang, M. (1988). In utero exposure to diagnostic ultrasound: A 6-year follow-up. *Radiology, 166*, 686-693.

Macklis, R. M. (1990). Radiothor and the era of mild radium therapy. *JAMA, 264*, 614-618.

Macklis, R. M., Bellerive, M. R., & Humm, J. L. (1990). The radiotoxicolgy of radiothor: Analysis of an early case of iatrogenic poisoning by a radioactive patent medicine. *JAMA, 264*, 619-621.

Martland, H. S. (1929). Occupational poisoning in the manufacture of luminous watch dials. *JAMA, 92*, 466-473.

McGivern, R. F., Sokol, R. Z., & Adey, W. R. (1990). Prenatal exposure to a low-frequency electromagnetic field demasculinizes adult scent marking behavior and increases accessory organ weights in rats. *Teratology, 41*, 1-9.

Milham, S. (1979). Mortality in aluminum reduction plant workers. *Journal of Occupational Medicine, 21*, 475-480.

Morgan, M. G., Nair, I., & Florig, H. K. (1989). *Biological effects of power frequency electric and magnetic fields.* Washington, DC: Office of Technology Assessment .

Morris, M. D., & Jones, T. D. (1989). Hematopoietic death of unprotected man from photon irradiations: Statistical modeling from animal experiments. *International Journal of Radiation Biology, 55*, 445-461.

Moskowitz, P. D., Pardi, R., DePhillips, M. P., & Meinhold, A. F. (1992). Computer models used to support cleanup decision-making at hazardous and radioactive waste sites. *Risk Analysis, 12*, 591-621.

Moure, R. (1981). The scientific rationale for a lower radon daughter exposure. In Gomez, M. (Ed.), *Radiation hazards in mining: Control, measurement, and medical aspects.* New York: American Institute of Mining, Metallurgical, and Petroleum Engineers.

Mur, J. M., Moulin, J., Meyer-Bisch, C., Massin, N., Coulon, J., & Loulergue, J. (1987). Mortality of aluminum reduction plant workers in France. *International Journal of Epidemiology, 16*, 257-264.

National Academy of Sciences. (1991). *Comparative dosimetry of radon in mines and homes.* Washington, DC: National Academy Press.

National Council on Radiation Protection and Measurements. (1987). *Exposure of the population in the United States and Canada from nat-*

ural background Radiation, NCRP Report No. 94. Bethesda, MD: Author.

National Council on Radiation Protection and Measurements. (1989). *Exposure of the U. S. population from occupational radiation* (NCRP Report No. 101). Bethesda, MD: Author.

National Research Council, Committee on the Biological Effects of Ionizing Radiation (BEIR IV). (1988). *Health risks of radon and other internally deposited alpha emitters.* Washington, DC: National Academy Press.

National Research Council, Committee on the Biological Effects of Ionizing Radiation (BEIR V). (1990). *The effects on populations of exposure to low levels of ionizing radiation.* Washington. DC: National Academy Press.

Neel, J. V. (1991). Update on the genetic effects of ionizing radiation. *JAMA, 266,* 698-701.

Nordstrom, S., Birke, E., & Gustavsson, L. (1983). Reproductive hazards among workers at high-voltage substations. *Bioelectro-magnetics, 4,* 91-101.

Office of Technology Assessment, U. S. Congress. (1991). *Complex cleanup: The environmental legacy of nuclear weapons production* (OTA-O-484). Washington, DC: U. S. Government Printing Office.

Office of Technology Assessment, U. S. Congress. (1993). *Hazards ahead: Managing cleanup worker health and safety at the nuclear weapons complex* (OTA-BP-O-85). Washington, DC: U. S. Government Printing Office.

Piccioni R. (1988). Food irradiation: contaminating our food. *The Ecologist, 18,* 48-55.

Rockette, H. E., Arena, V. (1983). Mortality studies of aluminum reduction plant workers: Potroom and carbon department. *Journal of Occupational Medicine, 25,* 549-557.

Rowland, R. E., & Lucas, H. F. (1984). Radium-dial workers. In J. D. Boice & J. F. Fraumeni (Eds.), *Radiation carcinogenesis: Epidemiology and biological significance.* New York: Raven Press.

Ruttenber, A. J. (1995). Evaluating health risks in communities near nuclear facilities. In J. P. Young & R. S. Yalow (Eds.), *Radiation and public perception: Benefits and risks.* Washington, DC: American Chemical Society.

Salzinger, K., Freimark, S., McCullough, M., Phillips, D., & Birenbaum, L. Altered operant behavior of adult rats after perinatal exposure to a 60 Hz electromagnetic field. *Bioelectromagnetics, 11,* 105-116.

Savitz, D. A. (1993). Health effects of low-frequency electric and magnetic fields. *Environmental Science and Technology, 27,* 52-54.

Savitz, D. A., & Calle, E. E. (1987). Leukemia and occupational exposure to electromagnetic fields: Review of epidemiological surveys. *Journal of Occupational Medicine, 29,* 47-51.

Schnorr, T. M., Grajewski, B., Hornung, R. W., Thun, M. J., Egeland, G. M., Murray, W. E., Conover, D. L., & Halperin, W. E. (1991). Video display terminals and the risk of spontaneous abortion. *New England Journal of Medicine, 324,* 727-733.

Shapiro, J. (1990). *Radiation protection: A guide for scientists and physicians.* Cambridge, MA: Harvard University Press.

Shimizu, Y., Schull, W. J., & Kato, H. (1990). Cancer risk among atomic bomb survivors: The RERF Life Span Study. *JAMA, 264,* 601-604.

Shleien, B. (1992). *The health physics and radiological health handbook* (revised ed.). Silver Spring, MD: Scinta.

Shore, R. E. (1992). Nonionizing radiation. In W. Rom (Ed.), *Environmental and occupational medicine* (2nd ed., pp. 269-291). Boston: Little, Brown.

Sliney, D. H., & Cuellar, J. (1992). Microwaves and electromagnetic fields. In M. Lippmann (Ed.), *Environmental toxicants: Human exposures and their health effects.* New York: Van Nostrand Reinhold.

Stark, C. R., Orleans, M., Haverkamp, A., & Murphy, J. (1984). Short- and long-term risks after exposure to diagnostic ultrasound in utero. *Obstetrics and Gynecology, 71,* 513-517.

Stevens W., Thomas D. C., Lyon J. L., Till, J. E., Kerber, R. A., Simon, S. L., Lloyd, R. D., Elghany, N. A., & Preston-Martin, S. (1990). Leukemia in Utah and radioactive fallout from the Nevada Test Site. *JAMA, 264,* 585-591.

Stewart, A. M. (1971). Low dose radiation cancers in man. In J. P. Greenstein & A. Haddow (Eds.), *Advances in cancer research* (pp. 359-389). London: Academic Press.

Stewart, A. M., & Kneale, G. W. (1990). A-bomb radiation and evidence of late effects other than cancer. *Health Physics, 58,* 729-735.

Telles, N. C., Thomas, L. B., Popper, H., Ishak, K. G., & Falk, H. (1979). Evolution of thorotrast-induced hepatic angiosarcomas. *Environmental Research, 18,* 74-87.

Turco, R. P., Toon, O. B., Ackerman, T. P., Pollack, J. B., & Sagan, C. (1983). Nuclear winter: Global consequences of multiple nuclear explosions. *Science, 222,* 1283-1292.

Till, J. E., & Meyer, R. H. (Eds.). (1983). *Radiological assessment: A textbook on environmental dose analysis.* Washington, DC: U.S. Government Printing Office.

U. S. Department of Energy. (1991). *Annual energy review, 1990* (DOE/EIA-0384[90]). Washington, DC: Author.

U. S. Nuclear Regulatory Commission. (1992). *Occupational radiation exposure at commercial nuclear power reactors and other facilities.* Washington, DC: Author.

Ubeda, A., Leal, J., Trillo, M. A., Jimenez, M. A., & Delgado, J. M. R. (1983). Pulse shape of magnetic fields influences chick embryogenesis. *Journal of Anatomy, 137,* 513-536.

Walter, S. D., Marrett, L. D., From, L., Hertzman, C., Shannon, H. S., & Roy, P. (1990). The association of cutaneous malignant melanoma with the use of sunbeds and sunlamps. *American Journal of Epidemiology, 131,* 232-243.

Wertheimer, N., & Leeper, E. (1986). Possible effects of electric blankets and heated waterbeds on fetal development. *Bioelectromagnetics, 7,* 13-22.

Wertheimer, N., & Leeper, E. (1989). Fetal loss associated with two seasonal sources of electromagnetic field exposure. *American Journal of Epidemiology, 129,* 220-224.

Wilson, B . W., Chess, E. K., & Anderson, L. E. (1986). 60 Hz electric-field effects on pineal melatonin rhythms: Time course for onset and recovery. *Bioelectromagnetics, 7, 239-242.*

Wilkinson, G. S. (1991). Epidemiologic studies of nuclear and radiation workers: An overview of what is known about health risks posed by the nuclear industry. *Occupational Medicine: State of the Art Reviews, 6,* 715-724.

Yamazaki, J. N., & Schull W. J. (1990). Perinatal loss and neurological abnormalities among children of the atomic bomb. *JAMA , 264*: 605-609.

SUGGESTED READINGS

American Conference of Governmental Industrial Hygienists. (1994). *1994-1995 threshold limit values for chemical substances and physical agents and biological exposure indices.* Cincinnati: Author.

Boice, J. D., & Fraumeni, J. F. (Eds.). (1984). *Radiation carcinogenesis: Epidemiology and biological significance.* New York: Raven Press.

Eisenbud, M. (1987). *Environmental radioactivity from natural, industrial, and military sources* (3rd Ed.). New York: Academic Press.

Hallenbeck, W. H. (1994). *Radiation protection.* Boca Raton, FL: Lewis.

Mettler, F. A., Kelsey, C. A., & Ricks, R. C. (1990). *Medical management of radiation accidents.* Boca Raton, FL: CRC Press.

National Research Council, Committee on the Biological Effects of Ionizing Radiation (BEIR IV). (1988). *Health risks of radon and other internal-*

ly deposited alpha emitters. Washington, DC: National Academy Press.

National Research Council, Committee on the Biological Effects of Ionizing Radiation (BEIR V). (1990). *The effects on populations of exposure to low levels of ionizing radiation.* Washington, DC: National Academy Press.

Murray, R. (1993). *Nuclear energy: An introduction to the concepts, systems and applications of nuclear processes.* Oxford: Pergamon.

Nazaroff, W. W., & Nero, A .V. (Eds.) (1988). *Radon and its decay products in indoor air.* New York: John Wiley.

Shapiro, J. (1990). *Radiation protection: A guide for scientists and physicians.* Cambridge, MA: Harvard University Press.

Shleien, B. (1992). *The health physics and radiological health handbook* (revised ed.). Silver Spring, MD: Scinta.

Soloman, F., & Marston, R. Q. (Eds.), *The medical implications of nuclear war.* Washington, DC: National Academy Press.

Turner, J. E. (1986). *Atoms, radiation, and radiation protection.* New York: Pergamon Press.

Wagner, H.N., & Ketchum, L.E. (1989). *Living with radiation.* Baltimore: The Johns Hopkins Press.

Young, J. P., & Yalow, R. S. (Eds.). (1995). *Radiation and public perception: Benefits and risks.* Washington, DC: American Chemical Society.

Part III

Routes of Exposure

Chapter 6

Air Pollution

Daniel S. Blumenthal and Harvey L. Ragsdale

The atmosphere is a chemically complex and changing air mass that exposes people to varying concentrations of air pollutants from local, regional, and global sources. Although most attention is paid to man-made pollutants, many naturally occurring substances compose the "background" pollutant levels of the atmosphere. Natural phenomena such as volcanic eruptions, plant pollination, and swamp gas emissions have always tainted the air. Naturally occurring forest fires inject oxides of sulfur and nitrogen—components of "acid rain"—along with soot into the atmosphere.

Organisms evolved in environments with these naturally occurring chemicals—sometimes in extremely high concentrations. Particles from exposed mineral soil and decaying vegetation are also natural components of the atmosphere. Ozone (O_3), another air pollutant, is generated naturally from both lightning discharges and through photochemical reactions. In the 20th century, however, these "natural" pollutants have become overshadowed by those that are man-made.

Concern about air pollution dates at least to the 13th century. In England, between 1285 and 1310, several governmental commissions were established to investigate the fouling of air that accompanied the switch from wood to coal as the principal fuel in lime kilns. This concern escalated during the Industrial Revolution in England and the

United States. During the 30-year period beginning in 1808, factories added more air pollution than had been generated by all previous agriculture and commerce.

The first smoke-control laws in the United States were established in Cincinnati and Chicago in 1881, and by 1912, 23 of the 28 largest cities had passed similar laws (Council on Environmental Quality, 1971). During the same period, agricultural crops and forests were severely damaged by high concentrations of sulfur dioxide from local sources such as smelters (MacKenzie & El-Ashry, 1988).

Air pollution damages the health and general well-being of people as well as the ecosystems that support their survival. These effects include:

1. *Human health.*   Air pollution can cause both acute effects from episodic releases of high concentrations of contaminants and chronic effects from continuous exposure to low levels of pollutants. Air pollution, moreover, may be indoors as well as outside a building. Pollutants in air have been implicated in such diseases as asthma, bronchitis, emphysema, cancer, and cardiovascular disease. Increased mortality rates have been attributed to the acute effects of air pollution in several severe episodes of urban smog. Urban O_3 concentrations often rise to levels high enough for health officials to recommend against strenuous outdoor activity in order to minimize health risks. Radioactive radon gas pollution in dwellings presents a risk for lung cancer and has stimulated monitoring and remedial actions in many countries. Air pollution also has been implicated as a cause of adverse health effects in animals.

2. *Ecosystems.*   Many different pollutants damage flowers, plants, crops, and forests. "Acid rain," the deposition of droplets containing sulfuric and nitric acids, is a threat to the health of soils and lakes. Crop damage was seen as early as the late 19th century, when factories released large amounts of sulfur dioxide. Luxuriant forests have been completely destroyed by sulfur dioxide fumes from copper smelters and from other industrial emissions such as fluorides. In the last 40 years, however, ozone has become the dominant air pollutant with respect to plant damage in forests and agricultural fields.

3. *Property.*   Materials such as paint on cars and houses are blackened or corroded by hydrogen sulfide; rubber and plastics are cracked by O_3; some metals are corroded by sulfur dioxide (SO_2); and "acid rain" destroys marble and limestone structures.

4. *Aesthetics.* Many pollutants are malodorous and some affect visibility. This may also be a safety hazard; particulate matter in the atmosphere and photochemical smog have impaired visibility badly at some airports. In developed countries the public is beginning to value the appearance of air; cities with "visible" pollution may become undesirable places to live even though the air quality is within regulatory limits. Visible pollution may also be a problem in natural scenic areas that are important sources of inspiration and recreation.

5. *Economy.* Air pollution can increase absenteeism, morbidity, hospitalization, and mortality, cause crop and property destruction, and decrease work efficiency. Governmental regulation of air pollution has had substantial economic impact on some industries, forcing some to shut down or move to areas with less stringent regulations. Air pollution and its regulation have also affected the lifestyles of community members and tourists—an impact that can also damage local economies.

6. *Weather.* Increased particulate concentrations in the atmosphere can "seed" clouds and increase rainfall. Air pollutants can also change local, regional, and global climates. The heating of the earth's surface is controlled in part by the reflectivity of clouds, which is affected by both sulfur dioxide and particulate concentrations. Urban areas store heat in buildings and pavement and radiate it back to the atmosphere. These "heat islands" can increase local precipitation when rising moisture-laden hot air expands, cools, and releases the moisture as precipitation.

Although not classified as an air pollutant, carbon dioxide (CO_2) is a major factor in the projected course of "global warming." Carbon dioxide is a by-product of combustion, as are pollutants such as sulfur dioxide (SO_2) and nitrogen dioxide (NO_2). Increased heating of the earth can occur when CO_2 and other gases trap the longer wavelength heat emitted from the earth (the "greenhouse effect"). Changes in local temperature, water supply, vegetation, and sea level are predicted if global warming occurs. Human health would be impacted by reduced food production in certain regions, migration of biota, and increases in the number of agricultural pests and insect disease vectors. Human settlements could be displaced from coastal land flooded by rising sea levels. The extent to which global warming has already begun is controversial.

WEATHER, CLIMATE, AND AIR POLLUTION

An understanding of the fundamentals of meteorology—in particular, the movements of air masses and the factors that influence them — is essential to an appreciation of the mechanisms by which air pollutants accumulate, disperse, and come into contact with humans.

Most meteorological events affecting air pollution take place in the troposphere (Chapter 1). Over 90% of the atmosphere's total air mass is concentrated in this 12-mile thick layer. The size of the troposphere, relative to the earth, is the size of the skin of an apple relative to the apple itself. It is somewhat thinner at the poles of the earth and thicker at the equator.

Movement of air within the troposphere and other layers is related directly to the ways that energy from the sun warms the earth's atmosphere. There are three mechanisms: radiation, conduction, and convection. Little of the sun's radiant energy is absorbed by the air directly; rather, it is absorbed by the earth and then radiated to the atmosphere. Much of the re-radiated energy is absorbed by the atmosphere, largely because of its water vapor content.

Conduction—the mechanical transfer of heat energy from one molecule to another—plays a larger role in warming the atmosphere. Heat energy is conducted from the warmed surface of the earth to the adjacent air layer and thence to air layers at higher altitudes.

Convection is the transfer of heat by the movement of air masses. Air warmed at the earth's surface expands, becomes lighter, and rises; the cooler air above it then sinks to take its place. Convection, in combination with the rotation of the earth on its axis, is responsible for the patterns of winds in the troposphere. By regularly presenting the sun with a different portion of the earth's surface, the earth's rotation gives rise to the prevailing winds (easterlies, westerlies, and trades).

The rate at which pollutants in the troposphere are dispersed is governed largely by the air's horizontal movement (wind) and its vertical movement (convection). As it rises and the atmospheric pressure drops, air expands and becomes cooler. The rate at which it cools is known as the *adiabatic lapse rate*. If this rate is high, warm air rises quickly; under such "unstable" conditions, pollutants are dispersed rapidly. Conversely, under "stable" conditions in which the adiabatic lapse rate is low, pollutants may accumulate.

The vertical distance through which warm air rises while undergoing adiabatic cooling, before it meets air of equal temperature, is the *mixing depth*. This represents the upper limit of pollution dispersion. At times when the earth and its adjacent air layer are relatively cool—as in winter or at night—the mixing depth is diminished and pollutants may be poorly dispersed.

An *inversion* represents a particularly stable situation in which the surface air is cooler than the layer of air above it and thus cannot rise (Figure 6.1). Pollutants concentrate in this surface layer because their molecules lack the kinetic energy to disperse vertically. Two types of inversion are of particular importance. A *subsidence inversion* is created when a high pressure air mass sinks, is compressed (and thus heated), and forms a layer above the cooler air beneath it. Subsidence inversions occur commonly on the west coast of the United States. The second type of inversion, a *radiation inversion*, occurs frequently on cool nights. As the ground cools (by radiating its heat), the air next to it also cools. This type of inversion is broken up as the sun warms the earth in the morning.

Season and topography affect the formation of inversions, which are most prevalent during the fall and winter; they are most frequent and persistent in valleys. Fog often forms in the cool surface air and can worsen coexisting pollution by, for instance, converting gaseous SO_2 to sulfuric acid mist.

Some special meteorological effects occurring in urban areas also deserve mention. The concrete surfaces of tall city buildings can become heat islands and generate a rising column of warm air that settles at the city's periphery. Particulates suspended in the air form a dome over the city that reflects the sun's heat and creates a system that tends to trap pollution in the urban atmosphere (Elsom, 1992; Figure 6.1).

These various meteorological phenomena, on several occasions during the past 50 years, have combined with periods of high pollution to create a number of major acute air pollution episodes. Some of these are described later in this chapter. The study of these episodes has contributed considerably to current knowledge of air pollution and its effects on human health.

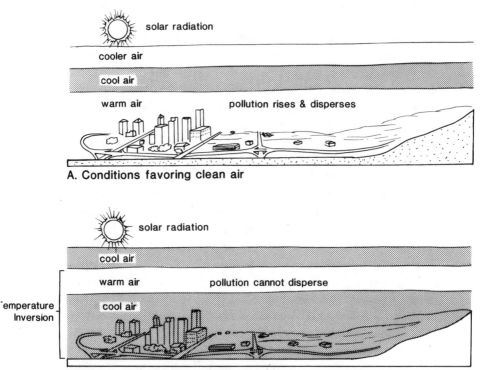

A. Conditions favoring clean air

B. Thermal inversion increasing pollution

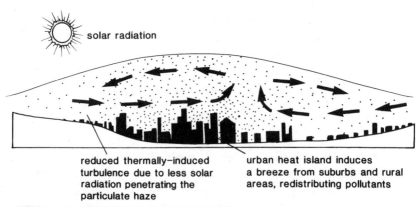

reduced thermally–induced turbulence due to less solar radiation penetrating the particulate haze

urban heat island induces a breeze from suburbs and rural areas, redistributing pollutants

C. Urban heat island increasing pollution

Figure 6.1 Factors that influence the concentration and distribution of air pollutants in urban areas. (Adapted from Chiras, 1994; Elsom, 1992.)

COMMON AIR POLLUTANTS

The 1970 amendments to the Clean Air Act require the U.S. Environmental Protection Agency (EPA) to establish National Ambient Air Quality Standards (NAAQS) for certain pollutants. These "criteria" pollutants are photochemical oxidants (specifically O_3), carbon monoxide (CO), SO_2, particulate matter, NO_2, hydrocarbons, and lead (Pb). For each of these pollutants the EPA has set a *primary standard* intended to protect human health within a reasonable margin of safety and a *secondary standard* designed to protect against adverse effects on human welfare such as crop and livestock losses, damage to vegetation and buildings, and reduced visibility (Table 6.1).

A second category of hazardous air pollutants is regulated by emission standards. These chemicals fall under the National Emission Standards for Hazardous Air Pollutants (NESHAPs), also created by the 1970 Clean Air Act. The law requires the EPA to set standards at levels that prevent any adverse effects to human health. Unable to determine such levels for all pollutants, the agency set standards for only eight: arsenic, asbestos, radionuclides, beryllium, mercury, vinyl chloride, benzene, and coke-oven emissions.

A third category of pollutants was created by the 1990 amendments to the Clean Air Act. Standards for controls on emissions of these substances are to be based not on health considerations but on "maximum achievable control technology." The 189 substances to be regulated are specified in the amendments (Quarles & Lewis, 1990; Centers for Disease Control [CDC], 1991a).

Ozone

Ozone is a molecule composed of three oxygen atoms and is the principal component of modern smog. It is by far the most plentiful photochemical oxidant, and the only one measured routinely by air-monitoring programs. Ozone and the other photochemical oxidants—including peroxyacetyl nitrates (PAN), formaldehyde, and peroxides—are called "secondary" pollutants because they are not emitted into the air directly. Rather, they are formed by chemical reactions between hydrocarbons and nitrogen oxides in the presence of sunlight (hence the term "photochemical smog").

Table 6.1   U.S. National Ambient Air Quality Standards (NAAQS) in Effect in 1993

Pollutant	Primary (Health related)		Secondary (Welfare related)	
	Type of average	Standard level Concentration[a]	Type of average	Standard level concentration
CO	8-hour[b]	9 ppm ($10 \ mg/m^3$)	No secondary standard	
	1-hour[b]	35 ppm ($40 \ mg/m^3$)	No secondary standard	
Pb	Maximum Quarterly Average	$1.5 \ \mu g/m^3$	Same as primary standard	
NO$_2$	Annual Arithmetic Mean	0.053 ($100 \ \mu g/m^3$)	Same as primary standard	
O$_3$	Maximum Daily 1-hour Average[c]	0.12 ppm ($235 \ \mu g/m^3$)	Same as primary standard	
PM-10	Annual Arithmetic Mean[d]	$50 \mu g/m^3$	Same as primary standard	
	24-hour[d]	$150 \mu g/m^3$	Same as primary standard	
SO$_2$	Annual Arithmetic Mean	$80 \ \mu g/m^3$ (0.03 pppm)	3-hour[b]	$1300 \ \mu g/m^3$ (0.50 ppm)
	24-hour[d]	$365 \ \mu g/m^3$ (0.14 ppm)		

[a]Parenthetical value is an approximately equivalent concentration.

[b]Not to be exceeded more than once per year.

[c]The standard is attained when the expected number of days per calendar year with maximum hourly average concentrations above 0.12 ppm is equal to or less than 1, as determined according to Appendix H of the Ozone NAAQS.

[d]Particulate standards use PM-10 (particles less than 10μ in diameter) as the indicator pollutant. The annual standard is attained when the expected annual arithmetic mean concentration is less than or equal to 50 μg/ m^3; the 24-hour standard is attained when the expected number of days per calendar year above 50 μg/m^3 is equal to or less than 1; as determined according to Appendix K of the PM NAAQS.

Source: EPA, 1993.

Automobiles, which produce both nitrogen oxides and hydrocarbons, cause high ozone concentrations in urban air. Generally, O_3 concentrations in cities rise rapidly in the morning, peak in the mid-to-late afternoon, and decrease to much lower levels at night. Ozone is also produced naturally through reactions with hydrocarbons released by plants, and by lightning passing through the atmosphere. Airplane cabins also have elevated concentrations of ozone.

Ozone is a respiratory irritant that rapidly oxidizes molecules in cell membranes. Acute exposures produce inflammation of mucous membranes and conjunctivae, whereas chronic exposure can produce a range of pathology—from fibrosis and thickening of the alveolar walls to chronic obstructive pulmonary disease. Ozone also exacerbates the course of chronic lung disease produced by other causes.

Older studies show that ozone concentrations of 0.15 parts per million (ppm) impair the activities of vulnerable individuals—children, the elderly, asthmatics, and persons who exercise outdoors. More recent research identifies acute effects in children at atmospheric concentrations as low as 0.11 ppm, lower than the current EPA maximum hourly average standard of 0.12 ppm (Sun, 1988). The American Academy of Pediatrics has recommended lower standards for both this pollutant and particulate matter (Committee on Environmental Health, 1993).

Carbon Monoxide

Incomplete combustion of a carbon-containing fuel produces CO, a colorless, odorless, poisonous gas. It is easily the most plentiful air pollutant. The U. S. Environmental Protection Agency (EPA) estimates that in the early 1990s, about 80 million metric tons of CO were emitted into the air each year in the United States (EPA, 1993). The major source, representing about two-thirds of CO emissions, is from internal combustion engines in motor vehicles (Table 6.2). Fortunately this toxic gas is quickly converted by natural processes to CO_2 and thus does not usually accumulate in the environment. However, it can accumulate in traffic tunnels and underground garages. Faulty furnaces or space heaters can result in deadly concentrations of CO in dwellings.

Table 6.2   U.S. Air Pollution Emissions[a] By Pollutant and Source 1992

Parameter	CO	Pb[b]	NO$_2$	VOC	PM$_{10}$	SO$_2$
Fuel Combustion	5.6	0.5	10.6	0.6	1.1	17.7
Industrial Processes	4.5	2.1	0.8	2.7	1.8	1.9
Solid waste	1.6	0.7	0.1	9.2	0.2	0.1
Transportation	63.5	1.4	9.4	7.5	1.7	1.0
Miscellaneous	3.9	0.0	0.1	0.5	0.7	0.0
Total	79.1	4.7	21.0	20.6	5.4	20.6

[a] Unless otherwise noted, quantities are in units of million metric tons per year; data for the sums of sources and totals may not be equal due to rounding; see text for abbreviations of air pollutants.

[b] Thousands of metric tons.

Source: EPA, 1993.

Carbon monoxide is an asphyxiant that binds with hemoglobin to form carboxyhemoglobin, thereby displacing oxygen from red blood cells (Chapter 4). At relatively low exposure levels, CO can decrease exercise tolerance in patients with coronary artery disease (Aronow & Isbell, 1973; Kleinman, Davidson, Vandagriff, Caiozzo & Whittenberger, 1989). At sufficiently high concentrations, CO can be rapidly fatal.

Sulfur Dioxide

Oxides of sulfur, primarily SO$_2$, are gases produced in the combustion of fossil fuels containing sulfur. Industrially generated SO$_2$, primarily from electric power plants, is the principal component of acid rain. Sulfur oxides are released to the atmosphere by coal-fired power plants along with particulates and are also released from pulp mills and paper production industries.

Sulfur oxides are highly soluble in water and form sulfurous acid on contact with moist membranes. Ninety percent of inhaled sulfur oxides are absorbed in the upper respiratory system, where they cause bronchoconstriction. Oxides of sulfur also impair mucociliary clearance. In lower airways they increase airway resistance and may exacerbate underlying asthma. Respiratory function is impaired in exercising humans at ambient SO$_2$ levels of about 1 ppm, or at lower levels in those with asthma (Schachter, Witek, & Beck, 1984).

Sulfur dioxide and particulates are sometimes grouped together as the sulfur dioxide/particulate complex. This is because the two pollutants usually are found together in urban settings and because SO_2 is transformed in the atmosphere into an aerosol of sulfate particulates. Fossil fuel combustion is the primary source of the SO_2/particulate complex. Its constituents have both irritant and toxic effects on the airways.

Particulates

Particulates include dust, soot, smoke, resuspended road sand and a number of chemicals of varying toxicity, including oxides of carbon, iron, aluminum, silicon, and phosphorus. Sources include motor vehicle emissions, residential wood burning, and smokestacks from factories and power plants. The EPA used to measure all particles in an air sample ("total suspended particulates"), but now measures PM_{10}, which includes only particles less than 10 microns (μm) in diameter—particles small enough to enter the lungs (EPA, 1993).

Fine particles and aerosols have an aerodynamic diameter ≤ 2.5 μm and include soot, condensates of acids, and particles composed of sulfate and nitrate compounds. Compared with larger particles derived from soil and crustal materials, fine particles are thought to pose a greater risk for respiratory damage because they are transported more deeply into the lungs.

Children living in cities with comparatively high concentrations of particulates have higher rates of reported respiratory illness than those in cities with low concentrations (Dockery et al., 1989), and atmospheric concentrations of sulfate particles have been correlated with respiratory complaints in adults (Ostro, Lipsett, Mann, Krupnick & Harrington, 1993). Epidemiologic studies have also correlated daily particulate concentrations with mortality from all causes in a number of cities (Schwartz, 1993; 1994), and a recent prospective cohort study that controlled for important confounding variables such as smoking showed an association between mortality and fine particulates in the adult subjects who lived in the six study cities (Dockery et al., 1993). Increased concentrations of SO_2 and particulates during acute air pollution episodes have also been associated with the exacerbation of cardiac and pulmonary disease.

Nitrogen Dioxide

High-temperature combustion in engines and boilers produces nitrogen monoxide (NO) from naturally occurring oxygen and nitrogen. Nitrogen dioxide is an oxidation product of NO. Motorized vehicles are the largest source of nitrogen oxides (primarily NO_2) in urban environments. In grain silos, NO_2 is produced by microbial decomposition of vegetation; silo workers may die from its irritant and asphyxiant effects. Fires and volcanoes are other important sources of nitrogen oxides.

Although NO_2 irritates and damages respiratory epithelium, it is less acutely toxic than O_3. Acute exposure to NO_2 causes bronchoconstriction if there is preexisting lung disease (Orehek, Massari, Gayrard, Grimaud, & Charpin, 1976). Chronic exposure causes histopathologic changes in animal models (Freeman, Stephes, Crande, & Furiosi, 1968) and may cause increased susceptibility to respiratory infections (Rutishauser, Ackermann, Braun, Gnehm, & Wanner, 1990).

Lead

Lead (Pb) is a toxic heavy metal that primarily affects the hematopoietic, renal, and central nervous systems. It accumulates in the body and is stored in bone. Exposure to air-borne lead occurs directly by inhalation of lead particles in air or dust, or indirectly by ingestion of lead-contaminated food, water, soil, and dust.

Vehicles burning leaded gasoline are a major source of atmospheric lead in countries than have not banned this additive. Certain industries—for instance, lead and copper smelters (Landrigan, Halpern, & Silbergeld, 1989) and battery recycling plants—are also important sources. Prior to 1975, gasoline combustion accounted for 90% of air-borne Pb. Environmental Protection Agency regulations reducing Pb content in gasoline and requirements for Pb-free gasoline-burning engines in the automotive industry have reduced Pb emissions from gasoline by 94% since 1977. Between 1983 and 1992, ambient atmospheric lead concentrations measured at urban sampling sites declined by 89% (EPA, 1993). The reduction in atmospheric lead content has been linked to a 78% decline (from 12.8 µg/dl to 2.8 µg/dl) in the mean blood lead level of the U.S. population between the sampling periods 1976–1980 and 1988-1991 (Pirkle et al., 1994).

Hydrocarbons

Hydrocarbons in the atmosphere are, by definition, volatile organic compounds (VOCs). Most of the estimated 20.6 million metric tons per year of hydrocarbons emitted to the U. S. atmosphere in 1992 came from incompletely burned gasoline in motor vehicles, from industrial processes, or from the use of solvents (EPA, 1993). There is epidemiologic evidence that exposure to VOCs from chemical industries increases the rates of chronic respiratory symptoms in children living nearby (Ware et al., 1993). Some hydrocarbons are known carcinogens and some are involved in the formation of ozone near the earth's surface. EPA-mandated controls on fuel combustion and tank storage of gasoline reduced VOC emissions by 11% between 1983-1992 (EPA, 1993).

Other Pollutants

A number of other substances with adverse effects on human health are released to the atmosphere from a variety of sources. Carbon dioxide, methane, nitrous oxide (N_2O), chlorofluorocarbons (CFCs), and other organic compounds are "greenhouse gases," which can trap heat energy that is radiated from the earth and cause global warming with the potentially disastrous effects mentioned previously. CFCs and other halogenated compounds such as the fumigant methyl bromide (CH_3Br) and the hydrochlorofluorocarbons (HCFCs, which are less ozone–destructive replacements for CFCs) also may deplete the stratospheric ozone layer that shields the earth from ultraviolet light, which causes crop damage and skin cancer (Chapter 5). The potential health and environmental effects of these gases are so great that they must be considered air pollutants.

Smoke from fires in buildings and forests contains a variety of respiratory irritants in particulate and gaseous form, several of which have been shown to cause bronchoconstriction, decrease in pulmonary function, and airway reactivity (Lipsett, Waller, Shusterman, Thollaug, & Brunner, 1994). In addition, forest and grassland fires produce large quantities of methyl bromide and methyl chloride, both of which have been shown to destroy ozone in the stratosphere (Cicerone, 1994), thereby increasing ultraviolet radiation at the earth's surface.

Bioaerosols are airborne particles that are either living organisms or the products of living organisms. They come from a wide variety of sources and are usually more of a problem for indoor environments, as discussed later in this chapter. The allergens produced by plant pollen are notable exceptions, as those with asthma and hay fever can attest. Recently, allergens on soybean particles have been associated with asthma epidemics in communities near a harbor where ships unloaded soybeans into storage silos (Anto et al., 1993).

ACUTE AIR POLLUTION EPISODES

Concern with the impact of air pollution on aesthetics dates back several centuries, but the first widespread appreciation that this environmental problem can threaten human lives stemmed from several acute episodes in the mid-20th century. Most of the adverse health consequences of these episodes have been attributed to high concentrations of sulfur dioxide and particulates produced by industry.

Meuse River Valley, Belgium

The first air pollution tragedy to arouse worldwide concern occurred in the Meuse River Valley, Belgium, where a heavily industrialized area extends for some 15 miles. Valleys are often subject to thermal inversions; it is not surprising, then, that the Meuse Valley became heavily polluted when, for a week in December 1930, Belgium was blanketed by a thick, cold fog. Pollutants accumulated in the stagnant inversion layer day after day. Thousands fell ill within a few days and 63 deaths were linked to the contaminated air. The dead were mostly elderly and had underlying heart or lung diseases. Those who were sickened by the polluted air primarily complained of coughing and shortness of breath (Firket, 1931).

Donora, Pennsylvania

Donora, Pennsylvania was the site of a similar tragedy in October 1948 (Schrenk, Heimann, Clayton, Gafafer, & Wexler, 1949). This heavily industrialized town is located in the Monongahela River Valley. An inversion that covered a wide area of the northeastern United States allowed pollutants to accumulate in the local atmosphere. Among a population of only 14,000, about 6,000 people fell ill complaining of coughs, sore throats, dyspnea, headaches, burning and tearing eyes, running noses, and vomiting. Instead of the expected two deaths for the period, 20 were recorded. As in the Meuse River Valley episode, the elderly and those with pre-existing heart or lung disease were disproportionately affected.

London, England

London has had several acute air pollution episodes but the worst of these occurred in December 1952 (Logan, 1953). For centuries Londoners heated their homes with open fireplaces that burned soft, high-sulfur-content coal. The smoke from these fires combined with the city's natural fog to create the original "smog."

During a 5-day inversion in 1952, residential smog combined with industrial emissions to produce an acute air pollution episode in which an estimated 4,000 people died and the weekly morbidity rate doubled. The normal number of weekly applications for emergency bed service in December was about 1,000, but during the 1952 episode the number of applicants rose to 2,500. The hospital bed demand did not subside to normal for two to three weeks afterward. As in other reported episodes, illness and death were more prevalent in the elderly and in those with existing heart and lung disease than in young healthy persons.

There had been six previous air pollution episodes recorded in London, the first dating back to 1873, when over 2,500 deaths were attributed to air pollution. In a December 1962 inversion about 750 deaths were attributed to polluted air (Scott, 1963). It is possible, therefore, that precautions instituted after the earlier tragedies kept mortality figures down.

New York City

In New York City, epidemiologic analyses of mortality rates and meteorologic patterns have revealed a number of acute air pollution events, including episodes in 1953, 1962, 1963, and 1966. These episodes were characterized by periods of high pollution, temperature inversions, and low winds. Because of the absence of accompanying fog, the severity of the pollution was not necessarily apparent at the time of their occurrence.

In 1953, 200 excess deaths were attributed to an air pollution episode (Greenburg, Jacobs, Drolette, Field, & Braverman, 1963). In 1963 there were 405 excess deaths (McCarroll & Bradley, 1966) and in 1966, 168 excess deaths. The fatalities in the 1966 episode were probably much lower than they might have been because the inversion occurred during a Thanksgiving weekend when many pollution-producing industries were closed, and because certain air pollution restrictions had been imposed by the city.

Copper Hill, Tennessee

The Copper Hill episode was not acute, nor was its primary effect on human health. It illustrates, however, the enormous potential that air pollution has for causing environmental damage. Rich copper ore discovered in Tennessee's 60,000-acre Copper Basin in 1843 led to intense mining between 1850 and 1878. Local smelting of the rich ore depleted the surrounding wood supply.

Active mining resumed in 1891 and ore was removed using open hearth or heap roasting. In this process alternate layers of ore and wood were stacked over an open hearth and ignited. Compared with the previous technique, the need for trees increased, resulting in the harvest of all timber within reasonable hauling range.

Fumes from the open roasting yards contained high concentrations of sulfuric acid, which destroyed virtually all remaining vegetation in the 7,000-acre area centered around Ducktown, Tennessee. The forest in an additional 32,000 acres of the basin was significantly damaged. The subsequent erosion filled the local creeks and the Ocoee River, producing massive fish kills. Continued erosion removed most topsoil, leaving a barren area of copper-colored, unweathered soil incapable of sustaining plant life (Seigworth, 1943).

Closed blast furnaces with stacks began operating in 1902. The sulfuric acid fumes were diluted and dispersed compared with the previous open hearth releases. However, the dispersed SO_2 fumes damaged vegetation, produced health complaints in the adjacent state of Georgia, and resulted in a law suit against the copper mining companies. In 1907 the Supreme Court ruled that the mining companies must control the sulfur fumes (Wallace, 1950).

The episode ended when the sulfuric acid in the region's contaminated soil was extracted and sold for commercial purposes, making the Copper Basin one of the nation's largest sulfuric acid producers. However, the events between the early 1900s and 1950 devastated the natural areas of the Copper Basin. Recent efforts to reforest the damaged areas of the Copper Basin are meeting with success (Witkamp, Frank, & Shoopman, 1966; Barnhardt, 1987), and the Ocoee River has become a popular site for whitewater boating.

THE HEALTH EFFECTS OF AIR POLLUTANTS

The adverse effects of acute exposure to air-borne pollutants have been demonstrated by animal experiments, studies on human volunteers, and morbidity and mortality data gathered during acute air pollution episodes. Adverse effects on humans from chronic low-level exposures have been more difficult to demonstrate. Epidemiologic studies of the toxic effects of air pollution suffer from a number of defects. These include the difficulty of documenting average or individual exposure levels in a given population over a long time period, the problem of identifying a nonexposed control group that is comparable to the exposed population under study, and the complexities of distinguishing ambient air pollution effects from those of concurrent exposures, such as cigarette smoking and occupational exposures.

However, a host of epidemiologic and experimental studies published over the last 30 years, when taken together, establish fairly conclusively a link between chronic low-level exposure to air pollutants and several identifiable chronic illnesses. Among the conditions associated with air pollution are chronic obstructive pulmonary disease, bronchial asthma, cardiovascular disease, and acute respiratory disease.

Associations between air pollution and mortality rates have also been demonstrated in epidemiologic studies. Whittemore (1981) summarized over a dozen such studies that, despite their many weaknesses, show a consistent pattern of increased mortality on days of increased SO_2 and particulate pollution. A more recent study by Schwartz and Marcus (1990), using more sophisticated statistical techniques, revealed similar trends, and a paper by Schwartz and Dockery (1992) suggests that particulates rather than SO_2 are related to mortality.

Mortality

One set of epidemiologic studies that demonstrates the air pollution hazard to human health focuses on correlations between levels of air pollutants and mortality rates from all causes. These studies analyze the changes in short-term mortality rates and correlate them with short-term changes in air pollution concentrations.

The method is well illustrated by a study of mortality rates in the New York metropolitan area (Buechley, Riggan, Hasselblad, & VanBruggen, 1973). On high pollution days (SO_2 levels of 1,000 to 1,300 $\mu g/m^3$), mortality rates averaged 2% more than expected. On low-pollution days (SO_2 less than 30 $\mu g/m^3$), mortality rates averaged 1.5% less than expected. Between these two extremes, the relation between mortality rates and SO_2 concentrations was almost linear. Similar findings appear in more recent studies of particulates and acid aerosols (Dockery, Schwartz, & Spengler, 1992), air pollution in London (Schwartz & Marcus, 1990), and air pollution in Los Angeles (Kinney & Ozkaynck, 1991).

An alternate epidemiologic approach is to compare long-term mortality rates in cities or communities with different levels of air pollution. Several such studies have been conducted using variations of this approach. Many studies show trends toward higher mortality rates in more polluted communities. However, a number of methodologic difficulties prevent clear-cut interpretation of these reports (Whittemore, 1981). For one thing, these studies do not test for links between specific pathologic processes and air pollution. Further, mortality rates for exposed areas can be affected by migration, leading to misclassification of exposure status. Other studies, however, have correlated atmospheric concentrations of specific pollutants with rates of specific diseases.

Chronic Obstructive Pulmonary Disease

Chronic obstructive pulmonary disease (COPD) is a general diagnostic term that comprises a variety of chronic respiratory conditions, including emphysema and chronic bronchitis. Epidemiologic studies of the relationship between air pollution and COPD date back to the 1950s when Fairbairn and Reid (1958) demonstrated a difference in the rates of sick leave, premature retirement, and death due to chronic bronchitis and pneumonia among British postal workers living in high pollution areas as compared with those living in low pollution areas.

Since then over a score of reports have revealed similar relationships (American Thoracic Society, 1978; Sunyer, Arito, Murillo, & Saez, 1991; Thurston, Ito, Kinney, & Lippman, 1992; Sunyer et al., 1993). Populations in Britain, Western Europe, Canada, the United States, and Japan have been studied and many of the analyses have adjusted morbidity rates for age, sex, smoking habits, and occupation. Most of these studies compared morbidity rates from COPD and related conditions between residents of more polluted and of less polluted areas. When specific pollutants were studied, the combination of SO_2 and particulates was implicated most often.

A question not completely answered regarding COPD and air pollution is what concentration of pollutants causes the disease as opposed to merely exacerbating preexisting disease. Clearly air pollution is not the only cause of COPD. Cigarette smoking is the leading culprit, and some persons are genetically predisposed to pulmonary disease. Bates (1972) proposed a model of the mechanism by which suspended particulates act in concert with pollutant gases (SO_2, NO_2, and O_3) to damage the lung and produce emphysematous changes. Lippmann (1989) reviewed research demonstrating chronic pulmonary epithelial damage and inflammatory changes in animal models with long-term exposure to O_3.

However, it also is apparent from studies correlating short-term morbidity and mortality from COPD with short-term changes in pollution levels that air-borne pollution does exacerbate preexisting disease. Air pollution is thus implicated as both a cause of COPD and a factor in acute exacerbations, although it is wholly responsible for neither (Waller, 1989).

Bronchial Asthma

Bronchial asthma, a chronic disease, is characterized by asymptomatic periods interrupted by acute attacks of variable frequency, intensity, and duration. The attacks typically consist of the rapid onset of bronchoconstriction and wheezing. These attacks may be mild or be severe enough to result in hospitalization or death. Asthma is an allergic response to sensitizing agents (Chapter 2), but increased levels of air pollution can precipitate acute attacks.

An early report on this phenomenon was a retrospective study of the Donora air pollution episode, which found that 88% of asthmatics reported symptoms (Schrenk et al., 1949). Numerous subsequent studies have demonstrated associations between increased pollution levels and increased incidence of acute asthma attacks (Pope, 1989; Berciano, Dominquez, & Alvarez, 1989; Schwartz, Slater, Larson, Pierson, & Koenig, 1993). Generally these studies have used self-reported symptoms or emergency room visits as markers of asthma attacks and have compared low-pollution with high-pollution days for one population at one location. Inspired pollutants have been shown to cause acute bronchoconstriction—even in non-asthmatic individuals (Schwartz, 1989).

No single pollutant has been implicated as the primary precipitant of acute asthma attacks. Moreover, a number of other factors have been found to be associated with an increased incidence of attacks, including season of the year, temperature, humidity, and even day of the week. Of particular concern is the finding that asthma prevalence (Taylor & Newacheck, 1992), hospitalization rates (Weiss & Wagener, 1990), and mortality rates (Gergen & Weiss, 1990) all increased throughout the 1980s. It is not clear whether this is related to air pollution or to some other cause.

Acute Respiratory Infections

In addition to the evidence linking air pollution and chronic noninfectious disease, numerous studies demonstrate a relationship between air pollutant exposure and acute episodes of infectious disease (American Thoracic Society, 1978). Presumably pollutants impair resistance to respiratory infection—an effect that has been shown for SO_2, NO_2, and O_3 in animal models.

Infectious respiratory disease and air pollution exposure have been linked for both adults and children. In both age groups, increased air pollution is associated with increased lower-respiratory infection (pneumonia and bronchitis), but the association is less clear for upper-respiratory infection (colds and pharyngitis). Two types of epidemiologic studies, one comparing disease rates in two or more different communities and the other based on changes in disease rates within a single population, have been used widely. The first has shown an increased incidence of acute respiratory infections among persons living in more polluted communities as compared to those in less polluted communities (Durham, 1974; Hammer, Miller, Stead, & Hayes, 1976; Dockery et al., 1989; Jaakkola, Paunio, Virtanen, & Heinonen, 1991). The other model demonstrated that in a given community the incidence of acute respiratory infections is greater during periods of increased air pollution (Levy, Gent, & Newhouse, 1977; Pope, Dockery, Spengler, & Raizenne, 1991).

Cardiovascular Disease

Air pollutants are not thought to directly cause cardiovascular disease, but it appears that some pollutants exacerbate the underlying coronary artery disease. Carbon monoxide is the air pollutant that has the greatest impact on the cardiovascular system. Aronow and Isbell (1973) and Kleinman et al. (1989) demonstrated that CO precipitates attacks of angina pectoris. Dockery and colleagues (1993) found an association between air pollution and death from cardiovascular disease in a study of 6 U. S. cities.

Lung Cancer

The role of air pollution as a factor in the etiology of lung cancer remains unclear. Cigarette smoking is well recognized as the most important cause of lung cancer, and occupational exposures also play a role. Air pollution must also be considered a cancer risk, since a number of carcinogens can be detected in ambient air, particularly around industrial facilities. However, attempts by epidemiologists to demonstrate the role of air pollution in lung cancer have yielded ambiguous results and the subject remains controversial (American

Thoracic Society, 1978; Vena, 1982; Buffler et al., 1988; Dockery et al., 1993).

Other Air Pollution Effects

Air pollution effects can be quite site-specific, as in industrial communities where the pollutant by-products of local industries may present special health hazards. Smelters, for example, may produce high levels of air-borne lead, causing neurological damage in residents of the surrounding community (Landrigan, Halpern, & Silbergeld, 1989). As noted above, various industries may emit potential carcinogens, such as other heavy metals, asbestos, hydrocarbons, or radionuclides. Air pollution is also a considerable nuisance. Irritation to the eyes and mucous membranes is noticeable in many communities on high-pollution days, and O_3 is often the primary cause. Objectionable odors from pulp mills, refineries, and a number of other sources may cause aesthetic and economic problems in areas where they are located (Shusterman, 1992).

Economic damage caused by air pollution is an issue in many communities. "Acid rain," the wet or dry deposition of acids, has been an international issue for over a decade because these pollutants often travel great distances from their sources (Schwartz, 1989). The emission of sulfur and nitrogen oxides into the atmosphere produces sulfuric (H_2SO_4) and nitric (HNO_3) acids when these compounds interact with water and sunlight. The caustic substances may be deposited on the ground as aerosols or particulates, or in rain, fog, dew, or snow (Council on Environmental Quality, 1982). In some areas of the United States, particularly the northeast, acid deposition is believed to have caused significant crop and forest damage and to have rendered some lakes uninhabitable by fish and other organisms.

INDOOR AIR POLLUTION

In recent years attention has focused increasingly on the quality of air inside buildings. The concentration of air pollutants inside a building may be the same as that outside, or higher or lower, depending on the building's ventilation system. Pollutants may also be produced inside dwellings, rendering indoor air considerably more hazardous than the air outside.

Pollution of indoor air may be a particularly important health problem for several reasons: (1) people spend most of their lives indoors and may spend large amounts of time in the same room; (2) indoor air is enclosed, so substances emitted into it may reach high concentrations; (3) many normal indoor activities (cooking, cleaning, and smoking, for example) may release hazardous substances into the air; and (4) building materials may release hazardous, volatile, or combustible substances, as well as radioactivity (Hinkle & Murray, 1981).

Indoor Air Pollutants

1. *Infectious agents.* Viruses, bacteria, and fungi in outdoor air are not usually considered to be an environmental health problem, except when they are associated with bodies of water (Rose, 1992). Because these agents are concentrated in indoor air, the chances of infection from the environment and of person-to-person transmission are accordingly greater than outdoors. Indeed, morbidity and mortality from influenza and pneumonia are greater during the winter months when people spend more time indoors. Legionellosis (Legionnaire's disease) is a pulmonary infection caused by the bacterium *Legionella pneumophila*; its reservoirs include hot water systems, air conditioning cooling towers, soil, and fresh water ecosystems. It is transmitted when contaminated water becomes aerosolized by a variety of mechanisms (Benenson, 1990), including the heating, ventilation, and air conditioning systems of buildings, indoor fountains (Hlady et al., 1993), and mist machines in the produce sections of grocery stores (Mahoney at al., 1992).

2. *Allergens.* Bioaerosols such as mold spores, animal danders, and dusts may occur in greater concentrations indoors than outdoors. Household items such as rugs and draperies serve as reservoirs for such particulate matter. Discarded or forgotten food items are sources of mold, and some household plants produce pollen. Each of these bioaerosols produces sensitizing antigens that can induce asthma.

3. *Combustion products.* Annually, approximately 4,000 deaths and 63,000 disabling illnesses in the United States are caused by inhaled products of indoor combustion (Hinkle & Murray, 1981). Most of the deaths are the result of fires in buildings and about 80% of these fire-related deaths result from inhalation of toxic gases—chiefly CO—rather than from burns or other causes.

Toxic concentrations of CO also may be produced by stoves, space heaters, other appliances, and by automobiles in garages. Carbon monoxide accumulates because of faulty devices or improper ventilation. Other gases may be produced in toxic concentrations by combustion in unventilated areas, including NO_2 from gas stoves and indoor ice skating rinks (Lee, Yanagisawa, & Spengler, 1993; Brauer & Spengler, 1994).

Passive cigarette smoking is recognized as an indoor health hazard. Cigarette smoke may irritate the mucous membranes or cause allergic reactions in nonsmokers. The nonsmoking spouses and children of smokers are at increased risk of lung cancer and other diseases (Department of Health and Human Services, 1987; Janerich et al., 1990; EPA, 1992).

4. *Household products.* The indoor use of cleaning fluids, paint and paint thinners, glues, and other volatile inorganic and organic substances, particularly with inadequate ventilation, can lead to toxic concentrations of their vapors.

5. *Building materials.* Potentially hazardous materials may be part of the construction of a domestic dwelling. These include asbestos used to insulate heating ducts, pipes, and attic spaces; radioactive radon gas from building stones; and particle board and urea foam insulation, which emit formaldehyde. Although asbestos is not used in new construction, many older dwellings contain asbestos in a variety of forms.

6. *Unknown pollutants.* During the past 15 years there have been widespread reports of headache, fatigue, and mucous membrane irritation among office workers in sealed air–conditioned buildings. These reports have led to the contemporary term *sick building syndrome.* Although the frequency and uniformity of the phenomenon has convinced most investigators that the syndrome is real (rather than psychogenic), extensive research often fails to implicate a particular pollutant (Kreiss, 1990).

In contrast to the sick building syndrome, *building-related illnesses* have identified causes. Building-related asthma has been associated with bioaerosols and biocides used in humidification systems, and hypersensitivity pneumonitis has been linked to several bioaerosols (Hoffman, Wood, & Kreiss, 1993; Kreiss, 1989). Several authors have shown that a variety of physical and behavioral signs and symptoms are produced by exposure to a low concentration (25 mg/m^2) of a mixture of 22 volatile organic compounds (VOCs) commonly found in buildings (Hudnell, Otto, House, & Molhave, 1992; Koren, Graham, & Devlin, 1992; Otto, Hudnell, House, Molhave, & Counts, 1992).

Although the hazards of many indoor air pollutants are well recognized, there is a scarcity of relevant epidemiologic data to define the magnitude of the indoor air pollution problem. Indoor air pollution ultimately may be as serious a problem as the better-studied outdoor air pollution.

REDUCING AIR POLLUTION AND ASSOCIATED DISEASES

Reduction of air pollutants is essential to both primary and secondary prevention of adverse human health effects, as is evident from the previous discussion. Clean air will prevent the development of significant numbers of cases of chronic obstructive pulmonary disease and possibly of cancer (primary prevention). Unpolluted air also will prevent morbidity and mortality in many preexisting cases of chronic obstructive pulmonary disease, bronchial asthma, coronary artery disease, and other disease conditions (secondary prevention).

National Ambient Air Quality Standards: Monitoring for Compliance

The National Ambient Air Quality Standards (NAAQS) written by the EPA establish, among other things, emission limitations for new pollutant sources such as factories and automobiles (Table 6.1). The *primary standards* are based on the levels required to protect public health. *Secondary standards* are levels set to protect the "public welfare," which includes protecting crops, painted surfaces, and other public concerns. States are responsible for implementing the new source limitations and for regulating existing sources to attain the NAAQS. Each state prepares its own implementation plan.

Air quality is monitored by a variety of sampling devices at over 7,000 stations across the United States. Most of these are operated by state or local pollution control agencies. The technology for measuring air pollutant concentrations is constantly improving. The values obtained at a sampling station depend on the location of the station relative to sources of pollution, the method used to measure pollutant concentrations, and other environmental factors.

The EPA obtains air pollution data from several sources. The National Air Monitoring Stations (NAMS) were established through regulations promulgated in 1979 specifically to provide the EPA with data that meet uniform technical criteria. The NAMS are located in areas with the highest pollutant concentrations and population exposures. Data from state and local air monitoring stations located in areas of high population and pollution concentrations and in other areas as well, along with data from special purpose monitors, are reported to the EPA. In 1992, data on the six NAAQS pollutants were reported to the EPA from more than 4,200 sampling sites (EPA, 1993).

The impact of multiple pollutants on air quality in metropolitan areas is commonly evaluated according to the Pollutant Standards Index (PSI), which was developed by the EPA, the Council on Environmental Quality, and the Department of Commerce (Federal Interagency Task Force on Air Quality Indicators, 1976). The formula for the PSI takes into account five of the seven criteria pollutants (all except hydrocarbons and lead) and yields a value of 100 or more (considered "unhealthful") if the concentration of any one of the pollutants rises to the level of its primary air quality standard at any monitoring station in a metropolitan area.

Air quality is deemed "good" (PSI less than 50) only when ambient concentrations of all five pollutants are less than half the primary standards at all monitoring stations. Index values are often reported by the media to enable persons with chronic respiratory or cardiac disease to avoid dangerously high levels of pollution.

Monitoring of pollution levels in recent years has demonstrated a steady improvement in metropolitan air quality, most of it attributed to the surveillance, regulations, and enforcement called for by the Clean Air Act and its amendments. For example, combined data from 716 sites in 23 cities show that the total number of days in which the PSI exceeded 100 declined from 1,019 in 1980 to 310 in 1992 (EPA, 1993) (Table 6.3).

Table 6.3 Number of PSI Days Greater Than 100 at Trend Sites, 1983–1992, and All U.S. Sites in 1992

MSA	# trend sites	Number of PSI days greater than 100 at trend sites /year										All active monitoring sites in MSA 1992[2]	
		1983	1984	1985	1986	1987	1988	1989	1990	1991	1992	Total # sites	PSI > 100
Atlanta	6	23	8	9	17	9	15	3	16	5	4	12	5
Baltimore	16	60	46	21	24	28	41	7	12	20	4	31	6
Boston	30	37	28	9	9	10	17	5	3	7	4	51	4
Chicago	58	23	18	16	15	21	30	6	7	15	8	95	8
Cleveland	29	17	4	1	2	10	18	8	1	5	3	48	5
Dallas	16	20	18	19	10	10	6	4	7	7	4	35	5
Denver	19	69	62	39	47	37	19	12	7	7	7	35	7
Detroit	28	18	7	2	5	9	18	10	3	7	0	45	1
El Paso	16	16	20	24	34	27	13	29	20	8	11	25	25
Houston	29	70	49	48	45	54	48	32	48	40	29	44	33
Kansas City	19	4	12	3	4	3	3	2	2	1	1	29	1
Los Angeles	85	194	225	205	218	199	240	231	180	177	183	142	187
Miami	13	3	2	5	4	4	4	4	1	2	0	37	0
Minneapolis —St. Paul	15	36	21	21	13	7	1	6	1	0	0	41	0
New York	70	89	140	88	72	64	58	27	24	30	10	119	13
Philadelphia	52	58	39	29	24	37	43	22	17	32	8	77	11
Phoenix	22	72	107	82	85	40	22	30	8	4	8	31	14
Pittsburgh	31	27	15	9	8	13	23	9	11	3	1	61	2
San Diego	21	60	51	54	45	41	49	61	39	25	19	34	19
San Francisco	52	26	33	31	16	15	11	17	7	12	2	82	2
Seattle	15	11	4	27	11	13	6	4	3	0	0	25	3
St. Louis	45	33	22	10	14	16	17	12	8	6	2	68	3
Washington	29	53	30	15	12	25	35	7	5	16	2	59	2
Total	716	1019	961	767	734	702	737	548	430	429	310	1126	356

Source: EPA, 1993.

Table 6.4   U. S. Annual Air Pollutant Emissions,[a] 1940–1993

Parameter	1940	1950	1960	1970	1980	1990	1993
Particulates	21.9	23.2	20.2	17.6	7.8	5.5[b]	5.4[b]
Sulfur Oxides	17.4	19.6	19.2	27.9	23.7	20.7	20.6
Nitrogen Oxides	6.5	9.3	12.7	18.5	20.7	21.4	21.0
Hydrocarbons (VOCs)	13.9	17.5	21.6	27.1	21.8	21.5	20.6
Carbon Monoxide	74.7	82.8	90.8	110.9	85.4	83.8	79.1

[a]Millions of Metric Tons
[b]PM-10 emissions from sources listed in Table 6.2
Source: Council on Environmental Quality (1982) EPA (1993).

Air pollution remains a major problem in many metropolitan areas, however. It is a particularly severe problem in Los Angeles, where the PSI exceeds 100 on around 180 days per year (Table 6.3). In 1992, 94 metropolitan areas did not meet primary EPA standards for O_3; 41 areas did not meet standards for CO; and 70, 46, and 13 did not meet primary standards for particulates, SO_2, and lead, respectively. More than 53 million persons in the U.S. lived in counties that exceeded at least one NAAQS (EPA, 1993).

For total pollutant emissions, Table 6.4 shows that air quality has been generally improving since 1970. In particular, significant strides have been made in the reduction of total suspended particulates and carbon monoxide. Longitudinal data are generally not available for documenting changes in health status that may correspond to these secular trends in air quality. As noted earlier in this chapter, average blood lead levels have declined, but morbidity and mortality from asthma have worsened in recent years.

Reducing Emissions to the Atmosphere

Two approaches have been used to lower air pollution levels. The first is reducing the production of pollutants. For instance, the mass of air pollutants can be reduced by using less energy or by burning cleaner fuels. The second is to limit pollutant emissions through the use of devices such as scrubbers and electrostatic precipitators.

Several international agreements have established goals for reducing or eliminating certain pollutants. The 24 nations signing the "Montreal Protocol" in 1987 agreed to reduce CFC emissions by about 35% by the year 2000, in recognition of the role CFCs play in depleting stratospheric ozone. In 1992 this treaty was strengthened at a meeting in Copenhagen, where over 70 nations agreed to virtually eliminate the production of CFCs and several other ozone–depleting compounds by 1996 and to eliminate HCFCs by 2030.

The 1992 Convention on Climate Change that emanated from the United Nations Conference on Environment and Development at Rio de Janiero calls for reducing CO_2 emissions to 1990 levels by the year 2000. At the insistence of the United States, however, the target was made voluntary rather than mandatory (Rogers, 1993).

In the United States, coal-fired electric generating plants have turned to coal with lower sulfur levels. In addition, EPA standards require all new plants to remove, through the use of scrubbers, 85% of potential SO_2 emissions, regardless of the sulfur level of the coal. These devices use water, limestone (calcium carbonate), or nahcolite (sodium bicarbonate) to absorb gaseous sulfates.

Electrostatic precipitators are installed on emission stacks to control particulate output and may reduce such emissions by 90% –99%. Other devices used to control industrial emissions include inertial and cyclone collectors, filters, scrubbers, and afterburners (Godish, 1991; Stern, Boubel, Turner, & Fox, 1984). Emissions of NO_2 from stationary sources have been reduced by the installation of more efficient equipment and by precise adjustments of flames and air flows on present equipment. Hydrocarbon emissions have been reduced, in part, by controlling the evaporation of volatile fuels and chemicals, by reducing leaks, and by finding alternatives to venting gases to the atmosphere.

Transportation remains the largest single source of air pollutants. Most cars produced in the United States since 1975 have catalytic converters installed in order to meet the EPA source emission standards, particularly for NO_2, CO, and O_3. Some smaller cars have used electronic fuel injection techniques to achieve similar results. Diesel automobile engines meet standards for the criteria pollutants, but they emit carcinogenic polycyclic aromatic hydrocarbons as particulates in their exhaust under fuel-rich driving conditions (Godish, 1991; Peterson, 1993).

The development of fuel-efficient engines has not been a priority for vehicle manufacturers, and advances in engine technology may never be adequate to achieve acceptable levels of air quality in many urban locations. Reducing automobile use by substituting urban rail and bus systems or other alternative transportation seems to be the only answer for these cities. Like other issues in environmental health, this problem is ultimately a social and political issue, rather than a problem that can be solved by technology or medicine.

Modeling the Dynamics and Distribution of Air Pollutants

Mathematical models of the atmospheric dispersion of pollutants are indispensable to scientists for understanding the dynamics of pollutants in the atmosphere and predicting their dispersal over space and time. Most of the predictions about the future effects of global warming and ozone depletion have been made with computer simulations of mathematical models (Trenberth, 1992). Today, air pollution models are used for a wide variety of purposes (Zannetti, 1990): to predict the maximum pollutant emission rates from an industry that will meet air quality standards; to evaluate pollution control plans; to locate industries in ways that will minimize air pollution; to warn the public of the times when air pollution is likely to be highest, so that they may reduce pollution-generating activities; and to estimate health risks from past, present, and future industrial activities.

Atmospheric transport and dispersion models combine data and equations from studies of the sources of pollutants, from the meteorology and chemistry of the atmospheric region to which the pollutants are released, and from the adverse effects of the pollutants. Models can be developed at a variety of scales, ranging from less than a kilometer from the source to the regional and global distribution of pollutants (Hansen et al., 1994).

The meteorologic component of a model comprises measurements of wind speed and direction, temperature, rainfall, and descriptions of the terrain over which air masses move (Stull, 1988). After fine-tuning a large complex of differential equations and validating the model with data collected for the problem of interest, meteorologic models can be used to predict the evolution of atmospheric systems over time.

By coupling a meteorologic model with data on pollution sources such as the exhaust stack height, temperature of exhaust gas, and quantity of pollutants released, modelers can predict pollution concentrations over space and time. Atmospheric modelers use a variety of ways to describe the transport of pollutants from a source, including straight-line gaussian plume models, puff diffusion models, gradient transport models, urban diffusion models, and particle models (Hanna, Briggs, & Hosker, 1982; Zannetti, 1990).

REFERENCES

American Thoracic Society Ad Hoc Committee on the Health Effects of Air Pollution. (1978). *The health effects of air pollution.* New York: American Lung Association.

Anto, J. M., Sunyer, J., Reed, C. E., Sabria, J., Martinez, F., Morell, F., Codina, R., Rodriguez-Roisin, R., Rodrigo, M. J., Roca, J., & Saez, M. (1993). Preventing asthma epidemics due to soybeans by dust-control measures. *New England Journal of Medicine, 329,* 1760-1763.

Aronow, W. W., & Isbell, N. W. (1973). Carbon monoxide effect on exercise-induced angina pectoris. *Annals of Internal Medicine, 79,* 392-395.

Barnhardt, W. (1987). The death of Ducktown. *Discover,* October, 35-43.

Bates, D. V. (1972). Air pollutants and the human lung. *American Review of Respiratory Disease, 105,* 1-13.

Benenson, A. S. (1990). Legionellosis. In A. S. Benenson (Ed.), *Control of communicable diseases in man* (pp. 235-238). Washington, DC: American Public Health Association.

Berciano, F. A., Dominguez, J., & Alvarez, F. V. (1989). Influence of air pollution on extrinsic childhood asthma. *Annals of Allergy, 62,* 135-141.

Brauer, M., & Spengler, J. D. (1994). Nitrogen dioxide exposures inside ice skating rinks. *American Journal of Public Health, 84,* 429-433.

Buechley, R. W., Riggan, W. B., Hasselblad, V., & VanBruggen, J. B. (1973). S02 levels and perturbations in mortality. A study in the New York-New Jersey Metropolis. *Archives of Environmental Health, 27,* 134-137.

Buffler, P. A., Cooper, S. P., Stinnett, S., Contant, C., Shirts, S., Hardy, R. J., Agu, V., Gehan, B., & Burau, K. (1988). Air pollution and lung cancer mortality in Harris County, Texas, 1979- 1981. *American Journal of Epidemiology, 128,* 683-699.

Centers for Disease Control. (1982). Blood lead levels in U.S. population. *Morbidity and Mortality Weekly Report, 31,* 132-134.

Centers for Disease Control. (1991a). Toxic air pollutants and noncancer health risks. *Morbidity and Mortality Weekly Report, 40,* 278-279.

Centers for Disease Control. (1991b). *Preventing lead poisoning in young children.* Atlanta, GA: U.S. Department of Health and Human Services.

Cicerone, R. J. (1994). Fires, atmospheric chemistry, and the ozone layer, *Science, 263,* 1243-1244.

Committee on Environmental Health (1993). Ambient Air Pollution: Respiratory hazards to children. *Pediatrics 91:*1210-1213.

Council on Environmental Quality. (1971). *Environmental quality 1970.* Washington, DC: U.S. Government Printing Office.

Council on Environmental Quality. (1982). *Environmental quality 1981.* Washington, DC: U.S. Government Printing Office.

Department of Health and Human Services. (1987). *The health consequences of involuntary smoking: A report of the Surgeon General* (Publication No. DHHS (CC) 87-8398). Washington, DC: U.S. Government Printing Office.

Dockery, D. W., Pope, C. A., Zu, X., Spengler, J. D., Ware, J. G., Fay, M. F., Ferris, Jr., B. G., & Speizer, F. E. (1993). An association between air pollution and mortality in six U.S. cities. *New England Journal of Medicine, 329,* 1753-1759.

Dockery, D. W., Schwartz, J., & Spengler, J. D. (1992). Air pollution and daily mortality: Associations with particulates and acid aerosols. *Environmental Research, 56,* 362-373.

Dockery, D. W., Speizer, F. E., Stram, D. O., Ware, J. H., Spengler, J. D., & Benjamin, G. F., Jr. (1989). Effects of inhalable particles on respiratory health of children. *American Review of Respiratory Disease, 139,* 587-594.

Durham, W. H. (1974). Air pollution and student health. *Archives of Environmental Health, 28,* 241-254.

Elsom, D. M. (1992). *Atmospheric pollution: A global problem* (2nd ed.). Oxford: Blackwell.

Fairbairn, A. S., & Reid, D. D. (1958). Air pollution and other local factors in respiratory disease. *British Journal of Preventive and Social Medicine, 12,* 94-103.

Federal Interagency Task Force on Air Quality Indicators. (1976). *A recommended air pollution index.* Washington, DC: U. S. Government Printing Office.

Firket, J. (1931). The cause of the symptoms found in the Meuse Valley during the fog of December 1930. *Bulletin of the Royal Academy of Medicine, 11*, 683.

Freeman, G., Stephes, R. J., Crande, S. C., & Furiosi, N. J. (1968). Lesion of the lung in rats continuously exposed to two parts per million of nitrogen dioxide. *Archives of Environmental Health, 17*, 181-192.

Gergen, P. J., & Weiss, K. B. (1990). Changing patterns of asthma hospitalization among children: 1979 to 1987. *JAMA, 264*, 1688-1692.

Godish, T. (1991). *Air quality* (2nd ed.). Chelsea MI: Lewis Publishers.

Greenburg, L., Jacobs, M. B., Drolette, B. M., Field, F., & Braverman, M. M. (1963). Report of an air pollution incident in New York City, November 1953. *Public Health Reports, 78*, 1061-1064.

Hammer, D. I., Miller, F. J., Stead, A. G., & Hayes, C. G. 1976, Air pollution and child lower respiratory disease. I. Exposure to sulfur oxides and particulate matter in New York, 1972. In A. J. Finkel & W. C. Duel (Eds.), *Clinical implications of air pollution research*. Acton, MA: Publishing Sciences Group.

Hanna, S. R., Briggs, G. A., & Hosker, Jr., R. P. (1982). *Handbook on Atmospheric Diffusion,* Technical Information Center, U.S. Department of Energy.

Hansen, D. A., Dennis, R. L., Ebel, A., Hanna, S. R., Kaye, J., & Thuillier, R. (1994). The quest for an advanced regional air quality model. *Environmental Science Technology, 28*(2), 71A-77A.

Hinkle, L. E., & Murray S. H. (1981). The importance of the quality of indoor air. *Bulletin of the New York Academy of Medicine, 57*, 827-872.

Hlady, W. G., Mullen, R. C., Mintz, C. S., Shelton, B. G., Hopkins, R. S., & Daikos, G. L. (1993). Outbreak of Legionnaire's Disease linked to a decorative fountain by molecular epidemiology. *American Journal of Epidemiology, 138*, 555-562.

Hoffman, R. E., Wood, R. C., & Kreiss, K. (1993). Building-related asthma in Denver office workers. *American Journal of Public Health 83*:89-93.

Hudnell, H. K., Otto, D. A., House, D. E., & Molhave, L. (1992). Exposure of Humans to a Volatile Organic Mixture, II. Sensory. *Archives of Environmental Health 47*:31-38.

Jaakkola, J. J. K., Paunio, M., Virtanen, M., & Heinonen, O. P. (1991). Low-level air pollution and upper respiratory infections in children. *American Journal of Public Health, 81*, 1060-1063.

Janerich, D. T., Thompson, W. D., Varela, L. R., Greenwald, P., Chorost, S., Tucci, C., Zaman, M. B., Melamed, M. R., Kiely, M., & McKneally, M. F. (1990). Lung cancer and exposure to tobacco smoke in the household. *New England Journal of Medicine, 323*, 632-636.

Kinney, P. L., & Ozkaynak, H. (1991). Associations of daily mortality and air pollution in Los Angeles County. *Environmental Research, 54,* 99-120.

Kleinman, M. T., Davidson, D. M., Vandagriff, R. B., Caiozzo, V. J., & Wittenberger, J. L. (1989). Effects of short-term exposure to carbon monoxide in subjects with coronary artery disease. *Archives of Environmental Health, 44,* 361-369.

Koren, H. S. Graham, D. E., & Devlin, R. B. (1992). Exposure of Humans to Volatile Organic Mixture, III. *Inflammatory Response Archives of Environmental Health* 47:39-44.

Kreiss, K. (1989). The epidemiology of building-related complaints and illness. *Occupational Medicine, 4,* 575-592.

Kreiss, K. (1990). The sick building syndrome: Where is the epidemiologic basis? *American Journal of Public Health, 80,* 1172-1173.

Landrigan, P. J., Halper, L. A., & Silbergeld, E. K. (1989). Toxic air pollution across a state line: Implications for the siting of resource recovery facilities. *Journal of Public Health Policy, 10,* 309-323.

Lee, K. Y., Yanagisawa, Y., & Spengler, J. D. (1993). Carbon monoxide and nitrogen dioxide levels in an indoor ice skating rink with mitigation methods. *Journal of the Air and Waste Management Association, 43,* 769-771.

Levy, D., Gent, M., & Newhouse, M. T. (1977). Relationship between acute respiratory illness and air pollution levels in an industrial city. *American Review of Respiratory Disease, 116,* 167-173.

Lippmann, M. (1989). Effects of ozone on respiratory function and structure. *Annual Review of Public Health, 10,* 49-67.

Lipsett, M., Waller, K., Shusterman, D., Thollaug, S., & Brunner, W. (1994). The respiratory health impact of a large urban fire. *American Journal of Public Health, 84,* 434-438.

Logan, W. P. D. (1953). Mortality in London fog incident. *Lancet, 1,* 336-338.

MacKenzie, J. J., & El-Ashry, M. T. (1988). *Ill winds: Airborne pollution's toll on trees and crops.* Washington, DC: World Resources Institute.

Mahoney, F. J., Hoge, C. W., Farley, T. A., Barbaree, J. M., Breiman, R. F., Benson, R. F., & McFarland, L. M. (1992). Communitywide outbreak of Legionnaires' disease associated with a grocery store mist machine. *Journal of Infectious Diseases, 165,* 736-739.

McCarroll, J., & Bradley, W. (1966). Excess mortality as an indicator of health   effects of air pollution. *American Journal of Public Health, 56,* 1933-1942.

Orehek, J., Massari, J. P., Gayrard, P., Grimaud, C., & Charpin, J. (1976). Effect of short-term, low-level nitrogen dioxide exposure on bronchial sensitivity of asthmatic patients. *Journal of Clinical Investigation, 57,* 301-307.

Ostro, B. D., Lipsett, M. J., Mann, J. K., Krupnick, A., & Harrington, W. (1993). Air pollution and respiratory morbidity among adults in Southern California. *American Journal of Epidemiology, 137,* 691-700.

Otto, D. A., Hudnell, H. K., House, D. E., Molhave, L., & Counts, W. (1992). Exposure of humans to a volatile organic mixture. I. Behavioral assessment. *Archives of Environmental Health, 47,* 23-30.

Peterson, J. E. (1993). Toxic pyrolysis products of solvents, paints, and polymer films. *Occupational Medicine: State of the Art Reviews,* 8, 533-547.

Pirkle, J. L., Brody, D. J., Gunter, E. W., Kramer, R. A., Paschal, D. C., Flegal, K. M., & Matte, T. D. (1994). The decline in blood lead levels in the United States: The National Health and Nutrition Examination Surveys. *JAMA, 272,* 284-291.

Pope, C. A. (1989). Respiratory disease associated with community air pollution and a steel mill, Utah Valley. *American Journal of Public Health, 79,* 623-628.

Pope, C. A., Dockery, D. W., Spengler, J. D., & Raizenne, M. E. (1991). Respiratory health and PM10 pollution: A daily time series analysis. *American Review of Respiratory Disease,* 144: 1123-1128.

Quarles, J., & Lewis, W. H. (1990). *The new Clean Air Act: A guide to the clean air program as amended in 1990.* Washington, DC: Morgan, Lewis, & Bockius.

Rogers, A. (1993). *The earth summit: A planetary reckoning.* Los Angeles: Global View Press.

Rose, C. S. (1992). Water-related lung diseases. *Occupational Medicine, 7,* 271-286.

Rutishauser, M., Ackermann, U., Braun, C., Gnehm, H. P., & Wanner, H. U. (1990). Significant association between outdoor NO_2 and respiratory symptoms in preschool children. *Lung, 168* (Suppl.), 347-352.

Schachter, E. N., Witek, T. J., & Beck, G. J. (1984). Airway effects of low concentrations of sulfur dioxide: Dose-response characteristics. *Archives of Environmental Health, 39,* 34-42.

Schrenk, H. H., Heimann, H., Clayton, G. D., Gafafer, W., & Wexler, H. (1949). *Air pollution in Donora, Pennsylvania. Epidemiology of the unusual smog episode of October 1948.* Washington, DC: U.S. Government Printing Office.

Schwartz, J. (1989). Lung function and chronic exposure to air pollution: A cross sectional analysis of NHANES II. *Environmental Research, 50,* 309-321.

Schwartz, J. (1993). Air pollution and daily mortality in Birmingham, Alabama. *American Journal of Epidemiology, 137,* 1136-1147.

Schwartz, J. (1994). Total suspended particulate matter and daily mortality in Cincinnati, Ohio. *Environmental Health Perspectives, 102,* 186-189.

Schwartz, J., & Dockery, D. W. (1992). Particulate air pollution and daily mortality in Steubenville, Ohio. *American Journal of Epidemiology, 135,* 12-19.

Schwartz, J., & Marcus, A. (1990). Mortality and air pollution in London: A time series analysis. *American Journal of Epidemiology, 131,* 185-194.

Schwartz, J., Slater, D., Larson, T. V., Pierson, W. E., & Koenig, J. Q. (1993). Particulate air pollution and hospital emergency room visits for asthma in Seattle. *American Review of Respiratory Disease, 147,* 826-831.

Schwartz, S. E. (1989). Acid deposition: Unraveling a regional phenomenon. *Science, 243,* 753-763.

Scott, J. A. (1963). The London fog incident of December 1962. *Medical Officer, 109,* 250.

Seigworth, K. J. (1943). Ducktown—a postwar challenge. *American Forests,* November, 521-524.

Shusterman, D. (1992). Critical Review: The health significance of environmental odor pollution. *Archives of Environmental Health* 47:76-87.

Stern, A. C., Boubel, R. W., Turner, D. B., & Fox, D. L. (1984). *Fundamentals of air pollution* (2nd ed.). New York: Academic Press, Inc.

Stull, R. B. (1988). *An Introduction to boundary layer meteorology,* Dordrecht, The Netherlands: Kluwer Academic Publishers.

Sun, M. (1988). Tighter ozone standard urged by scientists. *Science, 240,* 1724-1725.

Sunyer, J., Saez, M., Murillo, C., Castellsague, J., Martinez, F., & Anto, J. M. (1991). Effects of urban air pollution on emergency room admissions for chronic obstructive pulmonary disease. *American Journal of Epidemiology, 134,* 277-286.

Sunyer, J., Saez, M., Murillo, C., Castellsague, J., Martinez, F., & Anto, J. M. (1993). Air pollution and emergency room admissions for chronic obstructive pulmonary disease: A 5-year study. *American Journal of Epidemiology, 137,* 701-705.

Taylor, W. R., & Newacheck, P. W. (1992). Impact of Childhood Asthma on Health. *Pediatrics* 90:657-662.

Thurston, G. D., Ito, K., Kinney, P. L., & Lippmann, M. (1992). A multiyear study of air pollution and respiratory hospital admissions in three New York State metropolitan areas: Results for 1988 and 1989 summers. *Journal of Exposure Analysis and Environmental Epidemiology, 2,* 429-450.

Trenberth, K. E. (1992). *Climate system modeling.* Cambridge University Press, Cambridge, England.

U. S. Environmental Protection Agency. (1992). *Respiratory health effects of passive smoking: Lung cancer and other disorders.* (Publication No. EPA/90006F. Washington, DC: Author.

U. S. Environmental Protection Agency. (1993) *National Air Quality and Emissions Trends Report, 1992,* (Report No. EPA-454/R-93/031). Research Triangle Park, NC: Author.

Vena, J. E. (1982). Air pollution as a risk factor in lung cancer. *American Journal of Epidemiology, 116,* 42-56.

Wallace, R. W. (1950). The miracle of the Copper Basin. *The Tennessee Conservationist, 15,* 8-9.

Waller, R. E. (1989). Atmospheric pollution. *Chest, 96* (Suppl.), 363S-372S.

Ware, J. H., Spengler, J. D., Neas, L. M., Samet, J. M., Wagner, G. R., Coultas, D. C., Ozkaynak, H., & Schwab, M. (1993). Respiratory and irritant health effects of ambient volatile organic compounds. *American Journal of Epidemiology, 137,* 1287-1301.

Weiss, K. B., & Wagener, D. K. (1990). Changing patterns of asthma mortality: Identifying target populations at high risk. *JAMA, 264,* 1683-1687.

Whittemore, A. S. (1981). Air pollution and respiratory disease. *Annual Review of Public Health, 2,* 397-429.

Witkamp, M., Frank, M. L., & Shoopman, J. L. (1966). Accumulation and biota in a pioneer ecosystem of kudzu vine at Copper Hill, Tennessee. *Journal of Applied Ecology, 3,* 383-391.

Zannetti, P. (1990) *Air pollution modeling: Theories, computational methods and available software.* Van Nostrand Reinhold, New York, 1990.

SUGGESTED READINGS

Bitton, G. (1994). *Wastewater microbiology.* New York: Wiley.

Bolin, B. (Ed.), (1986). *The greenhouse effect, climatic change, and ecosystems.* Chichester UK: Wiley.

Cagin, S, & Dray, P. (1993). *Between earth and sky: How CFCs changed the world and endangered the ozone layer.* New York: Pantheon Books.

Committee on Advances in Assessing Human Exposure to Airborne Pollutants, National Academy of Sciences. (1991). *Human exposure assessment for airborne pollutants: Advances and opportunities.* Washington, DC: National Academy of Sciences.

Godish, T. (1991). *Air quality* (2nd ed.). Chelsea, MI: Lewis Publishers.

Elsom, D. M. (1992). *Atmospheric pollution: A global problem,* (2nd Ed.), Blackwell Publishers, Oxford, England.

Environmental Protection Agency. (1991). *Introduction to air quality: A reference manual,* (Report No. EPA-400/3-91/003).

James, A. (1993). *Introduction to water quality modeling* (2nd ed.). New York: Wiley.

National Research Council. (1985). *Epidemiology and air pollution.* Washington, DC.: National Academy Press.

Samet, J. M., & Spengler, J. D. (Eds.). (1991). *Indoor air pollution: A health perspective.* Baltimore, MD: Johns Hopkins Press.

Smith, K. B. (1987). *Biofuels, air pollution, and health: A global review.* New York: Plenum.

Seuss, M. J., Grefen, K., & Reinisch, D. W. (1985). *Ambient air pollution from industrial sources: A reference handbook.* Amsterdam: Elsevier.

Stern, P. C., Young, O. R., & Druckman, D. (Eds.). (1992). *Global environmental change: Understanding the human dimensions.* Washington, DC: National Academy Press.

Tomatis, L. (1990). *Air pollution and human cancer.* Berlin: Springer-Verlag.

Trenberth, K. E. (1992). *Climate system modeling.* Cambridge University Press, Cambridge, England.

U. S. Environmental Protection Agency. (1991). *Introduction to indoor air quality: A reference manual,* (Report No. EPA-400/3-91/003). Research Triangle Park, NC: Author.

Watson, A. Y., Bates, R. R., & Kennedy, D. (1988). *Air pollution, the automobile, and health.* Washington, DC: Academic Press.

World Health Organization. (1991) *Impact on human health of air pollution in Europe.* Copenhagen: World Health Organization Regional Office for Europe.

World Health Organization. *Estimating human exposure to air pollutants.* 1985. (WHO Offset Publication No. 69). Geneva: World Health Organization.

Zannetti, P. (1990) *Air pollution modeling: Theories, computational methods and available software.* New York: Van Nostrand Reinhold.

Chapter 7

Water: Pollution and Availability

A. James Ruttenber

Twenty years ago a chapter on water in an environmental health textbook would have focused on the microorganisms and toxic chemicals that contaminate water supplies. Today the simple availability of fresh water is just as important as water pollution. More and more, sources of fresh water have to be sought beyond the rivers and large aquifers close to consumers, and public health workers have to consult with ecologists and engineers to understand the issues involved in insuring water quality and availability.

Traditionally, fresh water has been defined as water with concentrations of salts (chiefly sodium chloride, but also salts of magnesium, calcium, and potassium) less than 5 parts per thousand by weight, or 5 ppt[w] (Mitsch & Gosselink, 1993). This definition is arbitrary, and it excludes many rivers and lakes that are usually considered to be bodies of fresh water, but that have salt concentrations from agricultural runoff or other sources.

In addition to rivers and lakes (surface water), sources of fresh water include soil, which holds water in spaces between particles, and *aquifers,* where water is stored underground in the pores of various rock formations. Large volumes of fresh water are also stored in ice and glaciers, but this water is generally unavailable for human use.

Salt water has salt concentrations above 5 ppt[w] and is found in oceans (average salt concentrations of 35 ppt[w], in lakes such as the

Great Salt Lake, where evaporation has concentrated salts over extremely long time periods, and in *estuaries,* which are coastal interfaces between rivers and *marine* ecosystems. The salinity of estuaries may vary considerably depending on changes in the volume of freshwater runoff and river flow that is mixed with sea water.

THE HYDROLOGIC CYCLE

Fresh water does not come from a single source, nor does it remain in one place for very long, unless locked within a glacier. Rather, water is part of the hydrologic cycle. In this cycle it assumes a variety of physical and chemical forms, is stored in many different locations, and has a variety of rates of transfer between sites of storage (Figure 7.1)

In the atmosphere fresh water is stored as vapor in clouds. Water remains in the air until various thermodynamic processes interact with the earth's topographic features to induce precipitation. The warmer the air, the more water it will hold in the vapor phase. When moisture-laden air cools, the result is rain if the air temperature near the ground is above 0°C (32°F), or snow and hail if the air temperature is lower. Moisture in the air also condenses at ground level to form dew at temperatures above 0°C, and frost if the air is below freezing. Snow provides water storage in the winter, when water is not in high demand by terrestrial vegetation, and becomes available in the spring when it melts.

When water reaches the ground, it travels vertically into the earth by *infiltration* and may also move horizontally along favorable topographic features by a process termed *surface runoff.* Water collecting in linear topographic depressions forms streams, which drain into larger collecting bodies such as lakes, rivers, or estuaries by *streamflow.* Hydrologists divide the earth's surface into different *watersheds* or *river basins.* These are regions bordered by elevated topographic features, which cause water to flow centrally into the same rivers, streams, and lakes. Pollution in a river can come from virtually anywhere within its watershed, but is unlikely to come from another watershed.

Water that has infiltrated the upper soil layer moves downward by gravity-induced flow (*percolation),* eventually reaching an aquifer.

This process is called aquifer *recharge*. Aquifers can be tapped with wells to provide large volumes for human use, but if consumption exceeds recharge, aquifers will ultimately be depleted. Such is the case in south Florida, where excessive consumption will ultimately damage the Biscayne Aquifer (Duplaix, 1990). The hydrologic cycle is completed when water is released back to the atmosphere by evaporation from soil and surface waters and by *evapotranspiration* (the combination of evaporation and transpiration) in plants.

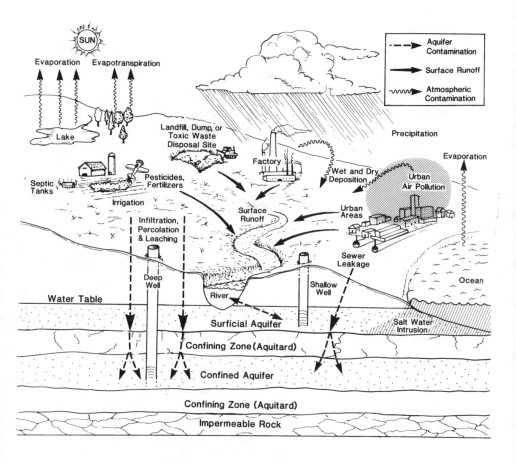

Figure 7.1   The hydrologic cycle and common sources of contamination for surface and ground water. Based on an illustration from U. S. Environmental Protection Agency (1990).

The volume of water available for human use is determined by regional rainfall and snowfall patterns, the topography that defines drainage basins, the extent to which local ecosystems capture and retain rainfall and snowmelt, and by the proximity of consumers to large aquifers, streams, and rivers. The illustration in Figure 7.1 can be converted to a systems model (Figure 7.2) in order to more clearly describe and quantify the processes that determine freshwater availability. In the model, pathway 1 depicts atmospheric circulation interacting with topography and solar radiation to produce the annual rainfall of a region. Rainfall provides water to terrestrial vegetation (pathways 2, 3, and 4), surface waters (pathway 5), and aquifers either directly (pathways 3 and 6), or via runoff into surface waters (pathways 3 and 7).

Precipitation is measured in units of inches or millimeters for an arbitrarily chosen area and for a specific time period such as a day, month, or year. All precipitation is not available for human use, as some runoff cannot be collected and stored for the future. The quantity of water actually available for human use is termed *stable runoff*. This measure is not always correlated with total runoff. Furthermore,

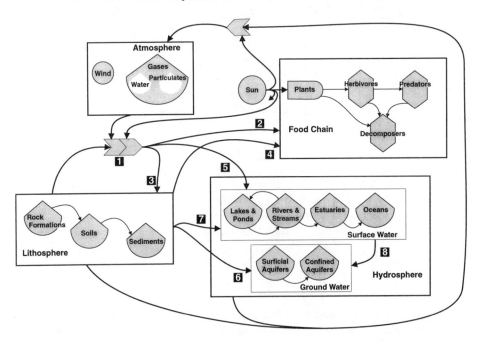

Figure 7.2   A model of the major pathways in the hydrologic cycle.

the size of the human population in a watershed may not be in balance with stable runoff. For instance, the volume of runoff in South America is one of the world's largest, but stable runoff on this continent is slightly above the average for all continents and its total population is one of the world's smallest (Postel, 1988). By contrast, the water consumption of the population in southern California far exceeds the regional stable runoff, and water must be piped in from the Colorado River, which is in another watershed.

SURFACE WATER

The volume, dynamics, and quality of surface water in a watershed are determined by spatial and temporal patterns of runoff. Surface water is affected by rainfall, geology, geography, and the stability of natural ecosystems. In forests about 85% of rainwater is absorbed by vegetation and soil. Deforestation and overgrazing remove the vegetation that traps water, thereby increasing runoff and relocating water to areas where it often cannot be recovered. Water not retained by damaged ecosystems may enhance the flooding of areas downstream. Reforesting, replanting with native vegetation, and regulating animal grazing help prevent this loss.

Engineering projects for flood control also influence the availability of water. In the United States extensive dam construction and modification of natural bodies of water have substantially altered surface water availability. In South Florida a system of over 1,400 miles of canals was designed to reduce flooding and to provide water for agriculture—particularly for sugar cane crops. When completed in 1971, fresh water flowed quickly through the canals on its way to the Atlantic Ocean, bypassing the ecosystems that once slowed and captured the water—including the vast expanse of wetlands in the Everglades. Much of the water that now moves through the canals into the Atlantic Ocean once recharged the Biscayne Aquifer—the only source of fresh water for South Florida residents. Since the 1970s the canal system has been linked to water shortages and periods of severe drought in the Everglades. The damage was so severe that parts of the canal system are being returned to their natural state—the first case of natural "retrofitting" in the United States (Duplaix,1990).

The locations of streams and rivers, as well as their surface flow rates, are also important determinants of freshwater availability to human communities. For many communities, these sources are not readily available. Colorado cities on the eastern slope of the Rocky Mountains do not have nearby rivers with adequate flow rates and must pipe water from lakes and rivers in the mountains. These lakes and rivers are fed by snowmelt—another important source of surface water. The city of Boulder actually owns the water rights to a nearby glacier, which provides a portion of its fresh water supply.

GROUND WATER

Historically, the first cities were located along the rivers that could provide ready access to water for personal, commercial, and industrial needs. By contrast, much of the economic development that occurred in the Third World following World War II was made possible by developing ground water resources (Heath, 1988). In the United States ground water supplies just over 50% of drinking water and between 20%–40% of all fresh water used (Heath, 1988; Jaffe & DiNovo, 1987; Solley, Chase, & Mann,1988).

Ground water is located in the spaces between rocks and soil at the earth's surface. The volume of water stored in the ground, its rate of flow, and its direction of flow depend on the size of these spaces, the degree to which they are interconnected, the rate of recharge from surface water, and on the elevation of the site where the water is stored. The spaces that store water range in size from extremely small ones in compacted clay to large caverns in limestone. The *water table* is the upper surface of water in the ground, and the *vadose zone* or zone of aeration extends from the water table to the ground surface.

Various geological formations separate aquifers. Consolidated sediment or rock below the water table retards the downward movement of water and forms a *surficial* or *unconfined* aquifer above. Surficial aquifers are not protected from surface soil and therefore can be readily contaminated.

Aquifers sandwiched between impermeable *confining beds* (also called *aquitards* or *aquicludes*) are termed *confined* aquifers. If water in a confined aquifer is under pressure, it can flow to the surface without pumping. Such aquifers are called *artesian* aquifers. Compared with surficial aquifers, confined aquifers are more protected but can be polluted when chemicals are carried through cracks or fractures in the confining layer, or intentionally injected in wells designed for waste disposal.

Ground water levels are important for maintaining the structural integrity of aquifers and for preserving water quality. In coastal regions the pressure of aquifers is determined by the height of the water table above sea level. This pressure helps keep salt water from migrating into the aquifer through the expanse of sand that separates aquifers from the sea. Periods of drought or excessive water removal can reduce aquifer pressure and facilitate the inland migration of salt water—a process called *salt water intrusion.*

Excessive volumes of water in surficial aquifers can lead to increased soil and water salinity when vegetation removes pure water through evapotranspiration and leaves the salts behind. This process occurs in agricultural areas where crops are intensively irrigated. In the former Soviet Republics of Kajakhstan and Uzbekistan, widespread irrigation of cotton crops has caused extensive salinization of soils. The diversion of water for irrigation from rivers flowing into the Aral Sea has also reduced the area of this inland body of water by 25%, destroying productive fisheries and polluting the air with windblown sediment from the dry sea bed (Perera, 1993).

Surficial aquifers are commonly used for drinking water and agriculture in the Third World because wells are more easily and cheaply installed in these aquifers than in deeper, confined aquifers. Areas without the economic resources for sewage disposal and industrial regulation are vulnerable to biological and chemical contamination of these shallow aquifers. For instance, septic tanks located too close to aquifers can contaminate drinking water with nitrates.

Another problem common to aquifers is *subsidence*—the caving in of surface soil that occurs when ground water is removed at a rate faster than the recharge rate, leaving no support for the surface soil. Subsidence is common in Florida, where "sink holes" can appear overnight and swallow household pets, automobiles, and houses.

DESALINATION

As sources of fresh water become scarce, alternatives to surface and ground water sources are required. Many cities on the coasts of the Mediterranean Sea and Persian Gulf depend heavily on desalinized sea water. In the Third World desalination of water in surficial aquifers may be the only inexpensive source of safe drinking water in the future.

In coastal regions *desalination* plants have been used to remove salt from sea water or brackish water—a process that requires considerable energy from fossil fuels and leaves concentrated salt solutions that damage coastal ecosystems unless properly treated. The technique is centuries old and was first used on board ships. It was then developed commercially in the 19th century, when persistent droughts and contamination of shallow coastal aquifers stimulated the search for alternate fresh water sources. Although desalination can provide a large percentage of the fresh water used in coastal communities, worldwide consumption of desalinized water accounts for only a fraction of a percentage of total water use.

Salts are most commonly removed from water by boiling and distilling the vapor or by *reverse osmosis*—the passing of pressurized salt water through a semipermeable membrane. Reverse osmosis is most effectively used with brackish water and, compared with distillation, is simpler and more energy efficient. The water from either process costs 4 to 5 times more than surface or ground water, and distillation uses large quantities of fossil fuels.

Other desalination techniques have been developed (Office of Technology Assessment [OTA], 1988a) and the new approaches are designed to maximize energy efficiency and environmental impact. The greatest challenge is to develop low cost desalination units that run on solar energy—these are desperately needed in Third World countries. Because efficient operation of desalination plants depends on relatively clean salt water, they are particularly susceptible to acts of "ecoterrorism," as demonstrated in the Persian Gulf War (Coghlan, 1991; Vesilind, 1993).

PATTERNS OF WATER USE

If human communities are allowed to expand beyond the capacity of nearby water sources, then the expense and environmental impact of engineering solutions has to be compared with the inconvenience and economic impact of conservation. As fresh water becomes scarce, the way people consume it becomes a concern to both environmental and public health scientists.

Water consumption is traditionally categorized as domestic, industrial, or agricultural. From a global standpoint, agriculture consumes the largest volume of fresh water—approximately three times the combined volume for domestic and industrial consumption. Nations such as Norway, Sweden, and Finland use the greatest percentage of their total water consumption for industry. Others—Greece, Japan, and Australia, for example—use far more for irrigating crops than for domestic or industrial purposes combined (van der Leeden, Troise, & Todd, 1991).

Per capita water use in the United States is higher than in any other country. Every day, each resident of the United States consumes between 40 and 130 gallons of water at home—50% of this water is used to flush toilets and water lawns (van der Leeden, et al., 1991). Per capita industrial use averaged 0.91 million gallons per day in 1985, and per capita use for crop irrigation averaged 0.58 million gallons per day (Solley, Merk, & Pierce, 1988). The total per capita water use in China and India is about one-fourth that of the United States, and in Switzerland and the United Kingdom, per capita use is about one-tenth the U.S. rate (van der Leeden, et al., 1991).

Predictions of future rates of water consumption suggest that in many areas of the world, consumption at current rates will result in lasting damage to rivers, aquifers, and ecosystems. One way to evaluate the adequacy of water supplies is to divide stable runoff by population size. As a rule of thumb, hydrologists consider countries with water supplies of 1,000–2,000 cubic meters per person to be "water stressed;" those with less than 1,000 cubic meters per person will be limited in their ability to produce food, develop economically, and protect natural ecosystems (Falkenmark, 1989; Postel, 1993). According to these criteria, there will be severe problems of water availability for some nations in northern Africa, the Middle East, and Eastern Europe (Table 7.1). Other nations are projected to have adequate stable runoff for all future needs.

Unused stable runoff can be captured with engineering approaches such as dams, reservoirs, and deep wells. Water can also be transported over long distances with pipelines. These solutions are costly, require fossil fuels for their operation, and may destroy productive ecosystems. Clearly, programs to reduce water consumption need to be considered as alternatives to removing water from aquifers and bodies of surface water at rates that exceed their recharge capacities.

Table 7.1 Water-Scarce Countries, 1992, with Projections for 2010[a]

Region/Country	Per capita renewable water supplies (cubic meters per person) 1992	2010	Change (percentage)
Africa			
Algeria	730	500	−32
Botswana	710	420	−41
Burundi	620	360	−42
Cape Verde	500	290	−42
Djibouti	750	430	−43
Egypt	30	20	−33
Kenya	560	330	−41
Libya	160	100	−38
Mauritania	190	110	−42
Rwanda	820	440	−46
Tunisia	450	330	−27
Middle East			
Bahrain	0	0	0
Israel	330	250	−24
Jordan	190	110	−42
Kuwait	0	0	0
Qatar	40	30	−25
Saudi Arabia	140	70	−50
Syria	550	300	−45
United Arab Emirates	120	60	−50
Yemen	240	130	−46
Other			
Barbados	170	170	0
Belgium	840	870	+4
Hungary	580	570	−2
Malta	80	80	0
Netherlands	660	600	−9
Singapore	210	190	−10
Additional Countries by 2010			
Malawi	1,030	600	−42
Sudan	1,130	710	−37
Morocco	1,150	830	−28
South Africa	1,200	760	−37
Oman	1,250	670	−46
Somalia	1,390	830	−40
Lebanon	1,410	980	−30
Niger	1,690	930	−45

[a]Countries with per capita renewable water suppplies of less than 1,000 cubic meters per year. Does not include water flowing in from neighboring countries.

Source: Worldwatch Institute, based on data from World Resources Institute. (1992). *World resources 1992–93* New York: Oxford University Press; and from Population Reference Bureau. (1992). *World Population Data Sheet* (Washington, DC: Author).

From Brown et al. (1993), with permission.

WATER CONSERVATION

The decreased availability of fresh water has stimulated efforts to reduce the volume required for agricultural, industrial, and domestic purposes. Because agriculture accounts for the largest volume of water used around the world, improvements in irrigation has the greatest potential for helping to achieve sustainable use (Postel, 1993). Currently available technologies for such improvement include better management practices, "microirrigation" (Pair, 1983), and irrigation with domestic wastewater (Biswas & Arar, 1988; Shuval, 1990).

Because industries mainly use water for cooling and processing, it can be recycled with closed-loop processes, which use the same water over and over. These have become more popular in industry and are one of the simplest ways to conserve water because only filtration and simple treatment techniques are required. Replacement of water used in industrial processes is another alternative. For example, the potato-processing industry used to remove skins with water, but now some facilities have changed to mechanical rollers (U. S. Environmental Protection Agency [EPA], 1988).

In many Third World countries large volumes of water are lost in distribution networks for agriculture, industry, and domestic uses. For instance, in the former Soviet Republics of Central Asia, current economic conditions preclude the maintenance of pipelines, faucets, and toilets, and large quantities of water are wasted. Because of these losses, treatment plants have to process larger volumes at an expense that would probably cover the costs of repairs to the distribution systems.

A similar situation exists for agriculture in Central Asia—extensive networks developed for irrigating cotton are leaking large volumes into the ground. In addition, field irrigation practices are extremely inefficient. Any attempt at restoring the Aral Sea to its natural state will require extensive repair and conservation in upstream areas (Perera, 1993).

As suggested by the wide range of estimates of per capita water use around the world, savings can also be realized by conserving water consumed for domestic purposes. This can be done by setting water efficiency standards for commonly used fixtures, replacing lawns with plants that need much less water (xeriscaping), and developing leak-detection systems for distribution systems. Regardless of the techniques used to implement conservation, the most effective way to achieve this goal is by raising the price of water to reflect its true cost (Postel, 1993). In many cities in the Third World and in the former Soviet Republics, however, there is no metering of water use and therefore little incentive to conserve.

INDUSTRIAL POLLUTION

The diagram of the hydrologic cycle in Figure 7.2 can be modified to describe the processes that impact the quality of surface and ground water (Figure 7.3). Industries introduce toxicants directly to surface waters (pathway 1), or indirectly by releasing them to soil, where they can be transported by surface runoff (pathways 2 and 3) soil. For example, underground mining often requires "dewatering"—the removal of ground water from mines that reach into the water table. This water is either pumped directly into surface waters, or to retention ponds for treatment before release to surface water. Toxic chemicals deposited on soil can percolate (pathway 4) or leach (pathway 5) into ground water.

The extent to which chemicals contaminate streams, rivers, and estuaries depends on their volumes and the rates of water flow. For lakes and reservoirs, pollutant concentrations depend on the rates of inflow and outflow of pollutants and fresh water, the extent to which water is mixed vertically, and the transfer of chemicals between sediments and the water column. In the past, industries depended on large volumes of surface water to dilute their wastes. In industrialized countries dilution is becoming less and less acceptable.

Industries also pollute water contaminating the atmosphere (pathway 6) and then soils (pathway 7) and surface waters (pathway 8) through rainfall or by the effects of gravity on small particles (*dry deposition*). For instance, acidic compounds released to the atmosphere by combustion have decreased the pH of many streams and lakes worldwide through wet (*acid rain*) and dry deposition.

Though aquifers can be contaminated by pollutants from surface waters, percolation and leaching (pathways 4 and 5) are the most common sources of aquifer contamination. Examples of contamination by these pathways include percolation of rainfall through land-

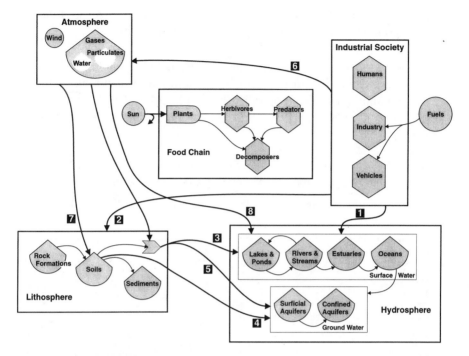

Figure 7.3   A model of the major pathways through which the hydrologic cycle is contaminated by industrial societies.

fills and leaking industrial retention ponds. In the past there was little regulation of retention ponds, but recently in the United States they have become an important reason for mandating cleanup of abandoned industrial sites under the Comprehensive Environmental Response, Compensation and Liability Act (CERCLA, or Superfund) legislation (Chapter 8). In agricultural areas heavy metals in fungicides and organic chemicals in pesticides and herbicides have contaminated ground and surface waters through these pathways.

COMMON WATER POLLUTANTS

Each pathway depicted in Figure 7.3 can transport any of the hundreds of agents that contaminate water. Water pollution can be classified by physical properties such as temperature, biological properties such as the concentration of viruses, bacteria, fungi, or parasites, and chemical properties such as the concentration of heavy metals, organic compounds, radionuclides, specific ions such as chloride or potassium, particulates, and pesticides.

The most common water pollutants are listed in Table 7.2. Each can pose a direct health problem by contaminating drinking water. Some contaminants also jeopardize human health indirectly by damaging aquatic ecosystems, resulting in loss or contamination of food supplies.

Table 7.2 Monitoring Variables Currently Included in the United Nations Global Environment Monitoring System for Water

	Rivers	L&R*	GW**		Rivers	L&R	GW
Basic Variables							
Temperature	×	×	×	Selenium	×	×	×
pH	×	×	×	Cyanide	×	×	×
Electrical conductivity	×	×	×	Fluoride	×	×	×
Dissolved oxygen	×	×	×	Nitrate	×	×	×
Nitrate	×	×	×	TOCl[a]	×	×	×
Nitrite			×	Dieldrin	×	×	×
Ammonia	×	×	×	Aldrin	×	×	×
Calcium	×	×	×	DDT	×	×	×
Magnesium	×	×	×	Copper	×	×	×
Sodium	×	×	×	Iron	×	×	×
Potassium	×	×	×	Manganese	×	×	×
Chloride	×	×	×	Zinc	×	×	×
Sulphate	×	×					
Alkalinity	×	×	×	Irrigation			
BOD	×						
Total suspended solids	×			Sodium	×	×	×
Chlorophyll a		×		Calcium	×	×	×
Transparency		×		Chloride	×	×	×
Orthophosphate	×	×		Boron	×	×	×
Total phosphorus	×	×					
Instantaneous discharge	×			General water quality[b]			
				Silica, reactive	×	×	
Use-Related Variables				Kjeldahl nitrogen	×	×	
				COD	×		
Drinking water supply				TOC	×		
Total coliforms	×	×	×	Chlorophyll	×	×	
Faecal coliforms	×	×	×	Hydrogen sulphide		×	×
Arsenic	×	×	×	Iron		×	
Cadmium	×	×	×	Manganese		×	
Chromium	×	×	×	PCBs	×	×	×
Lead	×	×	×	Aluminium	×	×	
Mercury	×	×	×	Sulphate	×	×	
				pH	×	×	

* Lakes and reservoirs.
** Ground waters.
[a] Total organochlorine compounds (TOCl), dieldrin, aldrin, and DDT are considered as representative of the major categories of organic pollutants.
[b] Such as aquatic life suppport, acidification, eutrophication, etc.; TOC = total organic carbon.

From Maybeck, Chapman, & Helmer (1989), with permission.

In order to predict the fate and toxicity of pollutants, their physical and chemical properties must be known. For instance, chemicals readily adsorb to organic and inorganic particles in aquatic systems, and the size of sediment particles determines where they will be deposited in surface waters. In addition, the reactivity and solubility of chemicals helps determine their concentration in detritus (decomposing plant matter), and sediments. The physical and chemical properties of surface and ground waters are also important determinants of pollution—pH and salinity, for instance, affect the solubility and movement of all chemicals.

The dynamics of ecosystems also help determine the fate of pollutants. For example, minute quantities of pollutants such as the pesticide dichlorodiphenyltrichloroethane (DDT) may be in low concentrations in water, but can accumulate in concentrations that are toxic to consumers at the ends of food chains.

Ecotoxicants

Water pollutants are toxic to a variety of aquatic organisms and can destroy or drastically alter stable ecosystems without becoming a direct threat to humans. Such ecological damage usually poses indirect risks to human health, however. For instance, increases in the nutrient load (particularly for nitrogen and phosphorous) or in the ratios of critical nutrients in coastal ecosystems—a process termed *eutrophication*— can cause algal or dinoflagellate "blooms" that destroy fish populations and reduce food supplies to human communities (National Research Council, 1993). In addition, certain dinoflagellates and bacteria produce neurotoxins that can poison humans who consume fish or shellfish contaminated during these blooms (Culotta, 1992; Chapter 4), although it is not clear exactly which nutrients are responsible for such blooms.

Algal blooms and organic wastes also deplete oxygen concentrations in the water column by stimulating the growth of microorganisms and plants and the deposition of detritus. The microbial decomposition of detritus, in turn, reduces oxygen concentrations in the water column.

The quantity of organic matter present in water and sediments helps determine the oxygen content of water, since microorganisms use oxygen to metabolize organic molecules. Water quality monitoring usually includes the determination of *biochemical oxygen demand (BOD)*—the concentration of oxygen dissolved in water needed by aerobic microorganisms to metabolize organic compounds in water. *Chemical oxygen demand (COD)* is another measure of the impact of organic contamination and is defined as the concentration of dissolved oxygen required to chemically oxidize organic and inorganic compounds in water. Decreases in oxygen concentration can reduce the survival of larval and adult fish and benthic invertebrates. The frequency with which reduced oxygen concentrations are detected in coastal ecosystems has been increasing throughout the world (National Research Council, 1993).

Algal blooms alter the taste, odor, and color of water; they also make recreational waters unattractive, increase the pH of water, and cause dermatitis and conjunctivitis in swimmers (Maybeck, Chapman, & Helmer, 1989). Eutrophication also enhances the growth of the algae and vascular plants that serve as habitats for the intermediate hosts of parasites such as freshwater snails, which harbor schistosomes.

The causes of eutrophication include sewage effluent, wastes from cattle, fertilizers, and deforestation. Excessive nutrient loads can be reduced by altering agricultural practices and by various engineered control measures. Because eutrophication is produced by a complex set of interacting processes, it can be studied with the aid of computer models that predict the effects of a variety of changes within aquatic ecosystems.

Suspended Particulates

Inorganic and organic particles are important components of all aquatic ecosystems. Erosion of rock and soil, removal of vegetation, intensive agricultural practices, steep topography, and heavy rainfall or snowmelt all contribute to the influx of suspended inorganic materials. Suspended organic material originates from decaying vegetation and aquatic organisms.

Processes that increase concentrations of suspended particles—reduced water flow during droughts and the dredging of channels and harbors for instance—also increase concentrations of toxic organic and inorganic compounds because chemicals adsorb to the suspended particles. In addition to contaminating drinking water supplies, suspended matter damages aquatic ecosystems by increasing turbidity and thereby reducing rates of photosynthesis and by interfering with the respiration of fishes and other organisms.

Inorganic Pollutants

Inorganic metals and ions affect water quality in many different ways. For instance, nitrogen is released to surface and ground water by a variety of natural, agricultural, and industrial processes. In addition to stimulating eutrophication, high concentrations of nitrates and nitrites in drinking water can cause methemoglobinemia. Outbreaks of methemoglobinemia in infants and young children have occurred in rural areas where streams and ground water have been contaminated by nitrate fertilizers (Centers for Disease Control and Prevention [CDC], 1993a). Because municipal distribution systems use large volumes of water that are unlikely to be contaminated with agricultural or industrial sources of nitrogen, they are rarely implicated in outbreaks of methemoglobinemia. Furthermore, these systems are routinely monitored for nitrates and can be shut down or obtain water from alternate sources in the event dangerous levels of nitrates are detected.

Oxides of nitrogen and sulfur from fossil fuel combustion are returned to the earth's surface by both wet and dry deposition. These gases also reach the ground by diffusion, where they can be oxidized to acids. The acidification of freshwater ecosystems has reduced fish and invertebrate populations worldwide—a problem that was first recognized in the 1970s. Marine ecosystems are protected from acidification by the buffering action of the bicarbonate ion. Acidification of surface waters increases the solubility of metals—many of which are toxic to both aquatic organisms and humans.

Salts of many light metals commonly contaminate water. Water leaching through mineral soils is the main source of both natural and anthropogenic salts in inland surface and ground water, whereas saltwater intrusion is a major source of natural salts contaminating coastal surface waters and aquifers. Mining, oil drilling, and highway deicing are also important anthropogenic sources. Salts damage aquatic vegetation, thereby disrupting aquatic food webs and salts in irrigation water build up in agricultural soils and reduce crop productivity. It is estimated that up to half the world's agricultural land has been damaged by salt deposition and waterlogging—the by-products of excessive irrigation (Meybeck et al., 1989). Careful design of irrigation systems can reduce both salinization and water loss through runoff into ditches and canals.

Salts usually make drinking water undesirable for human consumption at lower concentrations than those that produce acute toxicity. Some salts are toxic to humans in concentrations found in surface and ground waters. High concentrations of fluorides, for instance, cause teeth to become mottled, increase bone density, and are toxic to the kidneys (Felsenfeld & Roberts, 1991).

Heavy metals contaminate water through the weathering of soils, the mining and processing of ores and metals, the chemical wastes from manufacturing industries, animal and human excrement, and the leaching of metals from waste dumps (Meybeck et al., 1989).

Organic Pollutants

Organic compounds commonly contaminate surface and ground water. They can be grouped according to different criteria, including the type of source, the chemical composition of the compound, or the methods used to analyze the compound. The chemical properties and toxicity of many organic compounds that pollute water are described in Chapter 4.

Volatile Organic Compounds include the industrial solvents trichloroethylene and tetrachloroethylene. These solvents were used extensively in the semiconductor industry in the 1970s and 1980s and were often dumped in soil around industrial sites, thereby contaminating the ground water beneath. There is still debate over the extent to which these compounds are toxic to humans (Chapter 4).

A wide variety of pesticides and herbicides used in agriculture have polluted aquifers and surface waters. In the 1950s and 1960s, DDT was used so extensively that it severely contaminated estuaries and coastal marine ecosystems by transport from inland surface waters. Shallow aquifers are particularly susceptible to contamination from locally applied pesticides. Herbicides such as 2,4-D (2,4-dichlorophenoxyacetic acid) were commonly used to kill aquatic plants that had overgrown lakes and reservoirs. Recent evidence suggests this compound may be carcinogenic, and it has been banned for such uses in the United States (Chapter 4).

Polychlorinated biphenyls (PCBs) that were previously used in transformers and other electrical equipment have extensively contaminated the sediments of aquatic ecosystems. Like DDT, PCBs are fat-soluble and are concentrated in the adipose tissue of animals that consume them. They bioaccumulate in animals at the tops of aquatic food chains, posing risks to humans and other "top carnivores." This phenomenon has led to restrictions on fishing in many rivers and lakes in the United States, Canada, and other industrialized countries—restrictions that will remain in place as long as these chemicals remain in sediments. PCBs are toxic to humans and, because they alter concentrations of reproductive hormones in aquatic organisms, they may be a threat to the stability of aquatic ecosystems (Chapters 2 & 4).

Fuels also pollute ground water. A large number of filling stations have old, leaky storage tanks that have contaminated aquifers below them. Storage tanks have also leaked jet fuels into aquifers near airports and surface runoff from runways and maintenance surfaces has contaminated both surface and ground waters. In a similar way, a variety of organic compounds are released to surface and ground water by urban runoff.

Fuels also contaminate surface waters in "oil spills," which have increased in frequency over the years, and through acts of "ecoterrorism," as evidenced in the Persian Gulf War. Oil spills are acutely toxic to birds, marine mammals, fish and invertebrates by producing acute neurologic damage and by reducing buoyancy. They may cause irreparable damage to populations if large numbers of organisms are poisoned. It is not clear to what extent oil spills are toxic to humans. The economic impact of oil spills has been substantial, closing fisheries by reducing fish populations directly and through impacts on fish reproduction. Oil and other petroleum products comprise a large group of organic compounds that concentrate in fatty tissue and produce undesirable odors and tastes in aquatic animals and degrade natural areas that are important to tourist economies.

In treating drinking water with chlorine and bromine, many different volatile halogenated hydrocarbons, including chloroform ($CHCl_3$), bromodichloromethane ($CHBrCl_2$), and bromoform ($CHBr_3$), are produced if the untreated water has high concentrations of hydrocarbons (National Research Council, 1987). Because many of these disinfection by–products are suspected carcinogens and hepatotoxins, the EPA is considering regulations that will lower chlorine concentrations during treatment as well as the concentrations of disinfection by–products in treated water. There is a question, however, about the extent to which lowered chlorine concentrations will protect against outbreaks of diseases such as giardiasis and cryptosporidiosis. New treatment processes such as those using chloramine or ozone provide disinfection without forming halogenated hydrocarbons; these may provide a solution to disinfection without increasing risks for cancer.

Heated water released from industry does not affect human health directly. Increased temperature has serious implications for ecosystems by decreasing the concentration of dissolved oxygen and altering chemical reactions. Increased temperature also changes populations of microorganisms, aquatic vegetation, and fish by interfering with their reproduction and disrupting physiological processes that affect feeding and behavior.

TREATING WATER FOR DRINKING

Drinking water treatment ranges from removal of solids by gravity in rural areas and in cities of many Third World countries to sophisticated techniques in cities of industrialized nations. Municipal treatment systems first remove heavy solids by allowing them to settle in ponds or tanks. Smaller suspended particles are aggregated into larger clumps by adding chemicals such as alum (hydrated aluminum sulfate [$AlSO_4$]) and gently agitating—a process called flocculation. The clumps of particles are allowed to settle and the water is then filtered through sand or special filters that remove small particles. Special filters are required to remove the cysts of *Giardia lamblia, Cryptosporidium* species, and other parasites, but filters cannot remove bacteria or viruses. Filtered water is chemically treated with chlorine, ozone, bromine, chloramine, or ultraviolet light to destroy bacteria and viruses before it is pumped into distribution systems.

Activated carbon or charcoal can also be used to remove organic compounds that produce undesirable taste, odor, or color. Adding this processing step before chlorination helps remove organic compounds that react with chlorine to form carcinogenic organochlorine compounds. Organic compounds are also removed by aeration with special towers or basins that move air through water and allow the compounds to evaporate.

Hard water contains high concentrations of minerals, primarily salts of calcium and magnesium. Water softening removes these minerals and reduces the build-up of mineral deposits in distribution pipes, water heaters, and espresso machines. Many municipal distribution systems also add fluorine to drinking water up to a concentration of 1 ppm(w) to help prevent dental caries. Some areas have naturally high fluoride concentrations, and these must be reduced by special treatment with ion exchange columns or activated alumina to prevent fluorosis (an increase in bone density) and the mottling of teeth.

Advanced water treatment systems have allowed communities to exploit water resources that, without treatment, would pose clear risks to the public health. When the systems malfunction, or when the quality of raw water deteriorates substantially because of low stream flows during periods of low rainfall, then consumers are placed at risk for exposure to chemical and infectious agents. Although such problems occur infrequently (CDC, 1993b), when they involve large communities, the impact on public health and the economy can be substantial.

Municipal distribution systems can become contaminated with corroded metal from pipes, lead from solder, a variety of microbes from cross-connections with sanitary sewers, nitrates and microbes from animal wastes, and with a variety of chemicals from cross-connections with industrial waste systems.

SEWAGE AND WASTE WATER TREATMENT

As the human population increases, all areas of the planet are experiencing the impact of sewage generation. If sewage and waste water is not treated properly, human wastes pollute surface and ground water with organic compounds, bacteria, viruses, and parasites. *Pit privies* or *latrines* release feces and other wastes directly to the soil where they are degraded if bacteria are capable of metabolizing them. Rural areas in the Third World still rely heavily on this form of sewage treatment, which is better than no treatment at all in terms of ecosystem impact, and latrines have been shown to improve the health status of villagers who use them (Esrey, Habicht, & Casella, 1992).

In *septic tanks* solids settle to the bottom of large concrete tanks where they are metabolized by bacteria and liquids percolate through a drain field. This is the simplest form of *primary treatment.* Periodically the sludge in septic tanks has to be removed because microbial degradation is never complete.

Municipal sewage treatment may include: primary treatment by gravitational settling, screening, and other mechanical methods followed by the transport of solids to a sludge digester; *secondary treatment*—the bacterial decomposition of organic matter after primary treatment for the purpose of reducing BOD in waters that receive treated effluent; and *tertiary treatment,* which includes disinfection and removal of elements (such as nitrogen and phosphorous) that stimulate growth of algae and other undesirable organisms in the aquatic systems that receive sewage effluent. Tertiary treatment can be performed with chemicals, activated charcoal filtration, reverse osmosis, or by applying secondarily treated waste water to terrestrial or wetland ecosystems (Ewel & Odum, 1984; Shijun & Jinsong, 1989; Moshiri, 1993). Land application of secondarily treated effluent combines tertiary treatment with irrigation for lawns and golf courses, or for crops not destined for direct human consumption (OTA, 1988b).

Advanced waste water treatment integrates primary, secondary, and tertiary treatment with other processes designed to remove a variety of materials that still remain after tertiary treatment. These include metals and other inorganic compounds, complex organic molecules, and suspended solids. Such systems can produce effluent that meets primary and secondary drinking water standards.

Sludge, the solids remaining after municipal treatment, must either be transported to landfills for disposal or, preferably, recycled as fertilizer. Many advanced treatment systems use sludge to generate methane gas and then sell the remaining material for fertilizer—a process called *cogeneration.* In order to recycle sludge, it must be free of the many different heavy metals, such as zinc, copper, and cadmium, that are toxic to plants. Recently, there has been renewed interest in using treated sludge for fertilizers, particularly in coastal areas such as New York City, where sludge was formerly dumped in the ocean, but now cannot be disposed of in this way because of government regulations designed to protect marine ecosystems.

Alternative sewage treatment systems have been designed for small communities and even individual homes. On-site sewage treatment plants, or *package treatment plants,* provide primary and secondary treatment for small communities and are popularly used by hotels and commercial establishments located outside areas served by municipal waste water treatment plants. Small treatment systems for single dwellings have also been developed, as have plants for specific industries. Both types of treatment discharge waste water into surface water, wetlands, or terrestrial ecosystems. Because these systems are often not managed properly, they frequently malfunction and release improperly treated effluent to aquatic or terrestrial ecosystems.

Each of the above treatment systems can function effectively and safely under appropriate circumstances; however, each may be unsafe when used incorrectly or for treatment volumes beyond design capacity. Pit privies are not effective for high population densities, or in areas where shallow aquifers and surface waters can be contaminated. Septic tanks in coastal areas or river floodplains may be too close to the water table and may contaminate ground or surface water. They also require adequate drain fields and are therefore not suitable for high–density developments. Municipal sewage systems, though effective in treating sewage, sometimes malfunction and release large quantities of untreated or poorly treated sewage into surface waters.

Industry also poses problems for waste water treatment. Pollutants such as strong acids and bases and nutrients such as nitrogen and phosphorous can disrupt the microbial populations necessary for secondary treatment. Other pollutants such as lead, cadmium, and mercury can contaminate sludge and render it unusable for recycling in agriculture and landscaping. Many cities require *pretreatment* of industrial waste water, which removes contaminants before they are released to sewers. This is an effective alternative to the costly and perhaps ineffective measures that could be implemented at treatment plants. Pretreatment can also help keep toxic heavy metals out of sludge so that it can be recycled as fertilizer.

Urban runoff—rainwater that drains from buildings or pavement—also contaminates surface water directly with organic compounds and heavy metals. The worldwide trend toward urbanization is increasing surface water contamination by this pathway.

Another source of surface water pollution is runoff from rainwater that leaches toxic chemicals from industrial sites. Runoff from both urban and industrial areas can be treated before it is released to surface waters.

Surface runoff also leaches toxic chemicals from solid waste disposal sites, but proper location and design can minimize water pollution from these sites. For instance, fine-grained soils with low hydraulic conductivity are well suited for solid waste burial, as these soils are most effective in retaining and slowing the movement of toxic chemicals. Leachate from solid waste sites can also be collected and treated.

Treated waste water also poses health risks from microorganisms in the aerosols produced by a number of processes inside treatment plants, as well as from effluent released to the environment as aerosols—such as those produced by spray irrigation with treated sewage effluent. Aerosols pose health risks primarily through the inhalation route.

LAND USE AND WATER QUALITY

Water pollution problems are not confined to bodies of surface and ground water. The way humans use land also impacts water quality and as water resources become scarcer, suboptimal uses of land can have substantial public health impacts. For instance, forestry and agriculture increase the sediment loads in streams and rivers, thereby requiring additional filtration if water is to be used for drinking. Heavy metals and other toxic chemicals are leached from open-pit mines and mine tailings and may render rural water supplies unsafe for human consumption. Dams are attractive for hydropower, agricultural irrigation, and flood control. On the other hand, they destroy productive agricultural land and the reservoirs they create are subject to eutrophication. In tropical countries dams create habitats for the vectors of parasites such as the snails that transmit schistosomiasis and mosquitoes which transmit malaria (Council of Environmental Quality & The Department of State, 1988).

Wetlands retain soil in storm water runoff and filter water pollutants from surface waters. Wetland vegetation is also an important energy source for aquatic ecosystems. Past practices of filling wetlands for agriculture and urban land use have destroyed the "free" pollutant filtration these systems provide, as well as their contribution to coastal marine food chains. In the United States and other developed countries strict regulations have made such practices unattractive to developers, but extensive damage has already been done. In the Netherlands plans have been developed recently for returning wetlands that had been filled for agriculture to their natural state because agricultural chemicals and salts have damaged the ground water beneath these lands. Recognizing the services wetlands provide, environmental engineers are now creating new wetlands for tertiary water treatment and retention of runoff.

Animal wastes from feedlots contaminate surface waters in many agricultural areas, leading to eutrophication and reduced dissolved oxygen concentrations—particularly in fresh water ecosystems. These wastes can be recycled and used in cogeneration plants, instead of polluting water. Of course, the most sensible way to reduce such pollution is through source reduction—changing the diets of excessively carnivorous humans.

MODELING HYDROLOGIC PROCESSES

Practitioners in the field of environmental health are often called on to determine whether a source of water pollution needs to be cleaned up to avoid public health problems in the future. Likewise, they are asked to predict when contaminated waters may become safe for public use. Answers to these questions hinge on the complex dynamics of surface and ground waters and can only be approached with data from computer models (Anderson & Woessner, 1992; Calabrese & Kostecki, 1992).

Computer-based models are also used extensively by hydrologists and environmental planners. They incorporate information from topographic and geologic features as well as from ecosystem characteristics such as soil permeability, rates of evaporation and transpiration, and rates of stream and river flow. Hydrologic models for coastal areas incorporate the influences of waves, winds, and tides—physical energies that strongly affect the dynamics of coastal aquatic systems. In predictive models, mathematical equations are developed for conceptual models such as the one shown in Figure

7.3. The equations use hydrologic data to track all water inputs and outputs and to simulate the impact of the environmental factors that influence them.

Models are simulated on computers to explore the effects of changes in urban and natural environments. For instance, the impact of a large commercial development on water volume and quality in nearby streams and rivers can be explored by simulating a variety of weather conditions. Models are also used to assess the quantities of water remaining in an aquifer based on a variety of recharge and consumption alternatives.

WATER MONITORING PROGRAMS

Many countries have programs for surface and ground water monitoring. In the United States national, state, and local governmental agencies maintain programs for routine monitoring. The United Nations Environment Programme established the Global Environment Monitoring System (GEMS) in 1975—a project supported by a number of international agencies (Meybeck et al., 1989). The water monitoring component of this system—the Global Water Quality Monitoring Project—comprises more than 300 stations that monitor rivers, lakes, reservoirs, and ground water worldwide. Determining long-term trends in water quality is a major objective of this project.

To be used effectively for protecting public health, water monitoring data must be collected using standard protocols. Given the variety of methods for data collection and analysis, this is no simple task. Standard methods for collection and analysis of water samples have been developed by a number of governmental agencies—but even the standard methods are different from one country to another. For instance, many heavy metals and organic compounds adsorb to small particles in surface water. Unfiltered samples usually have higher concentrations of pollutants than filtered ones. Analysis of finely filtered samples may minimize the concentration of contaminants in a sample and actually misrepresent the environmental exposure to humans. Furthermore, samples collected in surface water disturbed by boat motors, wading in sediments, or by waves may inaccurately represent contaminant concentrations. Methods for sample preparation and analytical instruments used in the laboratory also vary considerably. It is important to take all these variables into consideration when comparing the results from data that were collected and analyzed by different laboratories and monitoring groups.

WATER POLLUTION REGULATIONS

Water pollutants are regulated worldwide, but countries vary with regard to permissible concentrations and the extent to which regulations are enforced. Regulations are established to protect ecosystems and to insure that water is safe for humans to drink. For pesticides which may also be toxic to important aquatic fauna, environmental regulations are stricter than those for drinking water. For other organic compounds and heavy metals, drinking water regulations are stricter.

In the United States there are federal drinking water regulations for *primary constituents*—those that could have any adverse effect on health; they include inorganic elements, radionuclides, organic compounds, coliform bacteria, and turbidity. Primary constituents are regulated by the EPA, which sets maximum levels that are not be exceeded. In the Safe Drinking Water Amendments of 1986, the EPA was directed to expand the list of primary constituents to a total of 86 chemical, radioactive, and biologic agents (Table 7.3).

Secondary constituents do not directly affect human health but may cause consumers to seek alternate sources that are less healthful. In the United States the federal government recommends standards for secondary constituents and individual states must enforce them.

U. S. water pollution regulations also prevent the release of any radiologic, chemical, or biological warfare agents into surface water and specify effluent standards for commonly used toxic chemicals. The EPA has enacted regulations that require industries and municipal waste water treatment plants to limit effluent concentrations to those that can be achieved by the best practical technology. The limiting of effluent releases is done through permits that are required for industries and municipal treatment facilities under the National Pollutant Discharge Elimination System (NPDES). EPA has used the same philosophy to develop performance standards for new industrial sources. Recent changes to the Clean Water Act (Chapter 8) now address the discharge of nonpoint source pollutants from urban runoff, storm water, mines, and sediment discharge to surface waters.

Table 7.3 Contaminants Required to be Regulated Under the Safe Drinking Water Act Amendments of 1986

Volatile organic chemicals	Beryllium
Trichloroethylene	Cyanide
Tetrachloroethylene	Organics
Carbon tetrachloride	Endrin
1,1,1-Trichloroethane	Lindane
1,2-Dichloroethane	Methoxychlor
Vinylchloride	Toxaphene
Methylene chloride	2,4-D
Benzene	2,4,5-TP
Monochlorobenzene	Aldicarb
Dichlorobenzene	Chlordane
Trichlorobenzene	Dalapon
1,1-Dichloroethylene	Diquat
trans-1,2-Dichloroethylene	Endothall
cis-1,2-Dichloroethylene	Glyphosphate
Microbiology and turbidity	Carboruran
Total coliforms	Alachlor
Turbidity	Epichlorohydrin
Giardia lamblia	Toluene
Viruses	Adipates
Standard plate count	2,3,7,8-TCDD (Dioxin)
Legionella	1,1,2-Trichloroethane
Inorganics	Vydate
Arsenic	Simazine
Barium	Polyaromatic hydrocarbons (PAHs)
Cadmium	Polychlorinated biphenyls (PCBs)
Chromium	Atrazine
Lead	Phthalates
Mercury	Acrylamide
Nitrate	Dibromochloropropane (DBCP)
Selenium	1,2-Dichloropropane
Silver	Pentachlorophenol
Fluoride	Pichloram
Aluminum	Dinoseb
Antimony	Ethylene dibromide (EDB)
Molybdenum	Dibromomethane
Asbestos	Xylene
Sulfate	Hexachlorocyclopentadiene
Copper	Radionuclides
Vanadium	Radium-226 and -228
Sodium	Beta particle and photon radioactivity
Nickel	Radon
Zinc	Gross alpha particle activity
Thallium	Uranium

From Calabrese, Gilbert, & Pastides (Eds.). (1989). *Safe Drinking Water Act: Amendments, Regulations, and Standards*. Reprinted with permission.

HAZARDOUS WASTE DISPOSAL

Considering the environmental pathways associated with the disposal of hazardous wastes, it is clear that one of the main reasons for controlling the disposal of hazardous wastes is to protect ground and surface waters.

Sources of hazardous wastes include underground storage tanks at industrial sites and filling stations, municipal landfills, wells that were used to inject wastes from industry into deep aquifers (*injection wells*), brine pits from petroleum extraction, and abandoned surface and underground mines.

Proper design of waste disposal sites is crucial for preventing ground and surface water contamination (OTA, 1989). Obviously, close proximity to shallow aquifers and to surface waters is not desirable. Liners made of clay and synthetic materials are commonly used to restrict the migration of wastes. Over long time periods, however, no barrier can be considered perfect. Backup systems, including monitoring wells and water processing plants, may be necessary.

REFERENCES

Anderson, M. P., & Woessner, W. W. (1992). *Applied groundwater modeling: Simulation of flow and advective transport.* San Diego: Academic Press.

Biswas, A. K., & Arar, A. (Eds.). (1988). *Treatment and reuse of wastewater.* London: Butterworths.

Calabrese, E. J., & Kostecki, P. T. (1992). *Risk assessment and environmental fate methodologies.* Boca Raton, FL: Lewis.

Centers for Disease Control and Prevention. (1993a). Methemoglobinemia in and infant. *Morbidity and Mortality Weekly Report, 42,* 217-219.

Centers for Disease Control and Prevention (1993b). Surveillance for waterborne disease outbreaks—United States, 1991-1992. *Morbidity Mortality Weekly Report, 42* (No. SS-5), 1-22.

Coghlan, A. (1991). Fresh water from the sea. *New Scientist,* August 31, 37-40.

Council of Environmental Quality & The Department of State. (1988). In D. H. Speidel, L. C. Ruedisili, & A. F. Agnew (Eds.), *Perspectives on water uses and abuses.* New York: Oxford University Press.

Culotta, E. (1992). Red menace in the world's oceans. *Science, 257,* 1476-1477.

Duplaix, N. (1990). South Florida water: Paying the price. *National Geographic,* July 1990, 89-112.

Esrey, S. A., Habicht, J-P., & Casella, G. (1992). The complementary effect of latrines and increased water usage on the growth of infants in rural Lesotho. *American Journal of Epidemiology, 135,* 659-666.

Ewel, K. C., & Odum, H. T. (Eds.). (1984). *Cypress swamps.* Gainesville, FL: University of Florida Press.

Falkenmark, M. (1989). The massive water scarcity now threatening Africa—Why isn't it being addressed. *Ambio, 18,* 112-118.

Felsenfeld, A. J., & Roberts, M. A. (1991). A report of fluorosis in the United States secondary to drinking well water. *JAMA, 265,* 486-488.

Heath, R. C. (1988). Ground water. In D. H. Speidel, L. C. Ruedisili, & A. F. Agnew (Eds.), *Perspectives on water uses and abuses.* New York: Oxford University Press.

Jaffe, M., & DiNovo, F. (1987). *Local groundwater protection.* Washington, DC: American Planning Association.

Meybeck, M., Chapman, D. V., & Helmer, R. (1989). *Global freshwater quality.* Oxford: Blackwell.

Mitsch, W. J. & Gosselink, J. G. (1993). *Wetlands* (2nd ed.) New York: Van Nostrand Reinhold.

Moshiri, G. A. (1993). *Constructed wetlands for water quality.* Boca Raton, FL: Lewis.

National Research Council. (1987). Drinking water and health: Disinfectants and disinfectant byproducts (Vol. 7). Washington, DC: National Academy Press.

National Research Council. (1993). *Managing wastewater in coastal urban areas.* Washington, DC: National Academy Press.

Office of Technology Assessment, U. S. Congress. (1988a). *Using desalination technologies for water treatment* (OTA-BP-0-46). Washington, DC: U. S. Government Printing Office.

Office of Technology Assessment, U. S. Congress. (1988b). Waste water reuse. In D. H. Speidel, L. C. Ruedisili, & A. F. Agnew (Eds.), *Perspectives on water uses and abuses.* New York: Oxford University Press.

Office of Technology Assessment, U. S. Congress. (1989). *Facing America's trash: What's next for municipal solid waste* (OTA-0-24). Washington, DC: U. S. Government Printing Office.

Pair, C. H. (Ed.). (1983). *Irrigation.* Silver Spring, MD: The Irrigation Association.

Perera, J. (1993). A sea turns to dust. *New Scientist,* October 23, 24-27.

Postel, S. (1988). Fresh water supplies and competing uses. In D. H. Speidel, L. C. Ruedisili, & A. F. Agnew (Eds.), *Perspectives on water uses and abuses.* New York: Oxford University Press.

Postel, S. (1993). Facing water scarcity. In L. R. Brown (Ed.), *State of the world 1993*. New York: W. W. Norton.

Shijun, M., & Jingsong, Y. (1989). Ecological engineering for treatment and utilization of wastewater. In W. J. Mitsch & S. E. Jorgensen (Eds.), *Ecological engineering: An introduction to ecotechnology*. New York: Wiley.

Shuval, H. I. (1990). *Wastewater irrigation in developing countries: Health effects and technical solutions*. Washington, DC: World Bank.

Solley, W. B., Chase, E. B., & Mann, W. B. (1988). Estimated use of water in the United States in 1980. In D. H. Speidel, L. C. Ruedisili, & A. F. Agnew (Eds.), *Perspectives on water uses and abuses*. New York: Oxford University Press.

Solley, W.B., Merk, C.F., & Pierce, R. R.(1988). *Estimated water use in the United States in 1985*, U.S. Geological Survey Circular 1004. Washington, DC: U. S. Geological Survey.

U. S. Environmental Protection Agency. (1988). Industrial waste water. In D. H. Speidel, L. C. Ruedisili, & A. F. Agnew (Eds.), *Perspectives on water uses and abuses*. New York: Oxford University Press.

U. S. Environmental Protection Agency. (1990). *National water quality inventory: 1988 report to Congress* (Publication No. EPA-440-4-90-003). Washington, DC: Author.

van der Leeden, F., Troise, F. S., & Todd, D. K. (1991). *The water encyclopedia* (2nd ed.). Chelsea, MI: Lewis.

Vesilind, P. J. (1993). The Middle East's water: Critical resource. *National Geographic*, May, 38-71.

SUGGESTED READINGS

Adler, R. W., Landman, J. C., & Cameron, D. M. (1993). *The Clean Water Act: 20 years later*. Washington, DC: Island Press.

Bitton, G. (1994). *Wastewater microbiology*. New York: Wiley.

Gustafson, D. I. (1993). *Pesticides in drinking water*. New York: Van Nostrand Reinhold.

Jaffe, M., & DiNovo, F. (1987). *Local groundwater protection*. Washington, DC: American Planning Association.

James, A. (1993). *Introduction to water quality modeling* (2nd ed.). New York: Wiley.

Laws, E. (1993). *Aquatic pollution: An introductory text* (2nd ed.). New York: Wiley.

Mitsch, W. J., & Jorgensen, S. E. (Eds.). (1989). *Ecological engineering: An introduction to ecotechnology*. New York: Wiley.

Mitsch, W. J., & Gosselink, J. G. (1993). *Wetlands* (2nd ed.). New York: Van Nostrand Reinhold.

National Research Council. (1977-1989). *Drinking water and health* (Vol. 1-9). Washington, DC: National Academy Press.

National Research Council. (1993). *Managing wastewater in coastal urban areas*. Washington, DC: National Academy Press.

Office of Technology Assessment, U. S. Congress. (1989). *Facing America's trash: What's next for municipal solid waste* (OTA-0-24). Washington, DC: U. S. Government Printing Office.

Speidel, D. H., Ruedisili, L. C. , & Agnew, A. F. (Eds.). (1988). *Perspectives on water uses and abuses*. New York: Oxford University Press.

van der Leeden, F., Troise, F. S., & Todd, D. K. (1991). *The water encyclopedia,* (2nd ed.). Chelsea, MI: Lewis.

Part IV

Environmental Health Practice

Chapter 8

Environmental Health Law

Andrew Robert Greene

There is no generally recognized definition of environmental health law. Descriptively, environmental health law is that component of environmental law that deals most directly with the impact of environmental contamination on human health. However, all environmental statutes have as primary goals both the protection of human health (public health goals) and the protection of the environment (ecological goals). The tension between these two sometimes competing sets of goals is reflected in governmental and programmatic priorities that may vary from year to year (Portney, Probst, & Finkel, 1991). This chapter provides an overview of the environmental health laws in the United States and a brief discussion of international laws and treaties concerned with the environment and its impact on human health.

HISTORICAL THREADS

In the United States, modern environmental law is woven from three distinct legal threads: the common law; public health protection; and the desire to bring man and nature into harmony—the "ecological tradition" (Council on Environmental Quality, 1987). Each thread has different premises and aims. Much of the current difficulty we experience in applying environmental statutes to real problems may be attributed to this interweaving of threads, with each tending to pull implementation in a different direction.

The Common Law

The first thread is the common law of property and tort (Thomas & Novick, 1992). Industrial pollution has long been known to damage property and health, and people have sued both to stop pollution and to obtain compensation for damages. The difficulty with common law suits against pollution damage has always been in demonstrating causation between the pollution and the damage. Such suits, however, became more popular in the 1950s as property owners became more conscious of the ill effects of pollutants—particularly those from air pollutants associated with postwar industrial expansion.

In response to the issues raised by these suits, states established scientific panels to determine "safe" levels for various pollutants, and these levels became the basis for laws that created environmental standards. These standards became administrative surrogates for court findings of damage or nuisance under common law. Pollution in excess of these standards was thus illegal without further proof of damage, and enforcement by state authorities could help resolve disputes between parties claiming damage and industries causing pollution.

In the 1960s, these state actions also increased pressure for uniform national standards. Industries wished to avoid the inefficiencies of differing standards in different states for the same pollutant; environmentalists wished to prevent states with less stringent standards from attracting industry away from states with more stringent ones. Thus, the development of national standards for air and water pollution is partially attributable to the desire to relieve common law courts of the responsibility for making individual determinations in an impractically large number of cases (Novick, 1987).

It is illustrative to note that the current debate on the allowability of risks from toxic substances is connected to the thread of a common law. Although risks have often been calculated to be extremely small, plaintiffs exposed to toxic agents rely on common law precedents to obtain redress for outrage or feelings of helplessness, as well as for actual harm (Dore, 1994).

Public Health Protection

In contrast to government action for redressing damage through common law is the thread of government action to *prevent* damage or illness (Hays, 1987). This is the essence of public health regulation, some elements of which date from ancient times—especially with respect to the environment. Modern laws against adulteration of food, against fouling the water with refuse or the air with smoke, and against the spread of contagion, all have ancient or medieval ancestry.

The modern public health movement, based on scientific observation, arose in response to the problems caused in late-eighteenth-century Europe by the enormous growth of urban populations and the beginning of the Industrial Revolution. The emphasis was first placed on prevention of water-borne diseases through the treatment of drinking water and the control of contamination of water and food supplies by human sewage and refuse.

Public health approaches to disease prevention are sometimes categorized as health promotion, health protection, and preventive services (U. S. Department of Health and Human Services, 1991). Environmental health laws are important components of health protection. Laws designed to prevent environmentally caused disease ideally establish strict standards based on scientific research. The practical problems of implementing public health measures has made it convenient to tie health protection standards to the particular engineering techniques that are available at the time a law is passed. This occurred first in sewage treatment and later in local ordinances controlling air pollution and the creation of so-called sanitary landfills.

In general, the public health approach to pollution control has not given heavy weight to cost, nor has it been concerned with measuring the degree of risk associated with public exposures to toxic agents. From the beginning the public health movement was uncomfortable with economic evaluations applied to various protective measures. To some extent this represents an ethical stance; to some extent it results from the fact that in the early days of the sanitation movement, quite modest expenditures produced enormous improvements in public health. In any case, from the public health perspective, a situation is either safe, or it is not, and laws following this thread reflect this view.

The Ecological Tradition

The third thread derives from the desire to preserve and protect the order of nature and to bring the human economic system into harmony with ecological systems (Anderson, Mandelker, & Tarlock, 1990). This is a particularly American tradition, with a number of complex nuances. One of these is the preservationist ethic—the sense that the earth is a kind of Garden of Eden subject to despoliation by human greed; it is the sense, too, that there is something in untrammeled nature that has a value that transcends health or economics—something that must be preserved for the future.

Modern ecological thinking also contributes to this tradition. From it, we get the concept that human actions may have unintended outcomes in the natural world, and that natural systems are in a balance that human activities may upset—sometimes with disastrous consequences. What we see as separate environmental media—air, water, and land—are interconnected, as are the organisms enmeshed in each. Survival, according to this perspective, requires adjusting human economic activity as much as possible to the dynamics of ecosystems. It follows from these arguments that a certain prudence is required when considering enterprises that may upset the natural order on which human life ultimately depends.

THE ENVIRONMENTAL PROTECTION AGENCY

The weaver of the threads, the National Environmental Policy Act of 1969, required that environmental values be weighed in all federal governmental decisions. However, no single agency was established as the conduit for federal environmental policy until 1970 when the Environmental Protection Agency (EPA) was created by presidential order. Before then, environmental responsibilities were scattered among many agencies. The Departments of Interior and Agriculture, the Army Corps of Engineers, and other federal agencies still retain some environmental responsibilities, but they cooperate with the EPA under a variety of agreements. For example, EPA and the Corps of Engineers jointly administer the Wetlands Protection Program of the Clean Water Act (Section 404).

The three threads of environmental health law are woven through the major national environmental statutes in different ways. This has presented the EPA with a regulatory mission of enormous complexity, as the aims and premises embodied in the several laws are often in conflict with one another. As a consequence, it has always been quite difficult for the EPA to set reasonable priorities based on a general vision. Protecting public health is sometimes different from protecting ecological systems, and often regulatory actions supporting one goal may have negative effects on the other (Science Advisory Board, 1990).

THEMES IN ENVIRONMENTAL LAWS

There is no one comprehensive environmental law. Rather, there is a series of laws enacted to address particular environmental issues. The laws themselves are probably a little easier to understand if one considers five major characteristics:

1. Each law represents an uneasy and sometimes conflicting alliance between public health advocates and conservationists.
2. Major statutes are very opportunistic—after years of debate, some external event will precipitate swift and, perhaps, ill-considered action.
3. Congress has historically been very reluctant to create a federal land-use plan. Therefore, environmental statutes have downplayed the role of planning.
4. The laws usually contain lofty goals and unrealistic timetables, and provide for broad agency discretion.
5. The laws rely on regulations rather than subsidies and they demonstrate a preference for delegation of responsibilities to the states (Percival, Miller, Schroeder, & Leape, 1992).

Although each law is somewhat different, several features are common and these are illustrated below as they apply to the EPA:

1. The laws provide national standards for regulating the handling, emission, discharge, and disposal of harmful substances.
2. Standards are applied through general EPA or state rules, through permits, or both.
3. The EPA is given authority to enter and inspect sites that release toxic agents to the environment and has authority to request or demand information, to monitor and test, and to report its findings.
4. The EPA is generally given authority to issue notices of violations and administrative compliance orders.
5. The EPA is generally given authority to seek injunctive relief through civil courts, by imposing it administratively, or both.
6. The EPA can usually seek administrative penalties and civil or criminal remedies. This authority generally allows the agency to eliminate, through penalty assessment, any economic advantage gained by a noncomplying source as a result of its noncompliance.
7. The EPA usually has the authority to address emergency situations.
8. The EPA may give states authority to administer and enforce programs; however, the EPA retains independent enforcement authority.
9. Federal facilities are generally required to comply with substantive provisions of EPA statutes, although enforcement raises other issues—for instance, the question of whether one federal agency can sue another.
10. EPA implements these laws through regulations that are assembled in Title 40 of the Code of the Federal Regulations (CFR) parts 1 through 799.

STANDARDS IN ENVIRONMENTAL LAW

Standards lie at the heart of virtually all the environmental regulatory programs, whether in the United States or in other countries. The term *standard* is many-faceted. In the context of occupational, product, and environmental health and safety laws, a standard is any of a great variety of requirements imposed under legislative authority, the purpose of which is to protect life, promote health, or prevent health- or life-threatening accidents. The different kinds of standards that are incorporated into environmental statutes are listed below (Anderson, 1982; Plater, Abrams, & Goldfarb, 1992):

Performance standards establish acceptable levels of protection or control without specifying the particular methods to be used for complying with them. Performance standards are particularly important in pollution control. Water and air pollution standards specify mean or maximum permissible discharges of pollutants from specific types of sources; for instance, air and water standards promulgated under the Clean Air Act and Clean Water Act may specify performance in terms of permissible concentrations of pollutants per quantity of discharge. Pollutants other than those in air and water—for instance, heavy metals in the soil—may also be regulated in this way.

Ambient standards specify the minimum conditions that must be met in an indoor or outdoor environment. Unlike performance standards that control actual discharges into the environment, ambient standards place quality requirements on the receiving water or air.

Design standards attempt to protect against health and safety hazards by specifying the manner in which equipment, structures, products, and production processes must be constructed or arranged.

Behavioral standards prescribe procedures intended to reduce the incidence of injury or illness.

Information standards require that information be supplied to affected parties or to the governmental agency charged with protecting the public. Information standards may be applied in circumstances where it is either difficult or impossible to enforce design and performance standards, but they may also be promulgated after a legislative or administrative judgment has been made that protection is unnecessary or paternalistic and that when suitably warned, persons can adjust their behavior to the risks involved.

REGULATING AIR POLLUTION

The first air pollution laws in the United States were passed by cities. In the 1880s, Chicago and Cincinnati initiated the earliest regulation of smoke emissions, followed in the 1890s by Pittsburgh and New York City. One of the earliest state air pollution laws was passed by Ohio in the 1890s to regulate smoke emission from steam boilers (Reitze, 1991). In 1959 Oregon became the first state to pass comprehensive statewide legislation and establish a state air pollution control agency.

Americans have long recognized dirty air as a serious problem but, initially, they paid little attention to the public health risks it presented. Air pollution was recognized as a serious health hazard when "killer fogs" in Donora, Pennsylvania in 1948 and in London in 1952 focused national and international attention on this aspect of air pollution (Chapter 6).

During the late 1940s, the state of California, Los Angeles County, and local industries began spending millions of dollars to study the causes and effects of smog. By the 1960s the necessity for an effective national approach to effective air pollution control was recognized. In 1963 Congress authorized the U.S. Public Health Service to study air pollution and to provide training grants to state and local agencies. This legislation was strengthened considerably when the Clean Air Act was enacted in 1970, making EPA the focal point of the federal effort (Reed, Wyckoff, & Dee, 1992).

The new act created a partnership between state and federal government. It gave state and local governments primary responsibility for preventing and controlling air pollution. The EPA had a leadership and support role: conducting research and development programs, setting national standards and regulations, and providing technical and financial assistance to the states.

As directed by the Clean Air Act, the EPA set national *ambient air quality standards* for those pollutants that pose the greatest overall threat to air quality (Chapter 6). These pollutants, termed *criteria pollutants*, include ozone, carbon monoxide, air-borne particulates, sulphur dioxide, lead, hydrocarbons, and nitrogen dioxide. For these pollutants, the act sets *primary standards* to protect human health and *secondary standards* to protect welfare — primarily crops, livestock, vegetation, buildings, and visibility. For some of these criteria pollutants, a single ambient standard has been established that protects both health and welfare.

In addition to the ambient air quality standards for the criteria pollutants, the Act also requires the EPA to set *emissions standards* for other particularly dangerous pollutants. These are the National Emissions Standards for Hazardous Air Pollutants, or NESHAPs. Hazardous pollutants are defined as those that can contribute to an increase in mortality or serious illness. The Clean Air Act Amendments of 1990 expanded the list of regulated hazardous air pollutants to 189, from the eight (asbestos, beryllium, mercury, vinyl chloride, arsenic, radionuclides, benzene, and coke oven emissions) the EPA had previously regulated.

REGULATING WATER QUALITY

The EPA, in partnership with state and local governments, is responsible for protecting and improving water quality. These efforts are organized around three themes. The first is maintaining the quality of drinking water. This is addressed by monitoring and treating drinking water prior to consumption, by minimizing the contamination of surface water, and by protecting against contamination of ground water. The second theme is preventing the degradation and destruction of critical aquatic habitats, including wetlands, coastal waters, oceans, and lakes. The third is reducing the pollution of free-flowing surface waters and protecting their uses.

The EPA is responsible for monitoring the quality of drinking water from both groundwater and surface water sources and for assuring compliance with standards, and the agency continues to establish standards for drinking water contaminants. It is also responsible for protecting wetlands, coastal waters, marine waters, and lakes that serve as breeding areas for commercial and sport fisheries and other wildlife, and as recreational areas for millions of residents and tourists. For a variety of reasons, some of these critical aquatic habitats have been significantly degraded or destroyed during our nation's history, and many more are threatened. The EPA places particular emphasis on protecting these resources.

In the early 1970s, the nation recognized the impact of sewage on surface water and developed programs for its control. The EPA and the states now have a major program for establishing standards for our surface waters and subsequent permitting and enforcement to safeguard those standards. We are also now aware of the impact of other toxic pollutants in surface water, including hundreds of organic compounds produced by industry. Protecting rivers, lakes, and streams is the third focus of EPA's effort to protect our nation's water resources.

Congress has given EPA, the states, and Indian tribal governments broad authority to deal with water pollution. The principal law is the 1972 Clean Water Act whose goal is to restore and maintain the chemical, physical, and biological integrity of the nation's waters (Andreen, 1987; Schoenbaum & Rosenberg, 1991). Under this mandate, EPA has developed regulations and programs to reduce pollutants entering all surface water, including lakes, rivers, estuaries, oceans, and wetlands. Amendments passed in 1977 and 1987 insured continued economic support for municipal sewage treatment plants, for accelerating control of toxic pollutants, and for initiating new federal and state programs to control non-point-source pollution (e.g., surface runoff). In this and other federal/state programs, regulations are formulated at the federal level but can be delegated to the states for enforcement.

In 1993 the Environmental Protection Agency revised state water quality standards under the Clean Water Act of 1987, using human health-based water quality standards. Generally, these standards are stricter than those based on toxicity to aquatic organisms. Also in 1993, Congress reauthorized the Clean Water Act and thereby required further reductions in industrial releases to surface and ground water, stricter control of storm water and sediment discharge to surface waters, more stringent wetland protection, and stricter water quality standards. Future revisions of the Clean Water Act are planned for late 1994 or 1995. They will address runoff from farms, preservation of existing wetland acreage, and restrict the discharge of certain chemicals.

The 1974 Safe Drinking Water Act created major legislative authority for protecting drinking water resources. Unlike the Clean Water Act, which protects all surface waters, the Safe Drinking Water Act applies only to surface and underground sources of drinking water. Amendments added in 1986 established two new major groundwater protection programs: The Well-Head Protection Program to protect areas around public drinking water wells and the Sole Source Aquifer Demonstration Program to protect underground water supplies that are the only source of drinking water for the communities they supply.

To protect the marine environment from the harmful effects of ocean dumping, Congress enacted the Marine Protection, Research, and Sanctuaries Act in 1972. This act established a permanent program to help insure that the dumping of waste in the ocean does not cause degradation of the marine environment.

Other environmental laws such as the Resource Conservation and Recovery Act (RCRA), the Comprehensive Environmental Response, Compensation and Liability Act (CERCLA) and the Toxic Substances Control Act, which are described later in this chapter, have also helped improve and protect our fresh water and marine ecosystems.

REGULATING TOXIC WASTES

More than 6 billion tons of agricultural, commercial, industrial, and domestic wastes are produced in the United States each year. Most waste presents few health or environmental problems. Half the total, for example, is agricultural waste, which is usually plowed back into the land. Other waste, particularly from industrial sources, can imperil the health of both the public and the environment. Leaks from underground storage tanks and chemical releases from industry also contaminate land and groundwater. If not properly disposed of, even common household waste can cause environmental problems (Office of Policy Planning and Evaluation, 1988).

Congress enacted several laws to regulate the generation and disposal of hazardous wastes. They have three basic objectives: (1) proper management and disposal of waste generated now and in the future; (2) cleanup of sites where the results of past disposal practices now threaten surrounding communities and the environment; and (3) minimizing the generation of waste and promoting the recycling of materials, where possible, to lessen the burden on the environment.

Developing methods for proper disposal of the waste Americans generate in their daily lives has been a focus of federal legislation for some time. In 1965, the Solid Waste Disposal Act was enacted to fund research and technical assistance for state and local planners. As the potential environmental problems posed by the disposal of chemical and other industrial waste became clearer, Congress amended these statutes by passing RCRA in 1976 (Stever, 1994a). This law promoted development of sanitary landfills and encouraged a shift from disposal toward conservation, recycling, and new control technologies. RCRA requires "cradle to grave" management of hazardous waste from its point of generation to its final disposal location. The program works by requiring written documentation of the generation, transportation, treatment, storage, and disposal of hazardous waste. Each hazardous waste container is accompanied by a manifest from its point of origin to its final point of disposal. It is therefore not possible to escape responsibility for the disposition of such waste simply by passing it on to another party.

The 1984 Hazardous and Solid Waste Amendments (HSWA) to RCRA altered the focus of waste management in many ways. HSWA required EPA to focus on issuing permits for land disposal facilities and eventually phasing out land disposal of some wastes. It also expanded the RCRA-regulated community to include businesses that generate small amounts of hazardous waste. Recycling and waste minimization incentives (for instance, mandates for federal procurement programs to use recycled materials) were also included in the Act as promising methods for reducing the overall amount of waste generated.

HSWA also addressed previously exempt underground storage tanks containing petroleum and other hazardous substances. With these provisions, Congress gave the EPA the responsibility for expanding its regulations of the storage of waste to include gasoline and other commercial products.

REGULATING HAZARDOUS WASTE SITES

The problems from hazardous waste disposal practices in the past were brought to national attention in a series of well-publicized incidents in the late 1970s. The first major incident occurred at the site of Love Canal in Niagara Falls, New York, where people were evacuated from their homes after hazardous waste buried for over 25 years rose to the soil surface and into the basements of homes. In Times Beach, Missouri, oil contaminated with TCDD was used on dirt roads to suppress dust and subsequently contaminated the soil and residences in the community.

It soon became clear that hazardous waste problems caused by past mismanagement were outside the purview of existing environmental statutes. A survey requested by a congressional committee found that one-third of the 3,380 waste disposal sites used since 1950 by the 53 largest chemical companies were not covered under federal regulations (Office of Policy Planning and Evaluation, 1988).

The Federal Water Pollution Control Act of 1972 established a fund of $35 million for the cleanup of hazardous substances and oil released into navigable waters. However, no similar fund existed for addressing hazardous waste releases that occurred solely on land. In response to this need, the Comprehensive Environmental Response, Compensation, and Liability Act (CERCLA) or Superfund was enacted in 1980 (Light, 1991; Stever, 1994b). CERCLA authorized $1.6 billion dollars over 5 years for a comprehensive program to clean up the worst abandoned or inactive waste sites in the nation. CERCLA funds used to establish an administrative cleanup program are derived primarily from taxes on the production of crude oil and 42 different commercial chemicals.

The re-authorization of CERCLA in 1986 is known as the Superfund Amendments and Reauthorization Act (SARA). These amendments provided $8.5 billion for the cleanup program and an additional $500 million for cleanup of leaks from underground storage tanks.

Under SARA, Congress strengthened the EPA mandate to focus on permanent cleanup of Superfund sites, involved the public in decision-making processes at sites, and encouraged states and tribes to actively participate as partners with EPA to address these sites. SARA expanded EPA's research, development, and training responsibilities. SARA also strengthened the EPA's authority to require others to clean up the hazardous waste problems for which they were responsible.

In the process of amending CERCLA, in 1986 Congress passed the Emergency Planning And Community Right To Know Act, known as EPCRA or Title III (Fogarty, 1993). Title III was enacted to promote public awareness of hazardous or toxic chemicals used or produced by industry. It also mandates that each community be prepared to respond to emergencies resulting from releases of chemicals. Industrial and commercial facilities are also required to report annually on the quantities of toxic substances present in their facilities and released to the environment on a routine basis and these data are summarized and published annually as the Toxic Release Inventory.

REGULATING PESTICIDES AND COMMERCIAL PRODUCTS

Pesticides and commercial chemical substances are regulated primarily through two laws: the Federal Insecticide, Fungicide, and Rodenticide Act of 1947 (FIFRA) (Lewis, 1993) and the Toxic Substances Control Act (TSCA) of 1976 (Stever, 1994c).

FIFRA applies to all pesticides used in the United States. When enacted in 1947, FIFRA was administered by the U. S. Department of Agriculture and was intended to protect consumers from fraudulent pesticide products. When many pesticides were registered, their potential for causing health and environmental problems was unknown. In 1970, EPA assumed the responsibility for enforcing FIFRA, and amendments to this act in 1972 shifted the emphasis to environmental protection. Under the law, EPA classifies pesticides according to their toxicity and regulates the quantity of various pesticides produced, as well as the ways they are used. The only aspect of pesticide control not included in FIFRA is the allowable levels of pesticides in food. These are specified under the authority of the Federal Food, Drug and Cosmetic Act of 1954 and are therefore regulated by the Food and Drug Administration.

TSCA authorizes the EPA to control the risks that may be posed by the thousands of commercial chemical substances and mixtures that are not regulated as either drugs, food additives, cosmetics, or pesticides. Under TSCA, the EPA can, among other things, regulate the manufacture and use of a chemical substance and require testing for cancer and other effects.

Under TSCA, the EPA must keep an inventory of all chemicals manufactured or processed in the United States. For selected substances, the manufacturer must submit a summary of proposed uses, estimates of production levels, a list of adverse health and environmental effects associated with each substance, a description of by-products, and an estimate of the number of workers exposed. Moreover, manufacturers must give the EPA 90 days' notice prior to beginning production of a new chemical substance; the notice must include all known data on health and environmental effects. EPA may also require the testing of a new or old substance.

FIFRA requires pesticides to be registered with the EPA in a manner similar to that required of other chemicals under TSCA; it also requires the manufacturer to show that the pesticide, when applied as directed, "will not generally cause unreasonable adverse effects on the environment."

Under both TSCA and FIFRA, the EPA is responsible for regulating certain biotechnology products, such as genetically engineered microorganisms designed to control pests or for use in industrial processes.

OTHER ENVIRONMENTAL LAWS IN THE UNITED STATES

This chapter has focused primarily on legislation passed specifically to protect the environment and to safeguard humans from environmental risks. However, some laws passed for other purposes also have environmental components. This includes legislation involving the Department of Transportation, the Department of Agriculture, the Department of Energy, and the Department of Defense. For instance, the 1991 Intermodal Transportation Act and the 1992 Energy Policy Act have strong environmental planning components.

INTERNATIONAL LAWS AND TRADE AGREEMENTS

Over the past 20 years, increased attention has been paid to problems of the international "commons" and to new forms of environmental pollution that cross national boundaries (transboundary pollution). This concern has resulted in a number of treaties based on compromises between the sovereignty of nations and the need to protect citizens and ecosystems from environmental agents that are generated outside state boundaries (Haas, 1993). International environmental health laws have addressed such issues as worker protection, pest control, water pollution, air pollution, and waste disposal.

Specific examples of international treaties include the Basel Convention on the Control of Transboundary Movements of Hazardous Wastes and Their Disposal (1989), which restricts the transport of hazardous waste among party countries; the Montreal Protocol on Substances That Deplete the Ozone Layer (1987), a treaty designed to reduce production and use of ozone-depleting chemicals (it was strengthened by the London [1990] and Copenhagen [1992] amendments); and the International Code of Conduct on the Distribution and Use of Pesticides (1985), designed to make nations responsible for notifying recipients of the export of restricted pesticides and for providing importing nations with information regarding domestic pesticide restrictions of exporters, as well as promoting safe handling of pesticides (Esty, 1994).

The United Nations Conference on Environment and Development (UNCED), held in Rio de Janeiro in June 1992, brought together representatives of 178 governments and produced five separate agreements (Grubb, Koch, Thomson, Munson, & Sullivan, 1993). Two of the agreements are legally binding: The Framework Convention on Climate Change established a legal framework for addressing human interference with the global and regional processes that determine climate, and the Convention on Biological Diversity developed guidelines for protecting species and ecosystems and the uses of biological resources and technology. The three nontreaty agreements are: The Rio Declaration on Environment and Development, which advocates sustainable development (a level of economic growth that can be maintained indefinitely without destroying a nation's environmental systems) that is protective of the environment; Agenda 21, a plan for attaining sustainable development; and the Principles of Forest Management, which contains general statements about exploiting forests within national boundaries while not adversely impacting other countries.

Trade agreements can also be used to protect health and the environment by regulating hazardous waste, regulating the production and sale of chemicals that deplete ozone or affect climate, and promoting sustainable development. However, trade agreements that promote economic growth can cause environmental harm by increasing economic development that can only be sustained by substantially depleting natural resources. Moreover, agreements that limit restrictions on trade, such as the General Agreement on Tariffs and Trade, could be used to override environmental regulations in the name of market access unless rules to assure environmental protection are included (Esty, 1994).

CONCLUSION

As environmental health law approaches the 21st Century, few absolute predictions are possible. But if history is a guide, some threads are likely to continue: regulation (or "command and control") will remain the preferred approach (rather than subsidization); fine-tuning rather than dramatic overhaul will be emphasized as the current laws are amended; and, as in the past, unexpected events will prompt reactive legislation.

Pollution control efforts will become increasingly proactive, emphasizing source reduction rather than waste management and pollution control. The Pollution Prevention Act of 1990 incorporates this philosophy (Plater, Abrams, & Goldfarb, 1992).

On the other hand, there will be some variation to the warp and woof: market incentives will be given a chance, international cooperation will become more important as we acknowledge both the global commons and intergenerational equity and, finally, governmental and other institutions may finally recognize that only by preventing pollution in the first place will we really protect environmental health.

REFERENCES

Anderson, R. (1982). Human welfare and the administered society: Federal regulation in the 1970s to protect health, safety, and the environment. In W. Rom (Ed.), *Environmental and occupational medicine* (1st ed.). Boston: Little, Brown.

Anderson, F., Mandelker, D., & Tarlock, A. (1990). *Environmental protection: Law and policy* (2nd ed.) (pp. 1-6). Boston: Little Brown.

Andreen, W. (1987). Beyond words of extortion: The congressional prescription for vigorous federal enforcement of the Clean Water Act. *George Washington Law Review, 55*, 202.

Council on Environmental Quality. (1987). *Sixteenth annual report* (pp. 4-6). Washington, DC: U. S. Government Printing Office.

Dore, M. (1994). *Law of toxic torts: Litigation/defense/insurance.* Deerfield, IL: Clark, Boardman, & Callaghan.

Esty, D. C. (1994). *Greening the GATT: Trade, environment, and the future.* Washington, DC: Institute for International Economics.

Fogarty, J. (1993). SARA Title III—The Emergency Planning and Community Right–to–Know Act. In S. Novick (Ed.), *Law of environ-*

mental protection (Vol. 3, sec. 13.07). Deerfield, IL: Clark, Boardman, & Callaghan.

Grubb, M., Koch, M., Thomson, K., Munson, A., & Sullivan, F. (1993). T*he Earth Summit agreements: A guide and assessment.* London: Earthscan.

Haas, P. (1993). Evolving international environmental law: Changing practices of national sovereignty. In N. Chourcri (Ed.), *Global accord: Environmental challenges and international responses.* Cambridge, MA: MIT Press.

Hays, S. (1987). *Beauty, health, and permanence.* New York: Oxford University Press.

Lewis, C. (1993). Pesticides. In S. Novick (Ed.), *Law of environmental protection,* (Vol. 3, Chap. 17). Deerfield, IL: Clark, Boardman, & Callaghan.

Light, A. (1991). *CERCLA law and procedure.* Washington, DC: Bureau of National Affairs.

Munoz, H., & Rosenberg, R. (Eds.). (1993). *Difficult liaison: Trade and the environment in the Americas.* Miami: North-South Center, University of Miami.

Novick, S. (1987). The goals of environmental protection. In S. Novick (Ed.), *Law of environmental protection,* (Vol. 1, sec. 2.04). Deerfield, IL: Clark, Boardman, & Callaghan.

Office of Policy Planning and Evaluation, Environmental Protection Agency. (1988). *Environmental progress and challenges, EPA's update,* Publication No. EPA-230-07-88-033. Washington, DC: U. S. Government Printing Office.

Percival, R., Miller, S., Schroeder, C., & Leape, J. (1992). *Environmental regulation: Law, science, and policy* (pp. 141-153). Boston: Little, Brown.

Plater, Z., Abrams, R., & Goldfarb, W. (1992). *Environmental law and policy: Nature, law, and society.* St. Paul, MN: West Publishing.

Portney, P., Probst, K., & Finkel, A. (1991). The EPA at "thirtysomething." *Environmental Law, 21,* 1461.

Reed, P., Wyckoff, P., & Dee, P. (1992). In S. Novick (Ed.), *Law of environmental protection,* (Vol. 2, Chap. 11). Deerfield, IL: Clark, Boardman, & Callaghan.

Reitze, A. (1991). A century of air pollution control law: What's worked; What's failed; What might work. *Environmental Law, 21,* 1575-1581.

Schoenbaum, T., & Rosenberg, R. (1991). *Environmental policy law* (2nd ed.). Mineola, NY: Foundation Press.

Science Advisory Board, Environmental Protection Agency. (1990). *Reducing risk: Setting priorities and strategies for environmental protection,* Publication No. SAB-EC-90-021. Washington, DC: Author.

Stever, D. (1994a). *Law of chemical regulation and hazardous waste* (Vol. 1, Chap. 5). Deerfield, IL: Clark, Boardman, Callaghan.

Stever, D. (1994b). *Law of chemical regulation and hazardous waste* (Vol. 1, sec. 6.04-6.09). Deerfield, IL: Clark, Boardman, Callaghan.

Stever, D. (1994c). *Law of chemical regulation and hazardous waste* (Vol. 1, Chap. 2). Deerfield, IL: Clark, Boardman, Callaghan.

Thomas, M., & Novick, S. (1992). Oregon's air pollution statute. In S. Novick (Ed.), *Law of environmental protection,* (Vol. 1, sec. 2.02[3][a]). Deerfield, IL: Clark, Boardman, & Callaghan.

U. S. Department of Health and Human Services. (1991). Healthy people 2000: National health promotion and disease prevention objectives, Publication No. (PHS) 91-50212. Washington, DC: Author.

SUGGESTED READINGS

Anderson F. R., Mandelker, D. R., & Tarlock, A. D. (1990). *Environmental protection: Law and policy.* Boston: Little, Brown.

Arbuckle, J. G., Brownell, F. W., Case, D. R., et al . (1993). *Environmental law handbook* (12th Ed). Rockville, MD: Government Institutes, Inc.

Baldwin, M., & Page, J. K., Jr. (Eds.). (1970). *Law and the environment,* New York: Walkevane Company.

Bonine, J. E., & McGarity, T. O. (1992). *The law of environmental protection* (2nd ed.). St. Paul, MN: West Publishing Co.

Bosselman, F., & Callies, D. (1971). *The quiet revolution in land use control.* Washington, DC: Council on Environmental Quality.

Bosselman, F., Callies, D., & Banta, J. (1973). *The taking issue.* Washington, DC: Council on Environmental Quality.

Campbell-Mohn, C., Breen, B., & Futrell, J. W. (1993). *Environmental law from resources to recovery.* St. Paul, MN: West Publishing Co.

Council on Environmental Quality (1971-1993). *Annual report 1970 –1992,* Washington, DC: Author.

Dore, M. (1987). *Law of toxic torts.* Deerfield, IL: Clark Boardman Callaghan. (Supplemented Periodically).

Findley, R. W., & Farber, D. A. (1992). *Environmental law in a nutshell* (3rd ed.). St. Paul, MN: West Publishing Co.

Gaba, J. M., & Stever D. W. (1992). *Law of solid waste, pollution prevention and recycling.* Deerfield, IL: Clark Boardman Callaghan.

Garrett, T. L. (Ed.). (1992). *The environmental law manual.* Chicago, IL: American Bar Association.

Grad, F. P. (1973). *Treatise of environmental law.* New York: Matthew Bender and Co. (Supplemented Periodically).

Hays, S. P. (1987). *Beauty, health and permanence*. Cambridge: Cambridge University Press.

Landy, M. K., Roberts, M. J., & Thomas, S. R. (1990). *The Environmental Protection Agency: Asking the wrong questions*. New York: Oxford University Press.

Machlin, J. L., & Young, T. R. (1988). *Managing environmental risk*. Deerfield, IL: Clark Boardman Callaghan. (Supplemented Periodically).

Novick, S. M., Stever, D. W., & Mellon, M. G. (Eds.). (1987). *Law of Environmental protection*. Deerfield, IL: Clark Boardman Callaghan. (Supplemented Periodically).

Percival, R. V., Miller, A. S., Schroeder, C. H., & Leape, J. P. (1992). *Environmental regulation: Law, science, and policy*. Boston: Little, Brown.

Plater, Z. J. B., Abrams, R. H., & Goldfarb, W. (1992). *Environmental law and policy: Nature, law, and society*. St. Paul, MN: West Publishing Co.

Rodgers, W. H., Jr. (1994). *Environmental law* (2nd ed.). St. Paul, MN: West Publishing Co.

Sax, J. L. (1970). *Defending the environment*. New York: Knopf.

Schoenbaum, T. J., & Rosenberg, R. H. (1991). *Environmental policy law* (2nd ed.). Westbury, NY: Foundation Press.

Selmi, D. P., & Manaster, K. A. (1989). *State environmental law*. Deerfield, IL: Clark Boardman Callaghan.

Stever, D. W. (1986). *Law of chemical regulation and hazardous waste*. Deerfield, IL: Clark Boardman Callaghan. (Supplemented Periodically).

Stone, C. D. (1987). *Earth and other ethics*. New York: Harper and Row.

Vincoli, J. W. (1993). *Basic guide to environmental compliance*. New York: Van Nostrand Reinhold.

Chapter 9

Occupational Health

Linda R. Murray

Occupational health is a field that addresses issues of worker health and safety. Like the field of environmental health, it comprises many different disciplines and is practiced by a variety of professionals. The astute practitioner of occupational health is ever alert for unusual or new diseases that suggest toxic exposures that must be controlled, and for hazardous conditions in the workplace that, if prevented, can prevent injury and disease.

Ramazzini's treatise, *Diseases of Workers*, published in 1700, stands as an excellent description of diseases observed among workers. As Ramazzini (1713/1940, p. 7) points out in his preface:

> For we must admit that the workers in certain arts and crafts sometimes derive from them grave injuries, so that where they hoped for a subsistence that would prolong their lives and feed their families, they are too often repaid with the most dangerous diseases and finally, uttering curses on the profession to which they had devoted themselves, they desert their post among the living. While I was engaged in the practice of medicine, I observed that this very often happens, and so I have tried my utmost to compose a special treatise on the disease of workers.

Estimates indicate that in the United States from 6,000 to 12,000 workers die each year from occupational injuries. This means that about 25 workers die on the job each working day (Office of Technology Assessment [OTA], 1985)—and these estimates are conservative.

It is much more difficult to arrive at an accurate estimate for morbidity and mortality from occupational diseases as they are difficult to differentiate from diseases with other causes. Often, symptoms from occupational diseases develop after the worker has become disabled or retired, making it difficult to link the disease to the workplace. The most common estimates are that in the U. S. workforce of 100 million workers, about 125,000 to 400,000 new illnesses and from 50,000 to 100,000 deaths from work related disease occur each year (Morris-Chatta & Rosenstock, 1994). The National Safety Council estimates that a work-related death occurs every 47 minutes and a work-related injury occurs every 17 seconds. Verifiable estimates of incidence and mortality are not available, however, as there are no national surveillance systems for workplace injuries (Cullen, Cherniack, & Rosenstock, 1990).

In today's industrialized world, man-made changes affect the environment of our planet in ways never before imagined. The substances that contaminate the environment are the same ones that affect workers. In the workplace, however, the levels of exposures are usually several orders of magnitude greater than those seen in the general environment. Like it or not, we have turned our workplaces into giant experimental laboratories. It is here that the impact of toxic substances and environmental stresses appears in its starkest form.

HISTORY

Coal miners used to take bird cages with canaries down into the mines. If a canary was exposed to a pocket of methane gas, it would fall off its perch and the miners would run out of the mine. If the miners were lucky, they escaped before experiencing the same fate as the canary. Unfortunately, this has too often been the approach society has taken toward health and safety in the workplace.

One of the worst occupational disasters in the United States occurred during the 1930s in West Virginia (Cherniack, 1986). During the height of the Great Depression, thousands of workers—disproportionately black—were hired to dig a tunnel through rock of almost pure silica at Gauley Creek, West Virginia.

Although the company hired to dig the tunnel was well aware that silicosis was killing its workers, it took no precautions to protect them. A congressional investigation in 1936 estimated that at least

476 workers died from acute silico-proteinosis and at least another 1,500 developed chronic respiratory disease.

Our attitudes towards work can be traced back to feudal times. The relationships between lords and serfs, masters and servants, employers and employees had, until recently, the same philosophical underpinnings. Each party had certain responsibilities and obligations. The lord was supposed to be kindly, fair, and make the appropriate decisions for his serfs. The serfs, in exchange, were tied to the land, not permitted to move about freely and required to work solely for the lord.

In the United States many of our traditions, as well as common and case law, reflect these feudal relations. Until the mid-1900s the employer provided the necessary conditions (tools, buildings, etc.) to perform work, and it was expected that no abuse of the worker would take place. In exchange, the worker accepted the "natural risks" of the job.

In the early twentieth century it was widely known that workers in the felt hat industry were at risk for a variety of neurologic problems (they were nicknamed "mad hatters" and immortalized by the character in *Alice in Wonderland*). This disease was an accepted risk for hatters until the U.S. Public Health Service related it to mercury vapor that was released from animal fur being treated with a mixture of nitric acid and elemental mercury in the early stages of the felt-making process (Neal & Jones, 1938).

Boilermakers' deafness (from the noise of making and repairing boilers), miner's knee (arthritic changes in coal miners), death from cave-ins, and the drowning of sailors at sea have all been viewed as "natural disasters"—provident events that were accepted (preferably quietly) by workers.

The old concept that occupational disease and injury are "just part of the job" is unacceptable today. The realization that an industrial "accident" can become a tragic environmental disaster for thousands of people in a few short hours has changed society's perception of these problems. Unfortunately, these major disasters are not *accidents* at all. They are the result of technology being used with inadequate attention to the health and safety of workers and the potential devastating effects on the environment.

Such large-scale disasters do not happen simply because of one error. They happen because of a systemic failure to consider health and safety issues. If action is to be taken to prevent these large-scale disasters, we must develop much higher standards for routine health and safety procedures.

Today, people who work in our factories, offices, and mines are the "miners' canaries" for the rest of society. They are exposed to toxic chemicals, physical agents, and psychosocial hazards at higher levels than the general public. When we see workers becoming ill in the workplace, we should be warned that something is amiss. Everyone has a vital interest in occupational health and safety; this is not an issue about which only labor needs to be concerned. Toxic agents are "equal opportunity dangers"—they can appear in the factory or in our drinking water. Efforts to clean up the workplace are of critical concern to everyone.

RECOGNIZING OCCUPATIONAL HAZARDS

Unfortunately, most occupational and environmentally related diseases go unrecognized. There are several reasons for this. In general, there are no unique biological characteristics of diseases with an occupational etiology. For instance, occupational asthma does not look clinically different from extrinsic asthma.

Even when occupational and environmental risk factors are suspected, they may not be the only causes of disease. Many chronic diseases are multifactorial in nature. It is well established that cigarettes and asbestos each cause lung cancer. When combined, these two agents have a multiplicative effect on the risk for lung cancer (Rom, 1992; Seidman, Selikoff, & Hammond, 1979; Selikoff & Hammond, 1979; Selikoff, Hammond, & Churg, 1968).

Most physicians have received no training in environmental and occupational medicine and may be intimidated by the multitude of different possible exposures and potential hazards. It is unrealistic to expect anyone to memorize the health effects of the hundred thousand commonly used industrial chemicals. Moreover, many industrial processes use chemicals and create by-products whose toxicities have never been fully documented or understood. Today a clinician's memory can be assisted by many clearly written reference books on diseases caused by occupational and environmental exposures, and by a number of computer databases and software packages.

Table 9.1   A General Classification of Occupational Hazards

Types of Hazards

Biological

Chemical

Dust & mineral

Physical

Ergonomic

Psychosocial

There are six basic types of occupational hazards (Table 9.1). When taking an occupational history or performing a workplace hazard evaluation, questions should be asked about each job to determine potential hazards facing workers. When doing this, thinking about these categories helps identify possible occupational causes of illness. Knowing about hazards commonly associated with specific industries (Table 9.2) is also useful in eliciting a thorough occupational history from a patient.

Biological hazards include microorganisms that contaminate plants and animals and cause diseases in handlers of these products. Bacteria and fungi are used in industry to produce alcoholic beverages and to synthesize chemicals and drugs; they also contaminate many damp areas in the workplace. Occupations at high risk for biological hazards include healthcare workers, laboratory workers, veterinarians, animal handlers, meat cutters, agricultural workers, outdoor workers, pharmaceutical workers, and brewers. For instance, hepatitis B infections are seven times more common among hospital laboratory workers than the general population. Office workers in buildings that use recirculated air are also at increased risk for exposure to airborne microbes.

Zoonoses are infectious diseases spread from animals to humans. Brucellosis (undulant fever) is a gram-negative bacterial infection acquired from cattle, sheep, goats, and other animals. About 50% of the reported cases in the United States are occupationally acquired. Other occupational zoonoses include tularemia, leptospirosis, and ornithosis (Donham & Horvath, 1988).

Table 9.2 Health Hazards In Selected Industrial Processes

Process	Exposure
Abrasive blasting Surface treatment with high velocity spray containing such materials as sand, steel shot, pecan shells, glass, and aluminum oxide	Inhalation of these materials and paint dust; noise
Degreasing Removing grease and dirt from objects using solvents and other cleaners	Inhalation of vapors; thermal degradation of chemicals may produce phosgene, hydrogen chloride, or other toxins
Cold Solvent Washing Aliphatic and aromatic solvents	Skin contact may cause dermatitis and absorption of toxic chemicals
Vapor Degreasing Methyl chloroform, trichloroethylene, ethylene dichloride	Fire and explosion
Electroplating Coating materials with thin layers of metals (e.g., gold, silver, copper, nickel, cadmium, chromium)	Inhalation of acid mists, hydrogen, cyanide, and other mists; skin contact with acids, alkalis; ingestion of cyanide
Furnace operations Melting and refining metals; boilers	Noise, heat stress; cataracts from infrared radiation, inhalation of dusts containing metals and abrasive compounds
Machining Metals, plastics, or wood are worked and shaped with lathes, drills, planers, and milling machines	Noise; skin contact with toxic cutting oils and solvents; inhalation of metal particles, cutting oil mists, and nitrosamines
Paint spraying Applying liquids to surfaces	Inhalation of mists and vapors containing organic mercury, lead, and other toxic chemicals; dermatitis from skin contact with these chemicals
Welding and metal cutting Joining or cutting metals by heating them to molten or semi-molten state (e.g., arc welding, resistance welding, brazing)	Inhalation of metal fumes and gases; noise; eye and skin damage from infrared and ultraviolet radiation

Reprinted from Smith & Schneider (1995).

Chemical hazards are seen in heavy industry as well as in office environments. Some six million chemicals have been identified in industrial processes, and at least 100,000 are used widely. Furthermore, several hundred new chemicals are introduced into the industrial environment each year.

Only a small fraction of these chemicals have been studied for possible environmental and health effects. The relation between organic solvents and health problems, for example, is not yet fully understood. On the other hand, chemicals like the heavy metals lead and mercury have been known for centuries to be poisonous, and their effects are fairly well understood.

Dust and mineral hazards include coal dust, asbestos, silica, cotton dust, and a variety of other substances. Many have caused debilitating chronic lung diseases in miners and factory workers. *Physical hazards* comprise ionizing and nonionizing radiation, heat, cold, humidity, noise, and vibration.

A wide range of problems that stem from the design and organization of work stations and production processes are classified as *ergonomic hazards*. For instance, computer work may cause back pain and a poorly designed hand tool may increase the risk for carpal tunnel syndrome.

Psychosocial hazards include issues of responsibility and autonomy in the organization and management of production. Occupationally related stress can be caused by the absence of worker representation by unions or other forms of worker representation, excessive reliance on part-time workers, and the single most prevalent occupational hazard in the United States—unemployment.

LEADING WORK-RELATED DISEASES AND INJURIES

The National Institute for Occupational Safety and Health (NIOSH) has developed a list of ten groups of diseases considered to be the leading causes of occupational morbidity and mortality (Table 9.3). This list is now being used to guide national research in safety and health.

Table 9.3   The National Institute of Occupational Safety and Health's Ten Leading Work-Related Diseases and Injuries

1.	Occupational lung diseases
2.	Musculoskeletal injuries
3.	Occupational cancers
4.	Occupational injuries
5.	Cardiovascular disorders
6.	Disorders of reproduction
7.	Neurotoxic disorders
8.	Noise-induced hearing loss
9.	Dermatologic conditions
10.	Psychological disorders

Occupational Lung Diseases

The respiratory tract is the major route of entry for most toxic agents. The damage suffered by the lungs can be acute and life threatening (asphyxiation, for example), or can result in chronic and insidious disabilities such as chronic obstructive pulmonary disease.

Asphyxiation.   Simple respiratory asphyxiants (Chapter 4) that are common in the workplace include carbon dioxide, nitrogen, and methane. Carbon dioxide (CO_2) is heavier than air and may build up in confined spaces. Methane (CH_4) is common in underground coal mines, and causes explosions as well as asphyxiation.

Chemical asphyxiants are also common in industry. Carbon monoxide is a ubiquitous product of combustion and is produced in many industries. Cyanide salts are commonly used in tanning, electroplating, metallurgy, and photography. Cyanide interferes with the cytochrome oxidase enzyme system, causing metabolic asphyxiation. Hydrogen sulfide is produced in the rubber industry, tanneries, coal mines, sewage treatment plants, commercial fishing, and petroleum refineries. It is toxic to the respiratory center of the brain and can cause respiratory paralysis.

Irritation.   Many gases and fumes are directly toxic to the cells that line the airways (Table 9.4). The actual symptoms they produce

Table 9.4   Chemicals That Produce Acute Airway Injury

Chemical	Occupations or Products
Acrolein	Plastics, rubber, textile
Ammonia	Chemical industry, fertilizer production
Chlorine	Pulp and paper mills, plastics, chlorinated hydrocarbons
Hydrogen chloride	Dye-making, chemical industry, petroleum refining
Hydrogen fluoride	Manufacture of solvents, refrigerants, plastics, photographic film, chemicals
Metallic mercury fumes	Mining, electrolysis
Nickel, nickel carbonyl	Electroplating
Osmium tetroxide	Chemical and metal industries
Ozone	Arc welding, air, sewage and water treatment plants
Phosgene	Chemical industry, dye making, pesticide manufacture
Sulfur dioxide	Chemical industry, refrigeration, bleaching
Vanadium	Iron, steel, and chemical industries
Zinc chloride fumes	Soldering, textile finishing

depend in large measure on their solubility in water, their concentration, and the duration of exposure. Gases that are highly soluble (e.g., ammonia, hydrogen chloride, and hydrogen fluoride) can produce irritation and edema in the upper airways. Moderately soluble gases like chlorine, fluorine, and sulfur dioxide usually affect the lower respiratory tract. Compared with soluble gases, those that are only slightly soluble (e.g., oxides of nitrogen, ozone, and phosgene) are more likely to cause extensive damage to cells.

One of the earliest examples of a disease caused by a pulmonary irritant is silo filler's disease, which was described by Ramazzini (1713/1940, p. 245):

> Another thing to wonder at is why such a noxious exhalation is given off from wheat that has been kept for a long time in a confined space.... It is enough to kill anyone who steps inside such a storage space to take out the corn, unless he leaves the cover open for a while and lets the poisonous air escape.

When grain is stored in silos or any confined space, microbial decomposition produces the irritant gas nitrogen dioxide (NO_2). This reaction runs its course in a few weeks, and the period of highest NO_2 concentrations is within two weeks after a silo has been filled.

Fume Fevers. Metal fume fever is caused by the oxides of metal fumes produced during welding, soldering, smelting, refining, and by furnaces. This syndrome has been linked to a wide range of metals, including zinc, copper, cadmium, and magnesium. Symptoms occur several hours after initial exposure, and include fever, myalgia, headache, and fatigue; they disappear in about 36 hours.

Polymer fume fever is caused by pyrolysis products of polytetrafluorethylene (PTFE), which is sold under the trade names Teflon, Fluon, and Halon. As with metal fume fever, the syndrome is characterized by a variety of symptoms, including chest pain, dry cough, myalgias, fever, chills, headache, and sore throat. The onset and duration of the acute phase of polymer fume fever are also similar to those for metal fume fever, but the former may cause severe pulmonary edema. Polymer fume fever may also produce interstitial fibrosis. The pathogenesis of both syndromes is poorly understood.

Interstitial Fibrosis. *Coal worker's pneumoconiosis* (CWP or black lung) is a fibrotic disease of the lung parenchyma produced by coal dust, graphite, or carbon black. The disease is most commonly seen in underground coal miners but has also been documented in surface workers. The early phases of simple CWP are usually asymptomatic. Gradually, symptoms of chronic bronchitis develop. With time, *progressive massive fibrosis* (PMF) may develop, and large irregular opacities may be seen on x-ray. Patients with PMF develop severe respiratory impairment, and eventually respiratory failure. There is a separate disability process for CWP under the Mine

Safety and Health Act of 1977, but many coal miners with CWP have been denied compensation.

Asbestos and crystalline silica (silicon dioxide) are among the best known causes of pulmonary fibrosis, however, a wide variety of other silicates (talc, kaolin or "china clay," and "ball clay," for instance) can also cause pulmonary fibrosis.

Crystalline silica produces silicosis, the oldest known occupational lung disease. Silica dust is a hazard in many kinds of mining, stone and quarry work, ceramics, foundries, abrasive blasting, and the production of refractory bricks for furnaces. Acute silicosis can develop and progress after only a few months' exposure. The chest X-ray of a patient with acute silicosis has a "ground glass" appearance. Chronic silicosis, classified as either simple or complicated, takes years to develop, and may first appear or progress even after exposure to silica has stopped. The radiographic features of simple silicosis include small opacities and eggshell calcifications of the hilar lymph nodes. In complicated silicosis, there is aggregation of small nodules into lesions that may encroach on airways or vessels.

Asbestos causes inflammation and fibrosis of the lung parenchyma and increases the risk for cancer of the lung, pleura, and peritoneum. This mineral fiber has been widely used in cement products such as pipes, tiles, and roofing in the construction industry for insulation and fireproofing, in heat-resistant textiles, in friction materials (brake linings and pads), and in paints and fillers. Although no longer used in shipbuilding and construction, many workers are still exposed, including those engaged in removing asbestos from old buildings.

Acute Airway Constriction. It is estimated that at least 200 compounds cause occupational asthma and bronchial hypersensitivity reactions (Bardana, Montanaro, & O'Hollaren, 1992). Such acute airway constriction can be divided into four general categories.

Reflex bronchoconstriction most often occurs in workers with preexisting asthma and is triggered by nonspecific stimuli (e.g., cold air or inert dusts). *Inflammatory bronchoconstriction* is usually a reaction to a high concentration of a chemical. Workers exposed to high levels of hydrogen sulfide, fumes from the production of plastics, diethylene diamine, chlorine, or ammonia sometimes develop inflammatory bronchoconstriction. Wheezing usually begins within hours of exposure and may last for several months.

The agents that produce *pharmacological bronchoconstriction* show a dose–response relation between the magnitude of exposure and the severity of bronchoconstriction. Such agents do not cause eosinophilia or nonspecific bronchial hyperactivity. Byssinosis, caused by the dust of cotton, flax, or hemp, is one example. The prevalence of byssinosis in the cotton industry depends on the dust levels generated in the different phases of production. For example, workers in the carding process where dust levels are high are more likely to develop byssinosis than those in other processes such as spinning.

In countries where the dust levels are higher than in the United States, as many as 90% of workers have been shown to have symptoms. The longer the exposure to cotton dust, the higher the prevalence of byssinosis. Organophosphate pesticides also elicit pharmacological bronchoconstriction.

Immunologic or *allergic bronchoconstriction* is caused by a diverse group of agents. Animal dander, grain dusts, certain enzymes (such as proteolytic enzymes used in detergents), metals (nickel and vanadium, for instance), urea formaldehyde, and many other agents cause occupational asthma. The percentage of the exposed workers who develop asthma varies, depending on the agent and the magnitude of exposure. For example, some surveys indicate the majority of bakers in family-owned bakeries eventually develop baker's asthma, whereas asthma is diagnosed in about 5%–10% of workers exposed to toluene diisocyanate (TDI).

Lung Cancer. Because the lung is the most common cancer site in the United States, it is worth noting some occupational causes (Table 9.5). Among the most notorious is asbestos. Other known pulmonary carcinogens and the workers exposed to them include chromium (metal workers), coal tar (chemical workers), arsenic (metal, glass, and pesticide workers) and radon gas (uranium miners). Secondary tobacco smoke may also be a factor in those workplaces that have not yet banned smoking in common areas.

Musculoskeletal Disorders

Ramazzini (1713/1940, p. 15) recognized occupationally related musculoskeletal disorders by noting that in one type of workplace there were "...certain violent and irregular motions and unnatural pos-

Table 9.5   Respiratory Carcinogens in the Workplace

Exposure	Process or Exposure Setting
Arsenic trioxide, arsenates, arsenites	Smelting (copper, lead, zinc); arsenical pesticide production
Asbestos	Insulation, construction, cement products
Chloroethers	Chemical production, fungicides, bactericides
Chromates	Mining, chromate production, chromate pigments, leather manufacturing, electroplating
Coal carbonization, coal tar pitch, volatile organics	Coke ovens, rubber production, roofing
Nitrogen mustard gas	Production of chemical warfare agents
Nickel dust and fumes	Nickel refining, smelting, electroplating
Radiation (radon daughters)	Uranium mining, hard rock mining

tures of the body, by reason of which the natural structure of the vital machine is so impaired that serious diseases gradually develop therefrom." Throughout the literature of medicine, fanciful names have been attached to a variety of cumulative trauma disorders such as coal miner's knee, cotton twisters hand, carpenter's elbow, and stitcher's wrist.

Musculoskeletal disorders rank second only to cardiovascular disease as the most frequent cause of disability. Moreover, they are the second most frequent reason for visits to physicians, the fifth most frequent reason for visits to hospitals, and the third most frequent reason for surgery. It is estimated that some 23 million American workers have some sort of musculoskeletal impairment (Parniapour, Nordin, Skovron, & Franklin, 1990). They are also the

Occupational *cumulative trauma disorders* have several common features. They are characterized by persistent or recurrent pain, fatigue, and eventually a decline in work performance. There are relatively few specific laboratory or radiographic features of findings for persons with these disorders and their treatment is uncertain and generally produces poor results. These disorders cause a great deal of absenteeism and often result in job loss for the worker (Putz–Anderson, 1988).

Cumulative trauma disorders have three clinical stages. In stage one, which usually lasts from weeks to months, workers note aching and fatigue during work, but these symptoms improve overnight or with rest. There are usually no physical signs of the disorder and no reduction in work performance. Damage in this first stage is likely to be reversible.

During stage two, aching and tiredness increase and persist for a longer period of time, often for months. Physical signs may be present and patients often complain of sleep disturbances. Rehabilitation is usually needed to return people to work.

The third clinical stage lasts from months to years. There is aching and fatigue at rest and chronic pain is a frequent complaint. Sleep disturbances and difficulty performing nonoccupational tasks are also common. There is often severe psychological stress and a disruption of social life. Medical treatment is palliative and workers are usually incapable of performing repetitive work.

Prevention of musculoskeletal disorders requires some understanding of their etiology. Causes include lack of appropriate supervision, inadequate training, and work that is performed without rest breaks (NIOSH, 1981). Piecework, bonus systems, and overtime incentives can also increase rates of cumulative trauma disorders.

The biomechanical contributory factors are posture, tool design, workplace design, rate of production, frequency of repetitive motions, and the force, speed and direction of movements. With a meat processor making 12,000 cuts per day, a data entry clerk typing 20,000 key strokes an hour, or an assembly line worker lifting above shoulder height 7,500 times a day, it is easy to appreciate how common musculoskeletal syndromes have become.

Carpal tunnel syndrome is the most common of the *entrapment disorders.* Any process that produces pressure on the median nerve as it passes through the carpal tunnel in the wrist will produce the syndrome. Other common entrapment syndromes include compression of the ulnar nerve in the cubital tunnel and the brachial plexus in the shoulder (Feldman, Goldman, & Keyserling, 1983).

Lower back syndromes affect the majority of the population at some time in their lives. Back pain accounts for about 25% of lost time among material handlers. However, it is possible to correlate an acute injury with only 15% of cases. Degenerative disc disease is probably the major etiological factor in occupationally related back disease.

Ergonomics is a multidisciplinary field that looks at the interaction of human movement with equipment and the work environment. Ergonomic principles can be used to design seats and work surfaces that are adjustable to fit different people (Moore & Garg, 1992).

Situations that require holding an object in a fixed position or sitting or standing in a fixed position should be eliminated. Furthermore, work positions can be designed so that most muscles are in neutral positions (Chaffin & Anderson, 1984). For example, work requiring the elbows to be above the mid-torso will cause pain and joint problems in the shoulders and wrists. Hand-held tools can be designed to be used with muscles and joints in neutral positions. Vibration can also be damped, and the amount of muscle force required to operate the equipment can be reduced.

CANCER

In 1775 Percival Pott reported an outbreak of scrotal cancer in young chimney sweeps in England. According to the tradition of the day, the chimney sweeps were all young boys who climbed inside the chimneys to clean. Generally they worked nude because this caused less wear and tear on what was often their only set of clothes.

Without epidemiologic studies, and with no idea of the carcinogenic agent, Pott was still able to make some suggestions to prevent scrotal cancer. First he suggested that the sweeps be given a second set of clothing and not be allowed to sweep nude. Second he suggested that the sweeps be allowed to wash after cleaning each chimney. Both of these suggestions met with great opposition in England and scrotal cancer continued as a significant cause of death among sweeps.

In Holland, however, these preventive measures were adopted and the incidence of scrotal cancer in chimney sweeps dropped. These early lessons in the prevention of occupationally related cancers are still important today. For example, workers in refineries and coke ovens continue to be exposed to the same carcinogen, benzo(a)pyrene.

Cancer is the second leading cause of death in the U.S., accounting for almost 475,000 deaths (about 20% of all deaths) annually. It has been estimated that the percentage of human cancer that may be attributed to environmental factors (i.e., those considered not genetic) is from 60%–90%. However, smoking, diet, and lifestyle are thought to be responsible for most of the nongenetic causes. The percentage of human cancer with an occupational etiology has been estimated to be between 1% and 10% (Hermo, 1987).

The International Agency for Research on Cancer has identified more than 50 chemicals or industrial processes for which there is sufficient evidence to support that they are causally related to human cancer and around 250 for which there is evidence that they are either probable or possible human carcinogens (Vainio & Wilbourn, 1992). Among the most notorious is vinyl chloride monomer, used in making plastic and a cause of liver cancer. Asbestos, in addition to causing lung cancer, causes mesothelioma, a tumor that is extremely rare in persons not exposed to asbestos.

Traumatic Injuries and Deaths

In the United States, the Bureau of Labor Statistics is charged with keeping account of occupationally related accidents. Despite the apparent ease of tracking deaths on the job, one–third of the occupationally–related deaths are missed by this surveillance system (Pollack & Keimig, 1987).

It is estimated that each year there are 400,000 occupational fractures, 21,000 occupational amputations, one million occupational eye injuries, and one million episodes of occupationally related back pain (NIOSH, 1989; OTA, 1985). Over the past decade, the number of deaths in private sector businesses employing more than 11 workers has varied between 3,000 and 5,000 fatalities per year. For those businesses that employ fewer than 11 workers the number is around

1,000. Annual estimates of occupational fatalities for the years 1979–1983 vary between about 3,700 and 12,200, depending on the data source and research methods (OTA, 1985). From 1980 to 1989, NIOSH reported 63,589 deaths from occupational injuries, an average of 17 per day (CDC, 1994; NIOSH, 1993).

Motor vehicle crashes are by far the leading cause of occupational fatalities, accounting for 23% of deaths from 1980 to 1989. Other frequent causes of death are machine-related injuries (14%), homicides (12%), falls (10%), electrocutions (7%), and being struck by a falling object (7%) (CDC, 1994; NIOSH, 1993). Four workforce sectors, together representing only 14% of all workers, accounted for 57% of all occupational fatalities in 1989. These sectors are: construction (20%), transportation and public utilities (13%), agriculture, forestry, and fishing (13%), and manufacturing (11%) (Moeller, 1992).

The most dangerous U. S. industries in the period 1981–1989, as measured by the number of deaths per 100,000 workers, were mining (31.9); construction (25.6); transportation, communication and public utilities (23.3); and agriculture, forestry, and fishing (18.3) (CDC, 1994; NIOSH, 1993).

Eye Injuries

Some surveys indicate that at least 70% of all eye injuries occur in the workplace. Industrial operations such as grinding and abrading often result in dust and debris entering the eye. Compressed air lines, if they rupture, can blow particles into the eye with great force. Most foreign body injuries are superficial and are caused by small particles lodged in the conjunctiva. These particles can abrade the cornea; if the abrasion covers a small area, complete healing usually occurs within 24–48 hours. Iron-containing foreign bodies can produce cataracts.

Blunt trauma can cause contusions to the eye, injury to the eyelids and surrounding tissue, corneal edema, and hemorrhage into the anterior chamber. Such injuries can also lead to glaucoma, dislocation of the lens, cataract formation, and retinal damage.

Penetrating injuries by foreign objects are serious emergencies and account for 1%–4% of all eye injuries. Acid or alkali splashes are also common industrial emergencies. The amount of damage depends on the pH of the liquid and the length of time it is in contact with the eye. Some acids are particularly dangerous; for example, concentrated nitric acid causes immediate opacification of the cornea.

Strong alkali burns are more dangerous than acid burns. Plasterers using a lime-based mixture are at particular risk because plaster is alkaline enough to cause severe tissue damage and clumps of plaster are difficult to remove from the eye with simple water irrigation (Pfister & Koski, 1982). Eyes must be flushed with water immediately if damage is to be prevented.

A wide range of other chemical substances such as detergents, ketones, and organic solvents can cause similar damage (Grant, 1986). Workplace eye injuries should be prevented rather than treated. Requiring and enforcing protective eyewear use and careful workplace design are the most effective preventive measures.

Exposure to infrared or ultraviolet radiation can damage the lens and produce cataracts. Glassblower's cataracts—a classic occupational disease—are caused by infrared damage to the anterior surface of the lens. Workers who view molten metal or molten glass for hours at a time are at risk for this type of cataract and require protective eyewear.

Photokeratoconjunctivitis (welder's flash) occurs when welders or other workers view ultraviolet light. Usually there are few, if any, symptoms in the first few hours following exposure; after this period, however, the damaged corneal epithelium sloughs and the worker experiences acute pain. Welder's flash can be prevented by using protective filters in eyewear; shields and curtains in the workplace protect neighboring workers. Exposure to bright visible light from welding arcs or bright sunlight may also produce retinal damage and visual impairment.

Cardiovascular Disease

The role that environmental and occupational toxicants may play in heart disease has not been well studied. Both halogenated and non-halogenated solvents have been implicated in cardiac arrhythmias and sudden death. Most of the evidence comes from studies of drug abusers who inhaled glue or solvents such as toluene or acetone, and from reports of single cases in occupational settings.

The halogenated solvents (e.g., 1,1,1-trichloroethane and trichlorethylene) and the chlorofluorocarbons (e.g., freon) are most often implicated in occupational arrhythmias. These solvents are used in a wide variety of cleansing and degreasing processes as well as refrigerants and propellants.

Some industrial chemicals, such as cadmium and lead, have been implicated in the development of hypertension (Batuman, Landy, Maesaka & Wedeen, 1983; Rosenman, 1979, 1984). Noise acutely raises blood pressure, though the role of chronic noise in hypertension is not fully understood.

Carbon disulfide is a widely used solvent that has been associated with atherosclerosis in both animals and humans. Workers exposed to carbon disulfide have a 2.5- to 5-fold increased risk for death from coronary artery disease (Beauchamp, Bus, Popp, Boreiko, & Goldberg, 1981; Sweetnam, Taylor, & Elwood, 1987).

Exposure to carbon monoxide or methylene chloride (which is metabolized to carbon monoxide in the body) may precipitate arrhythmias in patients with compromised coronary circulation. Carbon monoxide is perhaps the most ubiquitous of all occupational toxins, being present wherever combustion occurs. Mechanics, foundry workers, forklift operators, and garage attendants are some of the workers who are at high risk for exposure to this gas.

Nitrates, especially ethylene glycol dinitrate and nitroglycerin, have caused myocardial infarction and sudden death in ammunition workers. Nitrates induce vasodilation of coronary arteries and withdrawal produces compensatory vasoconstriction and coronary vasospasm. Young healthy workers exposed to nitrates during munitions manufacturing experienced chest pain (Monday-morning angina) and some had myocardial infarctions during vacations when they were away from nitrates for 48–72 hours. A cohort of Swedish workers had a 2- to 3-fold increase in the relative risk for death from heart disease after 20 years of exposure to nitrates, suggesting that cardiac damage was cumulative and permanent (Hogstedt & Axelson, 1977; Hogstedt & Andersson, 1979).

Arsenic, cobalt, and lead cause cardiovascular disease. Workers exposed to inorganic arsenic (for instance, while applying pesticides and working in smelters) also show increased rates of peripheral vascular disease (Rosenman, 1984).

Vibration produced by drills and other hand-held tools causes Raynaud's disease, a vasospastic disorder. The incidence of this disease ranges as high as 50–80% in some groups of workers. At greatest risk are lumbermen, jackhammer drillers in mines, chippers, and grinders. This problem can be greatly reduced or eliminated with better engineering to dampen vibrations.

Reproductive Disorders

Men working in industries with exposures to lead and synthetic estrogens have experienced suppression of testosterone secretion. Spermatogenesis is a continuous cycle, taking about 74 days and producing millions of sperm per day. This process can be disrupted or stopped by a number of occupational exposures, including those that alter hormone concentrations.

In the 1970s, azoospermia was documented in nine of 11 workers exposed to the nematocide 1,2-dibromo-3-chloropropane (DBCP) for more than 3 years. Follow-up studies indicated that most workers had not recovered even 5 to 8 years following exposure (Whorton & Foliart, 1983).

A number of studies suggest an inverse relationship between blood lead levels and sperm counts. Spermatogenesis has been shown to be adversely affected by carbon disulfide, naphthyl methylcarbamate, heat, and high doses of ionizing radiation. Animal studies have implicated an even longer list of chemicals that depress spermatogenesis, including arsenic, benzene, boron, cadmium, ethylene dibromide, ethylene glycol ethers, ethylene oxide, halothane, mercury, nitrous oxide, polybrominated biphenyls (PBBs), trichloroethylene, and others.

The risks to women from occupational hazards have been studied far less than those for men. Women working in hospitals are at risk of exposure to ethylene oxide—a gas used to sterilize instruments—or to anticancer drugs. Both of these agents have been shown to cause spontaneous abortions (Hemminki, Mutanen, Saloniemi, Niemi, & Vainio, 1982; Selevan, Lindbohm, & Hornung, 1985). In addition, anesthetic agents such as nitrous oxide have been linked to subfertility or spontaneous abortion (Gold & Tomich, 1994; Rowland et al., 1992). Women in other occupations may be exposed to known teratogens, such as PCBs, ionizing radiation, organic mercury, or solvents used in laboratories. Pregnant women exposed to PCBs have been shown to give birth to lower-weight infants than women not so exposed (Taylor, et al., 1984).

Historically, management response to the exposure of men to workplace reproductive hazards has been to remove the hazard. When women are exposed, however, the response used to be to remove the workers. Hence, women were sometimes excluded from certain jobs unless they had been sterilized or were otherwise infertile. In the United States, this type of discrimination has been determined to be illegal under the federal civil rights law (Filkins & Kerr, 1993; Perrolle, 1993).

Neurologic Disorders

Neurologic effects of occupational exposures have been known for centuries. Pliny described lead palsy in the first century A.D. Unfortunately, little is known about the neurotoxic effects of most industrial chemicals and even for those chemicals known to be neurotoxins (Table 9.6), there may not be agreement on the dose and length of exposure required to cause specific effects.

Chemical exposures usually cause a mixed sensorimotor neuropathy in the peripheral nervous system. The symptoms are nonspecific and include weakness, numbness, and tingling. Occasionally a chemical will cause a unique syndrome. For example, neurogenic bladder with retention and sexual dysfunction has been described in a group of workers exposed to dimethylaminopropionitrile (DMAPN), a chemical used as a catalyst in the chemical industry. Some symptoms, like motor neuropathy in lead-exposed workers, are seen only in workers with high body burdens of lead. Movement disorders such as parkinsonism may be produced by exposure to carbon disulfide, carbon monoxide, and manganese.

Over one million U.S. workers are exposed to organic solvents, which are widely used as degreasing and cleaning agents. Organic solvents are usually mixed with other chemicals, and exposures cause mild narcosis, irritability, and difficulty with concentration. Occasionally more severe impairments or encephalopathy may result.

Table 9.6 Health Effects of Selected Occupational Neurotoxins

Neurologic Effects	Toxins
Acute psychosis, marked emotional instability	Carbon disulfide, manganese, toluene
Ataxic gait	Acrylamide, chlordane, chlordecone (kepone), DDT, n-hexane, manganese, metallic and methyl mercury, methyl-n-butyl ketone (MBK), methylchloride, toluene
Bladder neuropathy	Dimethylaminopropionitrile (DMAPN)
Constricted visual fields	Metallic mercury
Cranial neuropathy	Carbon disulfide, trichloroethylene
Headache	Lead, nickel
Impaired psychomotor function	Carbon disulfide, lead, mercury, organophosphate insecticides, perchloroethylene and other solvents, styrene
Impaired visual acuity	N-hexane, mercury, methanol
Increased intracranial pressure	Lead, organotin compounds
Memory impairment	Arsenic, carbon disulfide, lead, manganese
Mixed sensorimotor neuropathy	Acrylamide, arsenic, carbon disulfide, carbon monoxide, DDT n-hexane and methyl-n-butyl ketone (MBK), mercury
Motor neuropathy	Lead
Myoclonus	Benzene hexachloride, metallic mercury
Neurasthenia, irritability, and other mild systemic symptoms	Acrylamide, arsenic, lead, manganese, metallic mercury, methyl-n-butyl ketone (MBK), organotin compounds, solvents, styrene
Nystagmus	Metallic mercury
Opsoclonus	Chlordecone (Kepone)
Paraplegia	Organotin compounds
Parkinsonism	Carbon disulfide, carbon monoxide, manganese
Seizures	Lead, organic mercury, organochlorine insecticides, organotin compounds
Tremor	Carbon disulfide,chlordecone (kepone), DDT, manganese

From Baker (1988).

Hearing Loss

Head trauma, explosions, and extremely loud noises can result in *acoustical trauma.* If the impacting sound is of sufficient energy, the tympanic membrane may be ruptured and ossicles of the middle ear fractured or dislocated. Immediate pain and loss of hearing usually follows such exposure.

After exposure to excess noise, workers often experience a *temporary threshold shift* (TTS) caused by metabolic fatigue of the cochlear hairs. This *noise-induced hearing loss* results in a temporary loss of hearing, and a number of hours may elapse before a return to baseline. A simple sign of TTS is the need for workers to turn up their car radios while driving home from work, even though they could hear the radio at a lower volume on the way in to work.

Chronic exposure to high noise levels causes gradual loss of hearing and communication ability. This often first appears as the inability to understand human conversation in the presence of background noise (e.g., at parties or in bars). As the hearing loss progresses, the ability to hear at conversational frequencies decreases. The earliest loss occurs between the frequencies of 3,000 and 6,000 Hertz. Once noise-induced hearing loss has occurred, it is irreversible.

The most effective method for preventing hearing loss is by reducing noise in the workplace with design changes in equipment and production processes. Machinery and operations can be designed to greatly reduce noise. In the case of older machines and operations, measures can be taken to isolate noise sources by enclosing them with baffles and other structures. The use of hearing protection (ear plugs and muffs) by individual workers is the least effective and least desirable method of preventing hearing loss but affords more protection than engineering solutions in some cases.

Protecting workers from hearing loss also depends on careful monitoring of noise exposure. Noise is defined as unwanted sound. Vibrations in an elastic media such as air transmit pressure variations that impinge on the eardrum and produce the sensation we call sound. Sound can be measured as pressure, intensity, and energy density. The most common measure of sound is the *sound pressure level.* The *decibel* (dB) is the unit of measure for sound pressure levels and is defined as ten times the logarithm (base 10) of the ratio between the measured sound pressure and a reference sound pressure, which is the average faintest sound that can be heard. Zero dB, therefore, is the faintest sound the human ear can detect. Because the decibel is a logarithmic measure, each increase in 3 dB represents a doubling of sound energy.

Because the human ear is more sensitive to high-frequency sounds than to low–frequency sounds, the high–frequency sounds are louder than lower–frequency sounds of the same sound pressure. Therefore, a weighting method has been devised to compare sound pressure levels at different frequencies. There are three different weighting schemes that have been accepted internationally: the A-network for low sound pressure levels, the B-network for medium sound pressure levels, and the C-network for high levels (Olishifski, 1988). The scaled sound pressure level is termed the *sound level*, the unit that is commonly used to measure noise in the workplace. Because it best represents the frequencies that damage human hearing, the A-weighted sound level measurement (in units abbreviated *dBA*) has been adopted by U. S. governmental agencies and professional associations.

The Occupational Safety and Health Administration (OSHA) has set the standard for the maximum allowable workplace noise as the noise dose that would result from continuous exposure to a sound level of 90 dBA for an 8-hour work day. To account for variable magnitudes in exposure throughout the work day, OSHA established a method for determining compliance with the 90 dBA permissible exposure level based on halving exposure time for each increase in 5 dBA above 90 dBA.

This approach allows a worker to be exposed for 4 hours to a sound level of 95 dBA, for 2 hours at 100 dB, or for 1 hour at 105 dB, as long as the exposures at other sound levels during the rest of the workday are below the specified exposure durations. It is not clear that this arbitrary dose–response relation is protective, and many have argued for halving exposure time in 3 dBA increments instead.

The OSHA Noise Standard also specifies that no worker can be exposed to a peak sound pressure level greater than 140 dB, no matter how short the period, or to continuous noise greater than 115 dBA. The Hearing Conservation Amendment to the OSHA Noise Standard requires that a hearing conservation program be implemented for employees who have exposures to sound levels that average 85 dBA. The amendment applies to all industries except those involved in drilling oil or gas wells, or in the servicing of such operations. The components of a hearing conservation program include audiometric testing, workplace monitoring of noise levels, the availability of hearing protectors, employee training, and record keeping (Olishifski, 1989).

For several years NIOSH and other organizations have recommended strengthening the noise standard to a time-weighted average of 85 dB for an 8-hour workday. Some studies estimate that over a working lifetime of 40 years, between 21% and 29% of workers would suffer significant hearing loss at 90 dB compared with between 5% and 15% at 85 dB and a negligible portion at 80 dB (Suter, 1988).

Dermatologic Disorders

The skin makes up about 6% of body weight and covers an average of 20 square feet. In 1991, skin diseases accounted for 16% of reported occupational diseases in the private sector according to the Bureau of Labor Statistics (1993).

Contact dermatitis appears as drying and cracking of the skin after a prolonged period of repeated exposures. The most common cause of occupational contact dermatitis is solvents, followed by soaps, detergents, and cleaners. Surfactants in cleaning solutions can dissolve skin lipids and keratin and erode the epidermis. Agents such as borax, sawdust, and pumice, which are added to cleaning solutions for their abrasive qualities, also damage the skin. Fiberglass can also irritate and inflame the skin.

Allergic contact dermatitis is an immunologically mediated reaction that accounts for as much as 20% of occupational contact dermatitis. There is a wide range of sensitizing agents. Rubber "accelerators" and antioxidants often cause problems for workers in the rubber and tire industries and for those who wear rubber protective clothing. Metal salts (gold, nickel, chromium, and cobalt) frequently sensitize workers in the electroplating and polishing industries, as well as cement workers, hairdressers, and electronic assemblers. A wide range of chemicals used in the plastics industry, particularly epoxy resins, also induce allergic contact dermatitis.

Contact urticaria (hives) may follow exposure to animal dander, urine, or saliva. Workers in shellfish processing commonly report this dermatologic disorder.

Occupational acne comprises common acne and the rarer *chloracne*, which is characterized by comedones, papules, milia and cysts. This disorder is seen after systemic exposure to chlorinated hydrocarbons—especially dioxins and polychlorinated biphenyls (PCBs) (Chapter 4). It is severe and often disabling, lasting for years after exposure has ended. Occasionally peripheral neuropathies and hepatotoxicity are seen with chloracne.

Oils and fats, particularly cutting oils, obstruct hair follicles and cause an acneiform rash in workers with chronic exposure. Mechanical pressure (e.g., truck drivers sitting for long periods of time) can induce acne lesions on the buttocks or other areas of the skin.

There are many *pigmentation disorders* (stains of the skin) that are traditional stigmata of certain occupations. Dyes, acids, and heavy metals used in such processes as smelting, roofing, construction, and tanning often stain the skin by binding with the keratin layer.

A variety of different agents cause hyperpigmentation. Furnace and oven workers often have dark and mottled skin in areas exposed to heat. Halogenated aromatic hydrocarbons, arsenic, and many phototoxins (tetracycline, polyaromatic hydrocarbons, and printing inks, for example) also cause a darkening of the skin. Hydroquinone (a chemical used in photography) and many phenols (used in resins and germicides) cause occupational vitiligo.

Agricultural and other outdoor workers are at high risk for skin cancer, as are X-ray and nuclear medicine technicians. Inorganic arsenic has also been shown to cause skin cancer in chemical workers and gold miners. Hair loss can be caused by chemicals such as thallium, sodium borate, ionizing radiation, trauma, and chemical burns.

Vibration-induced "white finger" occurs in workers with a history of exposure to vibration (e.g., lumberjacks, construction workers, foundry workers, and miners). The repetitive pressure from vibrating equipment compromises the microvasculature of the hand and fingers and alters control of local blood flow. Blanching usually occurs, but severe cases can lead to tissue destruction and loss of digits.

The most effective way to prevent skin injuries is to eliminate exposures by substitution or control. The use of protective clothing such as gloves and aprons is probably the most common method of prevention in industry. Such equipment may actually contribute to injury and disease, however. For example, rubber gloves may cause an allergic dermatitis, and increased sweat entrapment and friction can cause irritative dermatitis. Creams applied to the skin to form a "chemical barrier" have not proved effective.

Psychosocial Hazards

Unemployment and Underemployment. The most prevalent occupational hazard in most countries—particularly among minority groups—is unemployment. In countries with market-oriented economies, unemployment levels are allowed to rise and fall as a method of economic readjustment. Many economists and politicians prefer unemployment to inflation and consider moderate levels of unemployment necessary for economic stability. This is not the case, however, in some countries. Sweden, for example, has a long-standing policy of full employment. Even with generous pension, welfare, and unemployment benefits, Swedes remain concerned about the detrimental impact of unemployment on health.

Unemployment is a relatively new feature of human life. Although popular belief often places the blame for being unemployed on the individual, unemployment is a by-product of specific economic and social policies in industrial society. Moreover, high unemployment rates favor management and make it difficult for unions to effectively represent their members.

Workers who are unemployed, or threatened with unemployment, suffer from a number of health problems related to psychological stress. Studies have documented a greater prevalence of gastrointestinal symptoms, high blood pressure, headaches, insomnia, and cardiovascular problems among the unemployed than among the employed (Sperounis, Miller, & Levenstein, 1988). Brenner (1977, 1979) linked unemployment in the United States and Great Britain to increases in mortality from cardiovascular and liver disease, suicide, and murder, as well as to increases in admissions to psychiatric hospitals and prisons.

Kasl and Cobb (1980) conducted a series of studies on plant closings. They and other researchers identified the following stages of the unemployment cycle. The *preanticipation* phase begins with rumors of plant closing or layoffs circulating among the workers.

During this stage, researchers have measured increases in blood pressure that have persisted several months after new jobs have been found. Additionally, there are physiological responses associated with stress, including changes in blood sugar concentrations, increases in gastric acid secretion, and altered release of hormones and neurotransmitters.

The *point of separation phase* is the time when workers actually lose their jobs. At this time there may be a brief period of relief because the anxiety and uncertainty about losing a job has been settled. The *exhaustion of benefits phase* begins when a worker's family has depleted its unemployment benefits and resources. Separation, divorce, and other family crises are frequent during this phase.

In many ways, the *intensive job search phase* is the most damaging to the individual worker's well-being. The inability to find a job may radically devalue the worker's self-esteem. Some become *discarded workers*, who are unlikely ever to find jobs. Older and younger workers and minorities are at high risk for this category. During *adjustment to a new job*, at least half of workers on new jobs will be paid at rates lower than they formerly received. Some workers' families may never recover from the financial troubles incurred during unemployment.

From 1979 to 1984, some 11.5 million U. S. workers over the age of 20 lost jobs as a result of layoffs and plant closings. Some 5.1 million of these persons had worked at least 3 years on the same job. In the group of displaced workers with less than 3 years on the job (Flaim & Sehgal, 1985), black and Hispanic workers were overrepresented. Among those who remained unemployed, over half exhausted their unemployment benefits, lost their health insurance, or both.

In the 1980s unemployment among blacks was about 14%–15% and among Hispanics, about 10%, compared with about 6% among whites (Esutia & Prieto, 1987). Underemployment is also a growing problem in the United States. Increasingly, employers use part-time workers to help control costs. Part-time employees are generally paid less and often enjoy few or no fringe benefits. In a number of surveys among the nation's homeless, 5%–10% were employed full-time and another 10%–20% were employed part-time or episodically (Committee on Health Care for Homeless People, 1988).

Shift and Night Work. Over the past 25 years, the number of people engaged in night and irregular shift work has increased. In addition to jobs in public safety and industries with 24-hour production schedules, other workplaces, such as those in the financial sector, have begun night work. In the United States about 26% of men and 18% of women are employed in some form of variable shift work (Gordon, Clearly, Parker, & Czeisler, 1986).

It is well-established that a wide range of biological processes (e.g., hormone secretion, body temperature, and blood pressure) follow circadian patterns. However, the interaction between endogenous rhythms and workplace conditions is not well understood. Exposure to bright light has a strong influence on circadian rhythms and can be used to adjust them (Czeisler et al., 1990). The complaints of shift workers fall into three categories: sleep disturbances, health complaints, and psychosocial effects.

Perhaps the most common complaint of night and shift workers is disruption of sleep patterns. This may explain the shift differential seen in studies of injury rates. In a study of truck drivers, the risk of having a crash between midnight and 2:00 AM was twice the rate for other periods (Hamelin, 1987). Most workers sleep at night on their days off. Night-shift workers get the least amount of sleep, afternoon-shift workers sleep the most, whereas regular day-shift workers fall in between these two groups (Monk, 1990).

The most prevalent problem of shift workers is gastrointestinal complaints, which are estimated to be 34% more frequent in this group than in those who work regular daytime hours (Scott & LaDou, 1990). There is conflicting information on whether or not shift workers consume caffeine, alcohol, and tobacco more heavily than other workers.

Some studies suggest an association between shift work and cardiovascular diseases (Scott & LaDou, 1990). Furthermore, shift work disrupts social and family life and may contribute to divorce, social isolation, depression, malaise, and personality changes. These symptoms can appear suddenly, even in workers who are long-time shift workers. Perhaps the ability to adjust to night and shift work decreases with age.

Stress in the Workplace. Intuitively, people think that job-related stress has an impact on health. In fact, research in the area of stress is difficult to conduct and there is no consensus on the appropriate ways to measure stress. There are several competing models for describing occupational stress.

One model, the Person-Environmental Fit Model postulates that stress is produced as the subjective response of the individual worker to an objective relationship between the worker and the environment. Another model, the Job Demands Control Model suggests that stress is produced by the worker's inability to have control over work tasks (Baker & Karasek, 1994).

The strategies suggested for stress reduction and prevention by the two models are quite different. The Person-Environment Fit model suggests that stress is reduced by placing persons in jobs that are appropriate for their personalities, or by modifying the behavior of individual workers. The Job-Demand Model suggests that treating the organization of production is the best way to reduce stress.

Stressors in the workplace fall into three broad categories: job tasks, work organization, and extra-organizational factors. Stressors related to the job tasks include variable work schedules, length of work, pace of work, the degree to which a worker has control over his/her work, and physical conditions (heat, light, noise) on the job. Stressors related to the organization of work include interpersonal relationships among workers and the roles of workers in the management of production. Extra-organizational stressors include factors like the degree to which job security is assured and the extent to which workers can formulate and achieve their personal career goals.

REGULATING WORKPLACE HAZARDS

The attempt to control hazards in the workplace has a long and uneven history in the United States. One of the first measures to regulate health and safety was the introduction of standards for the manufacture of boilers. These regulations were put in place by the insurance industry and had to be met before it would insure a workplace against fire and explosion. The fact that workers were protected by this policy was merely a coincidence.

By the late 1800s, common law held that it was the duty of employers to furnish safe work tools, to exercise due care in production practices, and to warn workers of any "unusual" hazards. Even in those instances where workers attempted to go to court, employers were excused if they could show that there was negligence by other workers, that the injured worker knowingly accepted the risk, or that the injured worker was negligent.

In 1877 the State of Massachusetts passed the first factory inspection law in the United States. This legislation attempted to regulate fire exits, the safety of gears and belts, and inspection of elevators. In the early 1900s the social reformers of the Progressive Era and the growing labor movement began to agitate for improved working conditions. In 1907 a major mine disaster at Monongah, West Virginia resulted in the deaths of 362 miners. This disaster helped galvanize the pressures needed to create the U.S. Bureau of Mines in 1910.

Wisconsin passed the first worker's compensation legislation in 1911 and by 1921 most states had some kind of worker's compensation insurance. Under Roosevelt's New Deal, Frances Perkins was appointed Secretary of Labor and became the first woman to hold a cabinet-level post. During her term she established the Bureau of Labor Standards and directed this agency to address health and safety issues.

The Walsh-Healy Act was passed by Congress in 1936 to regulate workplaces with federal contracts that exceeded $10,000 and provided for direct federal involvement in the regulation of workplace safety and health. In 1968, 78 miners were killed by an explosion in a mine in Farmington, West Virginia. This tragedy and a resulting miner's strike for health and safety issues helped force stalled mine safety legislation through Congress, leading to the Coal Mine Health and Safety Act of 1969. It was amended in 1977 to create the Mine Safety and Health Administration (MSHA), which regulates radiation exposure and safety in mines and in the processing and milling of uranium ore.

The 1970 Occupational Health and Safety Act was passed in order to prevent occupational injuries and illnesses. This act assigns two basic duties to every employer: to comply with all standards created under the act and to maintain a workplace free from recognized hazards that are causing or are likely to cause death or serious physical harm to employees.

The Occupational Safety and Health Administration (OSHA) was created by the 1970 Occupational Safety and Health Act. OSHA is part of the U.S. Department of Labor and is charged with setting and enforcing occupational safety and health regulations and standards. It is empowered to engage in inspections and investigations, to require the maintenance of certain medical and industrial hygiene records, and to establish federal supervision of state workplace safety programs. The process of setting standards for specific hazards is long and cumbersome, and often controversial. Standards, of course, do not guarantee that workers will be free of disease.

NIOSH is a part of the CDC and is charged with the responsibility of leading national research efforts in occupational health and safety. In addition, this agency plays a major role in the training of safety and health professionals. NIOSH researchers also investigate safety and health hazards in U.S. industries and recommend standards to OSHA for implementation and regulation.

THE OCCUPATIONAL HEALTH OF SPECIAL POPULATIONS

Workers of Color

In the United States persons of color are disproportionately employed in the lowest paying jobs and industries, even when education, skills, and language are taken into account. In general, jobs in the service, agricultural, and production sectors are more dangerous than others, and African-American and Latino workers are overrepresented in each of these areas (Friedman-Jimenez, 1989).

One of the classic studies detailing occupational hazards among steel workers uncovered a significantly increased risk of lung cancer among African-American workers (Lloyd, 1971; Redmond, Ciocco, Lloyd, & Rush, 1972). The excess occurred primarily among workers in the coke oven department. Men who worked at the side of the ovens demonstrated a 1.7-fold increase in lung cancer compared with a seven-fold increase for those who worked at the top and a ten-fold increase for topside coke oven workers with more than 5 years of exposure. Working on top of coke ovens is one of the hottest, dirtiest, least desirable, and most dangerous jobs in a steel mill. Even though only one-third of steel workers in the coke oven department were classified as "nonwhite," 70% of the topside oven workers and 88% of topside oven workers with more than 5 years experience were black.

Similar patterns exist in other industries. In the rubber and textile industries, African-American workers disproportionately work in the dustier areas. About 50% of migrant farm workers are Hispanic and about 30% are African-American (Davis, 1980; Davis & Rowland, 1983).

On the basis of scarce data, the probability that minorities will be employed in hazardous jobs has been estimated to be between 37% and 52%. Studies suggest that black workers have a 37% greater chance of experiencing an occupationally related injury or illness, a 50% greater chance of being severely disabled from it, and a 20% greater risk for dying from it (Kottlechuck, 1977, 1979; Robinson, 1984).

Women

Eighty-four percent of all women workers are employed in the service sector. Over 50% of women over age 16 are in the workforce; they compose over 40% of the total workforce. About 20% of all working women are women of color. Almost a quarter of all working women work part-time, but it is estimated that 60% of these workers would prefer full-time employment.

Working women have several special occupational safety and health problems. Many experience hazards associated with jobs in which women are disproportionately represented (e.g., health care, teaching, laundry and dry cleaning, office work). Other hazards result from the use of tools and equipment that were designed for use by men (Klitzman, Silverstein, Punnet, & Mock, 1990).

Women are also subjected to a variety of work-related stresses. Many have chief or sole domestic family responsibilities, even though they are employed full-time outside the home. Women may be subjected to sexual harassment on the job; those in male-dominated occupations may suffer from gender discrimination. Occupations in which women predominate tend to be those in which workers have the least control over decision making, such as clerical and secretarial work. This lack of control may be the chief determinant of work-related stress (Baker & Karasek, 1994).

Agricultural Workers

In the United States there are from 2.5 to 4.1 million agricultural workers—most of whom are immigrants and people of color who perform seasonal work (Fenske & Simcox, 1994). According to some estimates, there may be as many as 500,000 to one million undocumented migrant workers in the U.S.

Workers in agriculture have a number of special health and safety problems related to such factors as climate, topography, specific crops, farming practices, and the economy. This population includes many women, children, and persons over the age of 65 who must work in jobs designed for young males.

Self-employed farmers often have no medical benefits and are not covered by workers' compensation. Farm workers are excluded from most labor legislation and protection, and only a small number are organized into labor unions. Rapid technological changes in farming adversely affect the social, economic, and political climates of farming communities and constantly create new health and safety hazards (Donham & Horvath, 1988).

In 1992 the rate of nonfatal occupational injuries among U. S. agricultural workers was 11.0 per 100 full-time workers—second only to the rate of 12.9 per 100 for construction workers (Bureau of Labor Statistics, 1993); and many experts think that farming injuries are underestimated by as much as 50%. Fatalities from farm machinery increased 44% in the 50-year period from 1930 to 1980. In 1991 the death rate for U. S. agricultural workers was 44 per 100,000—the highest for all industries, including construction (31 per 100,000) (National Safety Council, 1992). One of the leading causes of death among farmers is tractor roll-overs. In Sweden mandatory requirements for roll-over protection on tractors have resulted in a dramatic decline in fatalities from these accidents (Merchant, Kross, Donham, & Pratt, 1989).

Children under the age of 16 account for as much as 16% of the agricultural workforce in the United States (Fenske & Simcox, 1994). In agriculture, some 23,500 adolescents and children are injured each year and almost 300 die (Wilk, 1993). Injuries involving machinery, most commonly tractors, accounted for one-third of all deaths in children and almost 50% of the deaths in children under age ten (Rivara, 1985).

Several studies have documented increased noise-induced hearing loss among farmers and their families (Marvel, Pratt, Marvel, Regan, & May, 1991). Farmers are also exposed to whole-body vibration from heavy equipment. Studies in Sweden (Thelin, 1990) indicate that degenerative diseases, particularly of the upper extremities, the lower back, and knees are caused by this vibration. A recent study of U. S. farmers found cardiovascular diseases, arthritis, and amputations to be more prevalent among farmers than among other workers (Brackbill, Cameron, & Behrens, 1994).

Some studies indicate that suicide rates are highest in urban communities and isolated rural communities. High rates of depression and suicide may also be related to adverse weather and economic conditions. The close integration of home and business also may place special stress on farm families (Pratt & May, 1994).

Diseases transmitted from animals to humans (zoonoses) represent a special problem among agricultural workers. Agricultural workers—particularly those in Third-World countries—are also exposed to toxic fertilizers and pesticides. Although the acute effects of pesticides are usually well documented, the effects from chronic exposures are often not known—making it difficult to diagnose and prevent diseases from such exposures (Chapter 4).

PREVENTING DISEASE AND INJURY

Limiting Risks in the Workplace

Many environmental and occupational diseases are preventable. In the workplace there is a hierarchy of methods for controlling hazards, listed in order of their desirability and effectiveness:

1. Contain the hazard at its source or provide a safe substitute;
2. Interrupt the transmission of the hazard from its source;
3. Control the hazard in the local environment of the individual worker.

As specified above, the most effective way to deal with occupational and environmental health hazards is to eliminate them. For instance, asbestos can be replaced by less toxic materials. In the sandblasting industry, silica can be replaced with other materials, eliminating the risk for silicosis. Hazards like noise and vibration can be significantly reduced by changes in workplace and equipment design.

If a safer substitute is not reasonable, engineering controls may isolate or buffer the process from the worker. For example, a very dusty area like the shake-out department in a foundry may be automated and completely enclosed, eliminating silica exposure to workers and reducing their risk for silicosis. In a similar way, extremely dangerous work like handling radioactive materials can be performed with mechanical devices or robots in a completely enclosed setting.

Ventilation, special hoods, sound barriers, and sprinkler systems are examples of engineering controls that interrupt the transmission of hazardous materials from their sources to the workers. For example, local ventilation systems properly engineered and maintained can greatly reduce cotton dust levels and the incidence of byssinosis in the textile industry.

Attempting to control exposure at the level of the individual worker is the least effective approach. So-called "administrative" controls, where workers are rotated in and out of hazardous areas, are of questionable value and ethics. Such practices have been used in the nuclear industry to keep workers from receiving radiation doses higher than annual regulatory limits. Personal protective equipment such as gloves, respirators, goggles, and hard hats vary a great deal in their effectiveness and are often not used, or are misused, by workers.

Complying with regulations, installing engineering controls, and using appropriate protective equipment will not guarantee that workers are protected from occupational disease and injury. There is also a continuing need for research and surveillance to identify workplace hazards and for using the results to pass legislation to maintain and improve the health protection of workers.

Professionals in Occupational Health

The best way to assure health and safety in the workplace is by educating and training workers and making managers at every level responsible for promoting and enforcing safe work practices. Implementing this approach usually requires the combined efforts of a number of specialists in occupational health and safety. In large workforces, such specialists may be employed full-time; smaller businesses and industries may consult these professionals periodically.

Industrial hygienists are trained to recognize and measure workplace exposures to toxic agents and to determine the most effective ways to reduce exposures in order to comply with regulations and to minimize risks to workers (Berry, 1988; Smith & Schneider, 1994).

By understanding industrial processes and the ways by which they place workers at risk, industrial hygienists can also anticipate and prevent problems associated with new processes.

The role of the industrial hygienist in the workplace is similar to that of the environmental scientist who works on problems of reducing environmental contamination and human exposures to environmental agents. Industrial hygienists receive training in a variety of scientific fields including chemistry, physics, biology, engineering, and medicine (Berry, 1988).

Experts in occupational safety or *safety professionals* have a variety of educational backgrounds. To focus on preventing occupational injuries, they are trained in areas of systems safety analysis, human factors, engineering, biomechanics, ergonomics, and product safety (McLean, 1988). The work of safety professionals overlaps with that of industrial hygienists, though the former emphasize preventing unexpected incidents that result in injury, illness, or property damage. Safety professionals identify and assess hazardous conditions and practices, develop methods for controlling hazards, develop ways to communicate with workers and management on how to control hazards, and implement strategies to measure the effectiveness of a safety program.

Occupational health nursing is another profession dedicated to the health and safety of the worker (Cornyn, 1988). Occupational health nurses work on the front lines and may be the only medically trained personnel in the workplace on a routine basis; they are usually the first to evaluate occupational illnesses or injuries, and are often responsible for the day-to-day coordination of the services of other occupational health professionals—particularly for those services needed by individual workers. Occupational health nurses also coordinate and manage health education and counseling programs in the workplace.

Occupational medicine became a specialized discipline in the field of preventive medicine in the mid–1950s. It is estimated that of the 450,000 physicians in the United States, only about 10,000 (2.2%) work in the field of occupational health and safety. Of these, around 1,000 have had formal training or certification in occupational medicine. Specialists in occupational medicine are usually responsible for managing a team of health professionals and therefore must have in-depth knowledge of industrial hygiene, toxicology, epidemiology, and the environmental sciences, as well as the medical problems that are unique to workers.

In a survey of U.S. medical schools in 1982, only 66% offered course work in occupational medicine, and the median time a medical student spent studying occupational medicine was four hours (Levy, 1980, 1985). There is no indication that this training has been expanded in the 1990s. All physicians and nurses—especially primary care providers—see patients with occupational injuries and diseases. Whether or not they are able to recognize them as such may have a profound effect on diagnosis, treatment, and prevention.

REFERENCES

Baker, D. B., & Karasek, R. A. (1994): Occupational stress. In B. S. Levy & D. H. Wegman (Eds.), *Occupational health: Recognizing and preventing work-related disease* (3rd ed.) (pp. 381-406). Boston: Little, Brown.

Baker, E. L. (1994). Disorders of the nervous system. In B. S. Levy & D. H. Wegman (Eds.), *Occupational health: Recognizing and preventing work-related disease* (3rd ed.) (pp. 519-541). Boston: Little, Brown.

Bardana, E. J., Montanaro, A., & O'Hollaren, M. T. (1992). *Occupational asthma*. Philadelphia: Hanley & Belfus.

Batuman, V., Landy, E., Maesaka, J. K., & Wedeen, R. P. (1983). Contribution of lead to hypertension with renal impairment. *New England Journal of Medicine, 309,* 17-21.

Beauchamp, R. O., Bus, J. S., Popp, J. A., Boreiko, C. A., & Goldberg, L. A. (1981). Critical Review of the literature on carbon disulfide toxicity. *CRC Critical Reviews in Toxicology, 11,* 169-278.

Berry, C. M. (1988). The industrial hygienist. In B. A. Plog (Ed.), *Fundamentals of industrial hygiene* (3rd ed.).Washington, DC: National Safety Council.

Brackbill, R. M., Cameron, L. L., & Behrens, V. (1994). Prevalence of chronic diseases and impairments among U. S. farmers. *American Journal of Epidemiology, 139,* 1055-1065.

Brenner, M. H. (1977). Health costs and benefits of economic policy. *International Journal of Health Services, 7,* 581-623.

Brenner, M.H. (1979). Mortality and the national economy. A review, and the experience of England and Wales, 1936-76. *Lancet, 2*(8142), 568-573.

Bureau of Labor Statistics. (1993). *Occupational injuries and illnesses in the*

United States by industry, 1991. Washington, DC: U. S. Department of Labor.

Centers for Disease Control and Prevention. (1994). Occupational injury deaths—United States, 1980-1989. *Morbidity and Mortality Weekly Report, 43*, 262-264.

Chaffin, D. B., & Anderson, G. (1984). *Occupational biomechanics*. New York: Wiley.

Cherniack, M. (1986). *The Hawk's Nest incident: America's worst industrial disaster*. New Haven, CT: Yale University Press.

Committee on Health Care for Homeless People, Institute of Medicine. (1988). *Homelessness, health, and human needs*. Washington, DC: National Academy Press.

Cornyn, J. M. (1988). The occupational health nurse. In B. A. Plog (Ed.), *Fundamentals of industrial hygiene* (3rd ed.). Washington, DC: National Safety Council.

Cullen, M. R., Cherniack, M. G., & Rosenstock, L. (1990). Occupational medicine. *New England Journal of Medicine, 322*, 594-600.

Czeisler, C. A., Johnson, M. P., Duffy, J. F., Brown, E. N., Ronda, J. M., & Kronauer, R. E. (1990). Exposure to bright light and darkness to treat physiologic maladaptation to night work. *New England Journal of Medicine, 322*, 1253-1259.

Davis, M. E. (1980). The impact of workplace safety and health on black workers: Assessment and prognosis. *Labor Law Journal, 31*, 723 - 732.

Davis, M. E., Rowland, A. S., Walker, B., & Taylor, A. K. (1994). Minority workers. In B. S. Levy & D. H. Wegman (Eds.), *Occupational health: Recognizing and preventing work-related disease* (pp. 639-649). Boston: Little, Brown.

Esutia, M., & Prieto, M. (1987). *Hispanics in the workforce. Part III*. National Council of La Raza, Washington, DC.

Feldman, R. G., Goldman, R., & Keyserling, W. M. (1983). Peripheral nerve entrapment syndrome and ergonomic factors. *American Journal of Industrial Medicine, 4*, 661-681.

Fenske, R., & Simcox, N. J. (1994). Agricultural workers. In B. S. Levy & D. H. Wegman (Eds.), *Occupational health: Recognizing and preventing work-related disease* (3rd ed.) (pp. 381-406). Boston: Little, Brown.

Filkins, K., & Kerr, M. J. (1993). Occupational reproductive health risks. *Occupational Medicine: State of the Art Reviews, 8*, 733-754.

Flaim, P., & Sehgal, E. (1985). *Displaced workers, 1979-1983*. Washington, DC: Bureau of Labor Statistics, U.S. Department of Labor.

Friedman-Jimenez, G. (1989). Occupational disease among minority workers. *AAOHN Journal, 37*, 64-70.

Gold, E. B., & Tomich, E. (1994). Occupational hazards to fertility and pregnancy outcome. *Occupational Medicine: State of the Art Reviews, 9,* 435-469.

Gordon, N. P., Clearly, P. D., Parker, C. E., & Czeisler, C. A. (1986). The prevalence and health impact of shiftwork. *American Journal of Public Health , 76,* 1225- 1228.

Grant, W. M. (1986). *Toxicology of the eye* (3rd ed.). New York: Thomas.

Hamelin, P. (1987). Lorry driver's time habits in work and their involvement in traffic accidents. *Ergonomics, 30,* 1323-1333.

Hemminki, K., Mutanen, P., Saloniemi, I., Niemi, M-L, & Vainio, H. (1982). Spontaneous abortions in hospital staff engaged in sterilizing instruments with chemical agents. *British Medical Journal, 285,* 1461-1463.

Hermo, H. (1987). Chemical carcinogenesis: Tumor initiation and promotion. *Occupational Medicine: State of the Art Reviews, 2,* 1-25.

Hogstedt, C., & Andersson, K. (1979). A cohort study of mortality among dynamite workers. *Journal of Occupational Medicine, 21,* 553-556.

Hogstedt, C., & Axelson, O. (1977). Nitroglycerine-nitroglycol exposure and mortality in cardio-cerebrovascular diseases among dynamite workers. *Journal of Occupational Medicine, 19,* 675-678.

Kasl S. V., & Cobb S. (1980). The experience of losing a job: Some effects on cardiovascular functioning. *Psychotherapy and Psychosomatics, 34,* 88-109.

Klitzman, S., Silverstein, B., Punnet, L., & Mock, A. (1990). A women's occupational health agenda for the 1990s. *New Solutions, 1,* 7-17.

Kottlechuck, D. (1977). Work, race and health. *Health Pac Bulletin, No. 78* September-October), 19-20.

Kottlechuck, D. (1979). Occupational injuries and illness among black workers. *Health Pac Bulletin, Nos. 81-82,* 33-34.

Levy, B. (1980). The teaching of occupational health in American medical schools. *Journal of Medical Education, 55,* 18-22.

Levy, B. (1985). The teaching of occupational health in U.S. medical schools. Five year follow-up of an initial survey. *American Journal of Public Health, 75,* 79-80.

Lloyd, W. J. (1971). Long-term mortality study of steelworkers. V: Respiratory cancer in coke plant workers. *Journal of Occupational Medicine, 13,* 53-68.

Marvel, M. E., Pratt, D. S., Marvel, L. H., Regan, M., & May, J. J. (1991). Occupational hearing loss in New York dairy farmers. *American Journal of Industrial Medicine, 20,* 517-531.

McLean, W. T. (1988). The safety professional. In B. A. Plog (Ed.), *Fundamentals of industrial hygiene* (3rd ed.).Washington, DC: National Safety Council.

Merchant, J. A., Kross, B. C., Donham, K. J., & Pratt, D. S. (1989). *Agriculture at risk, a report to the nation; agricultural, occupational, and environmental health: Policy strategies for the future*, Washington, DC: National Coalition for Agricultural Safety and Health.

Moeller, D. W. (1992). *Environmental health*. Cambridge, MA: Harvard University Press.

Monk, T. H. (1990). Shiftwork performance. *Occupational Medicine: State of the Art Reviews, 5,* 183-198.

Morris-Chatta, R., & Rosenstock, L. (1994). Nature and magnitude of occupational and environmental disease. In L. Rosenstock & M. Cullen (Eds.),*Textbook of clinical occupational and environmental medicine* (2nd ed.). Philadelphia: Saunders.

Moore, J. S., & Garg, A. (Eds.). (1992). *Ergonomics:Low back-pain, carpal tunnel syndrome, and upper extremity disorders in the workplace.* Philadelphia: Hanley & Belfus.

National Institute for Occupational Safety and Health. (1981). *Work practices guide for manual lifting* (DHHS Publication No. NIOSH 89-122). Washington, DC: U. S. Department of Health and Human Services.

National Institute for Occupational Safety and Health. (1993). *Fatal injuries to workers in the United States, 1980-1989: A decade of surveillance, national and state profiles.* (DHHS Publication No. (NIOSH)93-108S). Morgantown, WV: Author.

National Safety Council. (1992). *Accident facts, 1992 ed.* Chicago: Author

Neal, P. A., & Jones, R. R. (1938). Chronic mercurialism in hatters' fur-cutting industry. *JAMA, 110,* 337-343.

Office of Technology Assessment. (1985). *Preventing illness and injury in the workplace* (Report No. OTA-H-256). Washington, DC: Author.

Olishifski, J. B. (1988). Industrial noise. In B. A. Plog (Ed.), *Fundamentals of industrial hygiene* (3rd ed.) (pp. 163-203). Washington, DC: National Safety Council.

Parniapour, M., Nordin, M., Skovron, M. L., & Frankel, V. H. (1990). Environmental induced disorders of the musculoskeletal system. *Medical Clinics of North America, 74,* 347-357.

Perrolle, J. A. (1993). Reproductive hazards: A model protection policy for the chemical industry. *Occupational Medicine: State of the Art Reviews, 8,* 755-786.

Pfister, R. R., & Koski, J. (1982). Alkali burns of the eye; pathophysiology and treatment. *Southern Medical Journal, 75,* 417-22.

Pollack, E. S., & Keimig, D. G. (Eds.). (1987). *Counting injuries and illnesses in the workplace: Proposals for a better system.* Washington, DC: National Academy Press.

Pratt, D., & May, J. (1994). Agricultural occupational medicine. In C. Zenz, O. B. Dickerson, & E. P. Horvath (Eds.), *Occupational medicine: Principles and practice* (3rd ed.). St. Louis, MO: Mosby.

Putz-Anderson, V. (Ed.). (1988). *Cumulative trauma disorders: A manual for musculoskeletal diseases of the upper limbs.* New York: Taylor & Francis.

Ramazzini, B. (1713). *De morbis artificum (Diseases of workers) (*1940 translation) W. C. Wright (Trans.). Chicago: University of Chicago Press.

Redmond, C. K., Ciocco, A., Lloyd, J. W., & Rush, H. W. (1972). Long-term mortality study of steelworkers. VI: Mortality from malignant neoplasms among coke oven workers. *Journal of Occupational Medicine, 14,* 621-629.

Rivara, F. P. (1985). Fatal and nonfatal farm injuries to children and adolescents in the United States. *Pediatrics, 76,* 567-573.

Robinson J. C. (1984). Racial inequality and the probability of occupation-related injury or illness. *Milbank Memorial Fund Quarterly; Health and Society, 62,* 567-590.

Rom, W. (1992). Asbestos-related diseases. In W. Rom (Ed.), *Environmental and occupational medicine* (2nd ed.), (pp. 269-291). Boston: Little, Brown.

Rosenman, K. D. (1979). Cardiovascular diseases and environmental exposure. *British Journal of Industrial Medicine, 36,* 85-97.

Rosenman, K. D. (1984). Cardiovascular disease and work place exposures. *Archives of Environmental Health, 39,* 218-224.

Rowland, A. S., Baird, D. D., Weinberg, C. R., Shore, D. L., Shy, C. M., & Wilcox, A. J. (1992). Reduced fertility among women employed as dental assistants exposed to high levels of nitrous oxide. *New England Journal of Medicine, 327,* 993-997.

Scott, A. J., & LaDou, J. (1990). Shiftwork: Effects on sleep and health with recommendations for medical surveillance and screening. *Occupational Medicine: State of the Art Reviews, 5,* 183-198.

Seidman, H., Selikoff, I. J., & Hammond, E. C. (1979) Short-term asbestos work exposure and long-term observation. *Annals of the New York Academy of Science, 330,* 61-89.

Selevan, S. G., Lindbohm, M-L, Hornung, R. W., & Hemminki, K. (1985). A study of occupational exposure to antineoplastic drugs and fetal loss in nurses. *New England Journal of Medicine, 313,* 1174-1181.

Selikoff, I. J., & Hammond, E. C. (1979). Asbestosis and smoking. *JAMA, 242,* 458-459.

Selikoff, I. J., Hammond, E. C., & Churg, J. (1968). Asbestos exposure, smoking and neoplasia. *JAMA, 204,* 106-112.

Selikoff, I. J., Hammond, E. C. & Seidman, H. (1979). Mortality experience of insulation workers in the United States and Canada, 1943-1976. *Journal of the New York Academy of Sciences*, 330, 91-116.

Smith, T. J., & Schneider, T. (1994). Occupational hygiene. In B. S. Levy & D. H. Wegman (Eds.), *Occupational health: Recognizing and preventing work-related disease* (3rd ed.) (pp. 125-144). Boston: Little, Brown.

Sperounis, F. P., Miller, L. M., & Levenstein, C. (1988). The American workplace: A sociological perspective. In B. S. Levy & D. H. Wegman (Eds.), *Occupational health: Recognizing and preventing work-related disease* (2nd. ed.) (pp. 15-26). Boston: Little, Brown & Co.

Suter, A. H. (1988). The development of federal noise standards and damage risk criteria. In D. M. Lipscom (Ed.), *Hearing conservation in industry, schools, and the military* (pp. 45-66). London: Taylor & Francis.

Sweetnam, P. M., Taylor, S. W., & Elwood, P. C. (1987). Exposure to carbon disulphide and ischemic heart disease in a viscose rayon factory. *British Journal of Industrial Medicine, 44,* 220-227.

Taylor, P. R., Lawrence, C. E., Hwang, H-L, & Paulson, A. S. (1984). Polychlorinated biphenyls: Influence on birthweight and gestation. *American Journal of Public Health, 74,* 1153-1154.

Thelin, A. (1990). Hip joint arthrosis: An occupational disorder among farmers. *American Journal of Industrial Medicine, 18,* 339-343.

Vainio, H., & Wilbourn, J. (1992). Identification of carcinogens within the IARC monograph program. *Scandinavian Journal of Worker and Environmental Health, 18*(Suppl.), 64.

Whorton, M. D., & Foliart, D. E. (1983). Mutagenicity, carcinogenicity, and reproductive effects of dibromochloropropane (DBCP). *Mutation Research, 123,* 13-30.

Wilk, V. (1993). Health hazards to children in agriculture. *American Journal of Industrial Medicine, 24,* 283-290.

SUGGESTED READINGS

Adams, R. M. (1983). *Occupational skin disease.* New York: Grune & Stratton.

American Conference of Governmental Industrial Hygienists. (1994). *1994-1995 threshold limit values for chemical substances and physical agents and biological exposure indices.* Cincinnati: Author.

Bardana, E. J., Montanaro, A., & O'Hollaren, M. T. (Eds.). (1992). *Occupational asthma.* Philadelphia: Hanley & Belfus.

Burgess, W.A. (1981). *Recognition of health hazards in industry.* New York: Wiley.

Checkoway, H., Pearce, N., & Crawford-Brown, D. J. (1989). *Research methods in occupational epidemiology.* New York: Oxford University Press.

Cralley, L. J., Cralley, L. V., & Harris, R. L. (Eds.). (1993). *Patty's industrial hygiene and toxicology, volume IIIA. Theory and rationale of industrial hygiene practice* (3rd ed.). New York: Wiley.

Finkel, A. J. (Ed.). (1983). *Hamilton and Hardy's industrial toxicology* (4th ed.). St. Louis: Mosby Year Book.

Grandjean, E. (1984). *Proceedings of the International Scientific Conference on Ergonomic and Health Aspects in Modern Offices, Turin, Italy.* New York: Taylor & Francis.

Haddad, L. M., & Winchester, J. (1990). *Clinical management of poisoning and drug overdose* (2nd ed.). New York: Saunders.

Hawkins, N. C., Norwood, S. K., & Rock, J. C. (Eds.). (1991). *A strategy for occupational exposure assessment.* Akron, OH: American Industrial Hygiene Association.

LaDou, J. (1990). *Occupational medicine.* Norwalk, CT: Appleton & Lange.

Levy, B. S., & Wegman, D. H. (Eds.) (1994). *Occupational health: Recognizing and preventing work-related disease* (3rd ed.). Boston: Little, Brown.

Maibach, H. I. (1986). *Occupational and industrial dermatology* (2nd ed.). Chicago: Year Book.

McCunney, R. J. (Ed.). (1994). *A practical approach to occupational and environmental medicine.* Boston: Little Brown.

Moeller, D. W. (1992). *Environmental health.* Cambridge, MA: Harvard University Press.

Monson, R. R. (1990). *Occupational epidemiology* (2nd ed.). Boca Raton, FL: CRC Press.

National Institute for Occupational Safety and Health. (1990). *NIOSH pocket guide to chemical hazards.* Washington, DC: U. S. Department of Health and Human Services.

Parkes, W. R. (1994). *Occupational lung disorders* (3rd ed.). Newton, MA: Butterworh-Heinemann.

Plog, B. A. (Ed.). (1988). *Fundamentals of industrial hygiene* (3rd ed.).Washington, DC: National Safety Council.

Proctor, N. H., Hughes, J. P., & Fischman, M. (1988). *Chemical hazards of the workplace* (2nd ed.). New York: Lippincott.

Raffle, P. A. B., Adams, P. H., Baxter, P. J., & Lee, W. R. (1994). *Hunter's diseases of occupations* (8th ed.). Boston: Edward Arnold.

Rom, W. N. (1992). *Environmental and occupational medicine* (2nd ed.). New York: Saunders.

Rosenstock, L. & Cullen, M. (1994). *Textbook of clinical occupational and environmental medicine.* Philadelphia: Saunders.

U. S. Department of Health and Human Services & U. S. Department of Labor. (1978, 1981, 1988). *NIOSH chemical hazard guidelines.* Publication Numbers DHHS (NIOSH) 81-123 and 88-118: Supplement I-OHG. Washington, DC: NIOSH.

Waldron, H. A. (1989). *Occupational health practice* (3rd ed.). Butterworths.

Weeks, J. L., Levy, B. S., & Wagner, G. R. (Eds.). (1991). *Preventing occupational disease and injury.* Washington, DC: American Public Health Association.

Zenz, C., Dickerson, O. B., & Horvath, E. P. (Eds.). (1994). *Occupational medicine* (3rd ed.). St. Louis, MO: Mosby.

Chapter 10

Environmental Epidemiology: Assessing Health Risks from Toxic Agents in the Environment

A. James Ruttenber

Questions about health risks from toxic agents in the environment are raised frequently by concerned citizens and scientists alike. How do we know whether exposures to chemicals pose dangers to workers in chemical industries or to residents of communities near industrial sites? Is an outbreak of a new disease due to an exposure from a nearby industry or to a communicable disease? Can we adequately protect human health by relying solely on data from studies of animals exposed in the laboratory? Do epidemiologic studies really provide the last word in the analysis of risk? And finally, are risks to human health the only risks we need to consider?

If corrective measures for environmental problems are implemented without good answers to these questions, the health of the public could be jeopardized rather than protected. For example, expensive remedial actions could be conducted in one community, whereas higher concentrations of a more toxic agent are permitted in another. Poorly designed or incorrectly interpreted studies of health risks can raise public anxiety unnecessarily, or lead to a false sense of security in a community that is really exposed to dangerous levels of an agent. Furthermore, chemical contamination (by greenhouse gases or ozone-depleting chemicals, for example) may cause widespread ecological damage without posing immediate risks to human health; but the ecological damage may, in time, produce substantial health risks.

We hope that decisions on issuing permits for industrial operations and initiating remedial actions following environmental contamination are based on valid assessments of all the dangers posed by toxic agents in air, soil, and water. Yet, it is often difficult to decide which methods should be used to characterize health risks from toxic exposures. This chapter describes a systematic approach for quantifying health risks to the public for exposures to toxic agents—one that selectively employs techniques from epidemiologic analysis and risk assessment.

RISK ASSESSMENT AND EPIDEMIOLOGY: AN OVERVIEW

Two types of studies have been popular in responding to questions of health risks from environmental exposures: risk assessment and epidemiologic analysis. Usually these methodologies are applied independently. That is, epidemiologic analysis has rarely employed the techniques of risk assessment, and risk assessment has mostly been used as an alternative to epidemiologic analysis.

In a risk assessment, health risks are estimated by first quantifying the cumulative intake or dose for the agent of interest and then predicting risk (the probability of experiencing an adverse health outcome) from epidemiologic studies of other human populations, from laboratory studies of animals, or from dose–response models (Chapter 2). For instance, a risk assessment for a community near an industry or a toxic waste site would not use disease data from the population actually at risk. Rather, disease rates for this group would be projected, based on the magnitude of the toxic exposure and estimates of toxicity reported from other studies (Paustenbach, 1989; U S. Environmental Protection Agency [EPA], 1989a, 1989b, 1989c).

The basic steps in risk assessment (Figure 10.1) are: (1) identify potential toxic agents (*hazard identification*); (2) estimate intakes or doses of these agents for the population of interest (*exposure assess-

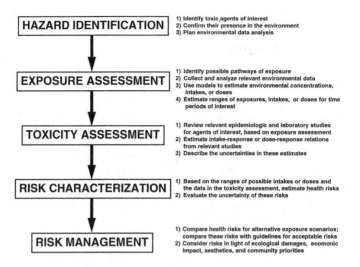

Figure 10.1   Steps in the risk-assessment process.

ment); (3) estimate the toxicity of these agents in terms of risk per unit intake or dose (*toxicity assessment*); (4) predict health effects that will result from the estimated intakes or doses (*risk characterization*).

Risk management—technically not part of the risk assessment—is the process through which regulatory and remedial options are developed, based on information from the risk assessment. Underlying the entire risk–assessment and risk–management process are questions about the meaning of the risk (Is it voluntary or involuntary? Which other health and environmental risks have not been evaluated?). Often such questions are overlooked, misunderstood, or intentionally restricted. Unless all potential health and environmental risks are identified and considered, risk assessment and risk management may produce results that are in error or that lead to ineffective remedial efforts. Moreover, the public may lose trust in the governmental agencies and scientists that fail to address these issues.

Because there are few rules specifying the types of data to be used or the assumptions to be made, risk assessments are particularly susceptible to manipulation by groups with special interests. Moreover, they involve complex chains of algebraic equations with estimates for terms that are based on sparse data and assumptions that have been poorly tested. Such analyses are difficult for many scientists to understand and evaluate critically. These factors make it easy to select data that support a predetermined position—as opposed to exploring risks impartially.

Epidemiologic analysis, on the other hand, employs health data collected directly through surveys of the exposed populations, from historical records, or from ongoing surveillance programs. Under the best conditions, an epidemiologic study tests a hypothesized relation between a toxic agent and a disease. Compared with risk assessment (Figure 10.1), analytic approaches in epidemiologic analysis involve steps that are less linear (Figure 10.2). The design of an epidemiologic study can begin with evaluating health data for a specific population, or by focusing on exposure to one or more toxic agents.

Interpreting the results from studies with crude measures of exposure or disease or flaws in their designs is a common problem in environmental epidemiology. Combining possible exposure to pollution with apparent elevations in disease rates makes for sensational press but may fail to convince the scientists, governmental regulators, and other interested parties who ultimately have the responsibility for reducing risks from environmental agents.

Although advocates of epidemiologic analysis and supporters of risk assessment get into debates over the relative merits of each technique, the real issue is: Which approach is the best for the problem at hand? In many cases, either technique could be applied. There are differences, however, between these methods. To conduct a risk assessment, the agent or agents implicated as health hazards must first be identified. An epidemiologic study, on the other hand, can be launched without having first identified an agent suspected of producing health risks. In fact, epidemiologic analysis is a powerful tool for investigating outbreaks of new diseases suspected to be related to previously unknown environmental exposures, such as the studies of the toxic oil syndrome of Spain and L-tryptophan-related eosinophilia-myalgia syndrome (Chapter 2).

Even though a specific agent has not been implicated in an outbreak of disease, identifying potential exposure pathways in the environment is necessary for developing hypotheses, formulating questions for interviews, and selecting the best ways to quantify exposure, intake, and dose (see Chapter 1 for an explanation of these terms). For this reason, risk assessment techniques are quite useful in the design phase of an epidemiologic study. The techniques of hazard

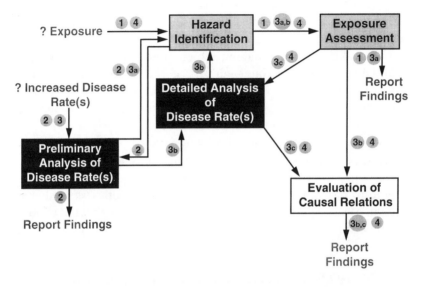

Figure 10.2   Steps in the process of epidemiologic analysis: (1) suspected exposure is not sufficient to justify analysis of disease rates; (2) suspected increase in disease rate(s) not confirmed by preliminary analysis and there is no evidence for exposure to toxic agents; (3) suspected increase in disease rate(s) is supported by preliminary analysis, leading to either a search for possible exposure(s) (3a), to a detailed analysis of disease rate(s) (3b), or both; if detailed analysis indicates an increase, then search for exposure(s) is initiated; if an exposure can be identified, then causal relations can be evaluated, provided that a detailed analysis of disease rates has been performed (3b,c); if an exposure is not identified, then the "negative" results are reported (3a); (4) suspected exposure is sufficient to justify analysis of disease rate(s) and evaluation of causal relations.

identification and exposure assessment are also needed to interpret preliminary analyses of epidemiologic data — such as those from surveillance programs or analyses of disease clusters (Aldrich, Drane, & Griffith, 1993).

The systematic approach to analysis of health risks presented in this chapter taps the most useful techniques of both risk assessment and epidemiologic analysis. It begins with identifying the specific toxic agents or, if this is not possible, the hypothesized agents. The sources of the agents and the environmental pathways through which humans could be exposed are then identified and diagrammed. Finally, the relative merits of risk assessment and epidemiologic analysis are compared and health risks are evaluated with one or both techniques.

In making decisions about which studies to conduct, keep in mind the goals for assessing health risks. The first goal is a quantitative estimate of the degree to which an exposure, intake, or dose increases the risk for disease. The second and most important is an analysis that can be understood, scrutinized, and discussed by the affected population and other interested parties. Members of the public who are subjects in an epidemiologic study or for whom a risk assessment is performed have personal interests in the data; they deserve to participate in the entire process of health risk evaluation (Brown, 1993). Workers who are studied because they were exposed to toxic agents in the workplace should receive similar consideration.

ASSESSING EXPOSURE, INTAKE, AND DOSE: A MODELING APPROACH

An ecosystem model such as the one in Figure 1.6 (Chapter 1) can help locate and describe important pathways of exposure and the natural processes that affect the dynamics of these pathways. The pathways in the model help identify data needed for quantifying exposures, intakes, and doses, which can be measured for current conditions or reconstructed from historical data (Ruttenber, 1993, 1995). Historical reconstructions are clearly less reliable than assessments made while an exposure is occurring. They are important, however, because many studies in environmental epidemiology involve diseases with long latent periods (Chapter 2)—diseases that could have resulted only from exposures that predated the occurrence of disease by many years.

As discussed in Chapter 1, the doses received by exposed persons are the best predictors of the health consequences of an environmental exposure. When data are inadequate to estimate dose, then various measures of exposure or intake can be used. Dose assessment involves estimating the intake and deposition of a toxic agent for the period over which exposure occurred. For an acute exposure, a single dose can be estimated for the entire exposure period. For chronic exposures, doses computed for specific intervals within the exposure period may be preferable because the exposure may have varied in intensity over time.

Doses are estimated with a set of equations that describe the transfer of the agent from the environment to the exposed human. These equations are usually called *environmental transport* or *dose models*. They are solved or simulated using computational techniques ranging from simple algebra performed by hand or with computer spreadsheet software to the mathematical solution of simultaneous differential equations by computers with more sophisticated software (Calabrese & Kostecki, 1992; Moskowitz et al., 1992).

To model the spatial distribution of a pollutant from its source, we must first estimate the quantity per unit time released to the environment. This measure, called the *source term*, can be estimated from industrial production records or obtained from monitoring devices placed in exhaust stacks or at points of liquid effluent release. The equations in environmental transport models link the source term to other "compartments" in the environment through a series of *transfer factors* that specify the rate of transfer from one compartment to another in an ecosystem model, from the ecosystem to humans, and ultimately to specific tissues or organs in exposed humans. When data for concentrations of a pollutant in environmental or human tissue samples are available, they can be used to check the predictions from the environmental transport model—a process called *model verification*. The more extensively a model has been evaluated and verified, the more reliable are its predictions.

For some exposures, data are not available for estimating source terms or transfer factors. In such cases, environmental monitoring data from compartments along the exposure pathway (Chapter 1) can be used instead. Actual measurements made in food, water, or air provide more accurate estimates of exposures and doses than predictions from models based on source terms. Such measurements are often unavailable—particularly for exposures that occurred in the past.

To estimate doses to humans, environmental transport models are coupled with models that predict the intake and distribution of toxic agents in the body (Chapter 2). They require data for the following: (1) rates of ingestion, inhalation, and dermal absorption; (2) rates of transport from the site of entry to the organs of interest; (3) rates of uptake, metabolism, and storage in specific organs; and (4) rates of elimination from the body. For pathogenic organisms, radionuclides, and some chemicals, data in the literature can yield reasonable estimates of these parameters.

Models vary with regard to the certainty of their predictions. The simplest employ source terms and environmental and physiologic transfer factors that maximize exposures and doses. These are called *worst-case* or *conservative models*. Estimates made for worst-case conditions are useful for making decisions in emergencies but they may be misleading when used to quantify risks from chronic exposures to low concentrations of a toxic agent or to evaluate the feasibility of an epidemiologic study. However, when worst-case estimates indicate that intakes or doses pose negligible health risks or risks that are so low that epidemiologic studies will not have adequate statistical power to detect a disease increase, more detailed assessments probably will not change these findings.

Models designed to predict the environmental distribution of toxic agents from a variety of industries—termed *generic* models—are useful for quick assessments (EPA, 1988), but may provide inaccurate results. Such models are not designed to handle unique environmental pathways and may not have been thoroughly tested in field situations. Accurate estimates require actual measurements of environmental transfer factors that have been determined for the specific agent of interest under relevant environmental conditions.

Because the methods used to model environmental concentrations, intake, and dose vary widely with regard to their accuracy of prediction, it is important to estimate the error associated with these calculations. *Uncertainty analysis* provides the methods for making such estimates (Burmaster & Harris, 1993; Hoffman & Hammonds, 1992). Uncertainty estimates should incorporate the propagation of errors made in environmental sampling, in detecting and performing quantitative analyses for estimating the intake, internal distribution, and dose of the agent, and in quantifying its risk. Recently computer software has been developed to make uncertainty analyses more feasible (Decisioneering, 1993). When such data are impossible to obtain, error estimates may have to be descriptive or qualitative (Hoffman & Gardner, 1983).

Another way to quantify doses to exposed humans is through analysis of biologic samples collected from exposed persons.

Concentrations of bacteria, viruses, parasites, and toxic chemicals can be measured directly in blood, urine, adipose tissue, or in organs. Metabolites or inducible enzymes can serve as indirect measurements of toxic chemical exposure. Tissue samples from biopsy, surgery, and autopsy can also be used to estimate doses. When biologic samples are used to estimate dose, the time between exposure and sample collection must be considered because many chemicals are stored in tissues for only short periods.

QUANTIFYING RISK

Estimating the probability of disease resulting from exposure to a toxic agent is termed *risk characterization*. Risk estimates can be made for many different outcomes, but are most often made for morbidity or mortality from acute and chronic diseases. The risk characterization phase of a risk assessment provides risk estimates similar to those obtained from an epidemiologic study. The difference between the two is that, in a risk assessment, data for relating health effects to exposures come not from the population of interest, but from studies of other populations of humans or animals. In an epidemiologic study, risk estimates are made directly for the specific population of interest.

In risk characterization, data from the exposure assessment are linked with those from the toxicity assessment. As discussed in Chapter 2, the toxicity assessment draws from all studies of the toxic effects of an agent, whether they were conducted on humans, other animals, or other organisms. The end result of a toxicity assessment is an estimate of risk per unit of cumulative intake or dose for the agent of interest. Quantitative measures of intake or dose are multiplied by estimates of disease risk per unit intake or dose from the toxicity assessment to obtain an estimate of the range of risk for the exposed population.

Disease risk from an environmental agent is expressed quantitatively as the number of adverse health outcomes (such as neoplasms, chromosomal mutations, diagnosed illnesses, or deaths) per unit intake or dose for an exposed person over a specified period of time. Often, the only evidence for the toxic effects of an agent comes from laboratory animals that received doses per unit of body mass that were far higher than those received by exposed humans. In such cases, disease rates from high doses are extrapolated to those for lower doses with various mathematical models for relations between dose and response. Frequently, there is debate over whether the risk for toxic effects should be extrapolated with a linear function, or whether a model with a threshold for toxic effects is more appropriate (Ames & Gold, 1990; Butterworth, 1990; Cohen & Ellwein, 1990; Upton, 1988).

The best data for assessing toxicity to humans are from disease rates measured in humans exposed to quantified doses of an agent. Such data are available for some common exposures, including the risk for lung cancer from cigarette smoking and the risk for cardiovascular disease from various diets. Data relating disease rates in the public to exposures from environmental chemicals are rarely available. Sometimes data exist for unique populations that have accrued high doses of specific agents, such as recipients of certain medical procedures and workers exposed in industry.

Quantitative health risks for chronic diseases have been determined for some occupational exposures: lung cancer in uranium and hard rock miners who were exposed to radon decay products (Hornung & Meinhardt, 1987); asbestosis and lung cancer in asbestos workers (Huncharek, 1994; Selikoff & Lee, 1978; Selikoff, Hammond, & Seidman, 1979), and for leukemia in persons exposed to benzene (Goldstein & Witz, 1992; International Agency for Research on Cancer, 1982). Quantitative risk estimates for cancers caused by exposure to ionizing radiation have been determined from studies of patients exposed during medical diagnosis and treatment and from studies of the survivors of the bombings of Hiroshima and Nagasaki (National Research Council [NRC], 1990; Shimizu, Schull, & Kato, 1990).

For many agents, only data from animal experiments are available for toxicity assessment. These data must be considered carefully because the ability of a chemical to cause disease in animals is sometimes not directly related to its human toxicity. In some cases there are clear-cut differences in susceptibility between species. For example, MPTP (1-methyl-4-phenyl-1,2,3,6-tetrahydropyridine), the neurotoxin that has produced parkinsonism in a group of California narcotics users (Langston, Ballard, Tetrud, & Irwin, 1983) produces different neurotoxic effects in different animal species (Jenner, Marsden, Costall, & Naylor, 1986).

The most toxic of the dioxins, 2,3,7,8 tetrachlorodibenzo-p-dioxin (TCDD), also causes a variety of tumors in different species at varying doses (Kociba, 1984). This variability makes it difficult to assign a quantitative estimate of human toxicity for this compound.

Scientists frequently disagree over the appropriate methodologies for calculating risk. Risk assessments made for carcinogens sometimes do not include the risks for benign neoplasia, even though benign tumors may be precancerous or provide evidence for a tumor-promoting effect (Landy, Roberts, & Thomas, 1990). Recently some scientists have argued that carcinogens that act as promoters should be evaluated differently from those that act as genotoxic initiators. They advocate less stringent regulations for promoters than for initiators and maintain that, for promoters, there are threshold doses below which there is no cancer risk (Leung & Paustenbach, 1989).

Laboratory data sufficient for risk assessments are available for only a few toxic agents and for a limited set of diseases and biologic effects. In spite of these limitations, risk estimates have been made for many environmental contaminants in order for the EPA and other regulatory agencies to conduct risk assessments (EPA, 1993a). These estimates should be used with caution.

Often the extent to which an agent is regulated by the government determines the quality of data available for risk assessment. For example, there are few regulations for neurotoxins in the environment, so few data have been gathered on the effects to the human nervous system from chronic exposure to environmental neurotoxins; compared with carcinogens, neurotoxins have rarely been the subject of risk assessment (Committee on Neurotoxicology and Models for Assessing Risk, 1992; U.S. Office of Technology Assessment, 1990), though there is now some evidence for progress (EPA, 1993b). These circumstances have created an unfortunate paradox: data needed to determine the need for regulation are not collected on agents that are not already regulated.

SCIENTIFIC CRITERIA FOR RELATING EXPOSURE TO DISEASE IN EPIDEMIOLOGIC STUDIES

Epidemiologists may initiate studies of the health effects of environmental exposures because of scientific interest in the toxicity of a specific agent, because a community has been exposed to an agent and wants their health risks explained, or because surveillance data suggest an increased rate of disease in a community. Studies of communities exposed to toxic agents are invariably controversial. Debate has usually focused on the conclusions of these studies, often with little consideration for the methods used to collect and analyze the data, or the guidelines by which the data were interpreted.

Because studies in environmental epidemiology frequently involve poorly measured exposures and diseases that are not clearly defined, it is important to interpret them with caution. Epidemiologic criteria for establishing causal relations are helpful in this regard (Hill, 1965). These criteria (often called Hill's postulates) are meant to be general guidelines, and the extent to which they, as a group, are fulfilled is a measure of the quality of evidence for a hypothesized relation between an environmental exposure and disease. In general, environmental epidemiologists have not paid much attention to Hill's postulates, as evidenced by the large number of studies that seemingly enhance rather than reduce debate (Shleien, Ruttenber, & Sage, 1991). Many recent texts and articles (Elwood, 1988; Kline, Stein, & Susser, 1989; Rothman, 1982, 1988) have clarified and extended Hill's original criteria, which are outlined below.

The *strength* of an association between exposure and disease is a measure of the extent to which exposed persons have a disease, as compared with the disease rate in an unexposed population. Strong associations support causality and are less likely to be due to other factors. *Consistency* between studies is a determination of whether the results of one study are congruent with those of similar studies of different populations.

The *specificity* of a relation between exposure and disease pertains to its uniqueness. A causal relation between a disease that appears only after exposure to a single agent or class of agents is easier to support than one for a disease that can be caused by many different agents, or for an agent that causes many different diseases. For example, an epidemiologist is likely to find it easier to determine the cause for an unusually large number of cases of mesothelioma in a county than for a "cluster" of lung cancer cases. This is because only a single class of agents (asbestos and asbestos-like fibers) has been shown to cause mesothelioma in laboratory studies of animals and epidemiologic studies of humans. On the other hand, many classes of chemical and physical agents have been shown to cause lung cancer. Therefore, an epidemiologic study of mesothelioma can focus on environmental and occupational exposures to fibers, whereas a study of lung cancer must consider many different possible causes.

Hill's point about specificity is more relevant to studies of infectious diseases and environmental exposures to biologic agents than to studies of cancer and environmental exposures to carcinogens. This is because evidence for infection by biologic agents can usually be obtained and because such agents often cause diseases with unique features.

If an exposure precedes disease, the principle of *temporality* has been established—an obvious prerequisite for causation. Adherence to temporality is particularly important when evaluating the relation between environmental exposures and cancer and other slowly developing chronic diseases. For cancer to have been caused by an environmental exposure, the exposure must have occurred sometime before the beginning of the hypothesized latent period.

A *biological gradient* or *dose–response* relation exists when persons with comparatively low exposures, intakes, or doses have disease rates lower than those with high exposures, intakes, or doses and when a similar relation exists for the entire spectrum of exposure. Because epidemiologists usually cannot manipulate environmental exposures to test hypotheses, as done in controlled experiments and clinical trials, examining dose–response relations is quite difficult. Quantitative estimates of environmental exposures are usually of poor quality or not available at all, and dose–response relations are often not evaluated in environmental epidemiology.

METHODOLOGIC AND STATISTICAL CONSIDERATIONS

The design of an epidemiologic study also helps determine the extent to which it can be regarded as evidence for a causal relation between an exposure and a disease. Well-designed studies account for possible biases in obtaining exposure data and diagnosing disease, and evaluate possible measurement errors in determining exposures and outcomes. Bias and systematic errors in measurement lead to erroneous interpretations, and random measurement errors attenuate associations, making it difficult to detect relations between exposure and disease (Elwood, 1988; Rothman, 1986). The inclusion of an adequate number of study subjects is also an important feature of study design, as discussed below.

Statistical Power: How Good Are Negative Results?

Epidemiologic studies of environmental exposures frequently involve small populations with exposures that are not large enough to cause widespread disease—even though the exposures may pose health risks to the populations. Under these conditions, it is more likely than not that epidemiologists will find no statistically significant relation between exposure and disease (studies with such findings are termed "negative studies")—even when a relation exists. For this reason, it is important to determine the likelihood that a nonsignificant relation between exposure and disease is actually correct (Susser, 1988). *Statistical power* (Schlesselman, 1982) is the probability of detecting an association, assuming the association actually exists. It is calculated by subtracting the ß(Type II) error from one and multiplying the difference by 100% ([1 - ß] × 100%). The higher the statistical power of a study, the less likely its negative results are incorrect. Studies with low statistical power provide poor evidence for arguing that no causal relation exists.

To calculate statistical power, one must know: (1) the size of the exposed and unexposed populations for cohort studies or the number of cases and controls for case-control studies; (2) the estimated rate of the disease in the unexposed population; and (3) an estimate of the extent to which the exposure elevates the disease risk in exposed persons. Computer software for estimating statistical power is now readily available (Dean, Dean, Burton, & Dicker, 1994; Statistics and Epidemiology Research Corporation, 1993).

Computing the statistical power of a study in its design phase helps determine whether there is an adequate number of subjects, provides important information for determining the cost-effectiveness of epidemiologic research, and clarifies the reliability of any negative results that may be reported. There is no universally accepted level of adequate statistical power for an epidemiologic study. Mausner and Kramer (1985) suggest that the ß error should be less than four times the α (Type I) error. That is, if an a error of 0.05 is used to determine significance, then statistical power should be 80% or greater. In environmental epidemiology, power less than 50% is undesirable. There are, however, many published studies with power lower than this minimum.

Studies of environmental exposures with predictably low statistical power are sometimes useful, particularly when data on the human toxicity of an agent are limited. If a negative finding is produced under these conditions, it should be reported along with the highest risk that could have existed without being detected by statistical analysis.

Interpreting Positive Findings

A statistically significant relation between exposure and disease is not, by itself, evidence for causation. There are a number of ways in which a study can produce false-positive results (Type I errors). These can be classified as either errors in measuring the true value of the exposure or in diagnosing the disease, or as bias (Elwood, 1988). *Confounding* is a type of bias that occurs when the apparent effect of the exposure of interest is actually caused by an extraneous variable. A confounding variable is correlated with both the exposure of interest and the disease and is associated with the exposure of interest but is not a consequence of this exposure. Confounding can also obscure a true relation between an exposure and a disease, causing a Type II error.

Age is a common confounding variable in epidemiologic studies of environmental exposures. If the age structure is different for exposed and unexposed populations or for cases and controls, and the incidence of the disease under study is affected by age (cancer, for example), then it may appear that a hypothesized exposure is related to a disease when the relation is really due to a higher proportion of older subjects in the exposed group. There are a number of analytic strategies available for controlling the influence of confounding variables (Elwood, 1988; Rothman, 1986).

Type I errors can also result from analyzing many different relations between variables—a situation common in exploratory studies of risks from environmental agents. When several hypotheses are tested in the same study (a practice termed "multiple comparisons"), the likelihood of a false-positive error increases as a function of the number of hypotheses tested. The significance of positive results from such studies can be adjusted to account for this effect (Wakeford, Binks, & Wilkie, 1989).

Another problem in environmental epidemiology is interpreting data from many different studies of the same exposure-disease relation. If one or more of the studies has either a flawed design or lacks statistical power, then it may be misleading to draw inferences about causal relations based on the "weight of the evidence." Meta-analysis is a methodology for increasing statistical power and reconciling differences in results between studies by analyzing data compiled from many different ones. Meta-analysis will not, however, fix the design flaws in the individual studies—although there are methods for assessing the impacts of such flaws.

An example of the problems faced in reconciling the results from many different studies is the interpretation of the findings from studies of cancer in communities near nuclear facilities (Shleien et al., 1991). Most studies have combined residence within geopolitical units and distance from a nuclear plant to represent exposure to ionizing radiation—thus providing potentially flawed estimates of dose-response relations and, because exposures were so crudely defined, precluding a meta-analysis of the combined results from different studies. Moreover, each study examined many different hypotheses and most lacked adequate statistical power.

Because at least one positive finding (more cases of cancer than would be expected in an exposed area) was reported in almost every study, it may seem reasonable to conclude that there is a much higher risk for cancer from environmental exposure to low levels of ionizing radiation than has been previously recognized—even though this conclusion conflicts with a large body of evidence from well-designed studies that found no such relation for the levels of exposure that have been measured around most nuclear plants. So far, the "weight of the evidence" from the community studies has not changed the estimates of risk made by the groups of scientists that develop recommendations for radiation protection standards. This example supports the concept that results of well-designed studies are given more attention that those from poorly designed ones.

Whereas estimates of statistical power are crucial to the interpretation of "negative" epidemiologic studies, evaluations of the important features of study design—such as confounding, other types of bias, the effects of multiple comparisons, and evidence for causal relations—are necessary to correctly interpret the results of "positive" studies.

STUDY DESIGNS IN ENVIRONMENTAL EPIDEMIOLOGY

Cohort Studies

When an epidemiologist can identify a group of people who were exposed to a toxic agent, a *cohort* study can be considered. With this study design, rates of diseases in a population exposed to a toxic agent are compared with rates in a demographically similar, but unexposed group (Breslow & Day, 1987). The disease rates for the unexposed population can be national or state averages for the entire population from which the exposed subjects are drawn, or they can be based on data collected from a population unexposed to the agent of interest. The association between exposure and disease in these studies is commonly expressed as the *relative risk* (the risk of disease in the exposed cohort divided by the risk in the unexposed cohort) for a particular toxic agent or dose level of a toxic agent.

The criteria for exposure in a cohort study can be broad or narrow, depending on how accurately exposures or doses can be quantified, and the degree to which one desires the results to be generalizable. A cohort study can be restricted to a highly exposed group in order to maximize the chances of detecting an exposure–disease relation; or it can include a large group with a wide range of exposures in order to produce results that are more generalizable or data that can be examined for exposure–response or dose–response relations with statistical models. There is no limit to the number of diseases that can be assessed in a cohort study, as long as the problem of multiple comparisons is addressed. The cohort design is useful for studying a toxic agent that is suspected to cause more than one disease. Cohort studies are also useful for studying the acute effects of environmental exposures that may not be severe enough to be recorded by disease surveillance systems.

Examples of cohort studies in environmental epidemiology include the study of cancer incidence in persons exposed to dioxins and other chemicals from an explosion at a chemical plant is Seveso, Italy (Bertazzi et al., 1993), and studies of thyroid disease in children exposed to fallout from atmospheric tests of nuclear weapons at the Nevada Test site in the United States (Kerber et al., 1993). Cohort studies in environmental epidemiology are usually retrospective or historical—that is, the cohort is defined after the exposure has occurred. Prospective cohort studies are rare, primarily because health agencies limit environmental exposures that are suspected to cause disease. However, when they can be done, prospective cohort studies can be quite effective, as evidenced by the study of the relation between air pollution and lung disease performed by Dockery et al. (1993).

Case-Control Studies

The *case-control* or *case-comparison* study is another commonly used research design (Breslow & Day, 1980; Schlesselman, 1982). This approach compares a group of case subjects who have a disease with a group of control subjects who do not have the disease. Subjects in both groups are evaluated for exposure to one or more toxic agents, and the association between exposure or dose and disease is estimated with a statistic called the *odds ratio*, which, under appropriate conditions, approximates the relative risk.

Case-control studies are particularly useful for studying rare diseases such as cancer. Because exposures are assessed after the occurrence of disease, they must be measured carefully to avoid bias due to differing measurement protocols for cases and controls. Studies comparing exposures to electromagnetic fields in children with cancer to those in control groups are examples of case-control studies (Savitz, Wachtel, Barnes, John, & Tvrdiik, 1988).

Ecologic Studies

A study that assigns a single measure of exposure to a group of subjects is termed an *ecologic* study (English, 1992; Morgenstern, 1982)—much to the dismay of ecologists. Geopolitical boundaries are commonly used to define exposures in ecologic studies. In the United States, researchers choose counties, cities, or census tracts to define the boundaries for exposed and unexposed areas, and then compare disease rates for the populations within these boundaries.

Data from an ecologic study must be interpreted with caution, because persons within geographic units are usually not exposed to the same degree. Ecologic studies may include persons who have immigrated after the exposure occurred, and exclude persons who were exposed but emigrated before diseases were enumerated. Furthermore, environmental exposures are rarely homogeneous within geopolitical boundaries. Elevated disease rates produced by exposure to a toxic agent in a small section of a geographic area can therefore be diluted by many unexposed and unaffected subjects—an example of misclassification bias. The confounding effects of variables other than the exposure of interest can lead to inaccurate estimates of the toxicity of environmental agents (Greenland & Morgenstern, 1989); some of these effects can be controlled for by such methods as stratifying disease rates by specific time periods and by accounting for latent periods between the onset of exposure and the time of diagnosis or death.

Mapping Exposures and Diseases

Exposures and disease rates for geopolitically defined areas can also be mapped (Boyle, 1989; Briggs, 1992; Cliff & Haggett, 1990; Mason, Fraumeni, Hoover, & Blot, 1981; Pickle, Mason, Howard, Hoover, & Fraumeni, 1987). In the past, important theories on the relation between the environment, insect vectors, and infectious diseases were based on such maps (Cliff & Haggett, 1990; Howe, 1989). To date, this type of analysis has failed to uncover new exposure-disease relations for cancer and other chronic diseases. Studies of mapped disease rates have mainly confirmed associations already known to exist, such as the relation between lung cancer and asbestos exposure in shipyards located in coastal counties of the United States (Blot & Fraumeni, 1982; Enterline & Henderson, 1987), and between solar radiation and skin cancer in the southern United States.

Improvements in computer technology have eased the mapping of multiple data sets for environmental monitoring results, geologic factors, and disease rates. These *geographic information systems* (Antenucci, Brown, Croswell, & Kevany, 1991; Taylor, 1991) may be useful in graphically relating the distribution of toxic agents in the environment to the location of specific populations and in selecting remedial options for the cleanup of environmental contaminants that are most likely to reduce health risks (Nuckols, Berry, & Stallones, 1994). Whether such systems will improve current analytical approaches in environmental epidemiology remains unclear, however.

Mapped disease rates and ecologic studies have both been of limited use for the same reason: When geopolitical boundaries define exposures, persons with diseases caused by toxic exposures are mixed with those who have no exposure or disease and with those who have diseases caused by ubiquitous exposures, such as smoking. Furthermore, geopolitical boundaries are not very useful for evaluating dose–response (or exposure–disease) relations.

The distance between a suspected source of exposure and the place of residence at the time of diagnosis or death is commonly used in mapping, cohort, and case-control studies. Distance may not correlate with intensity of exposure, and place of residence at the time of diagnosis may not reflect earlier exposures at other residences. Results from studies with such crude measures of exposure must be confirmed with more detailed estimates of exposure or dose if they are to be accepted as evidence for causal relations.

In spite of the forementioned limitations, members of the public and practitioners of public health are seemingly infatuated with the distribution of diseases around potential sources of environmental exposure. If geographic information systems are used to construct maps of exposures and diseases for purposes of discussion and hypothesis generation, then they can provide useful information. Knowledge that disease rates in the community of interest are not ten times higher than the average for other areas can be helpful, as can the confirmation of a suspected increase in disease incidence or prevalence for a particular area. To evaluate causal relations, however, epidemiologists must employ other designs such as cohort and case-control studies with data for exposures or doses that are more accurate than those used in mapping studies (Blot & Fraumeni, 1982; Bolviken & Bjorklund, 1990; Carstensen, 1989; Howe, 1989).

Cluster Analysis

One of the most common problems environmental epidemiologists encounter is determining whether reported cases of disease in an area are more numerous than would be expected by chance alone, and if so, whether there is an environmental exposure responsible for the "cluster." Determining whether a cluster is a statistically significant elevation in incidence or prevalence can be done using a fairly logical sequence of analyses, as outlined below. Whether a cluster is related to an environmental exposure is, however, far more difficult to determine (Neutra, 1990; Rothman, 1990).

The first and most important step in investigating a cluster is to learn as much as possible about how the cluster was discovered and whether possible causes of the cluster have been identified. Invariably, the news of a disease cluster in a community causes public concern, and members of the public can become quite angry with those who are thought to be responsible for its cause as well as with government officials and scientists who are perceived to work too slowly, to be insensitive to community concerns, or to be covering up the cause of the cluster.

Listening to those who are concerned about the cluster will help researchers design their investigation so that it will produce results that are relevant to the public's questions. Discussions of research goals will also inform the public about the limitations of epidemiologic analysis. In addition, these discussions help identify the exposure(s) thought to be responsible for the cluster—information that is extremely important for evaluating causal relations if the cluster is real. This information can also be used to address the problem with methods of risk assessment if there is not a statistically significant elevation in the incidence or prevalence of disease.

The second step in a cluster investigation is to determine whether the reported cluster represents a true increase in the usual occurrence of one or more diseases. Clusters can occur at random in space or in time, and there are statistical techniques for determining whether reported disease rates are significantly higher than rates expected by chance alone (Aldrich, Drane, & Griffith, 1993; Elliott, Cuzick, English, & Stern, 1992). Recently, software has been developed to make a variety of these techniques accessible to epidemiologists (Aldrich & Drane, 1993). The rapid advances in software development for geographic information systems should favorably influence the design of even better cluster analysis software in the future. Remember, however, that all techniques depend on reliable data for disease rates, which should be collected and verified for both the alleged cluster and for comparison groups before they are analyzed.

A statistically significant cluster of disease does not, by itself, confirm a proposed exposure-disease relation. Nor does the absence of a cluster mean the suspected source of exposure poses no health risk. If statistical analyses suggest a true increase in disease and if there are exposures that have been proposed as possible causes, then investigators can determine the feasibility of a cohort or case-control study, as described later in this chapter.

In situations in which there is a statistically significant cluster but no hypothesized cause, a careful search for possible causes is necessary before planning an epidemiologic study. The search should involve a review of all agents known to cause the disease and possible sources of such agents, as well as the consideration of agents to which diseased subjects were exposed but which have not previously been associated with the disease. If there is no evidence for a disease cluster, then the previously described techniques of risk assessment can be used to estimate health risks.

Although the outlined procedure seems pretty straightforward, conducting a cluster investigation can be quite frustrating (Caldwell, 1990). This is particularly true for investigations of cancer, because exposure data for the prelatent period are frequently unavailable and there are many lifestyle and dietary factors that could confound the effects of environmental exposures. Cluster investigations of acute diseases (called outbreak or epidemic investigations) are central to the practice of public health (Goodman, Buehler, & Koplan, 1990) and have revealed the causes of many diseases. Clusters of chronic diseases with poorly understood etiologies also deserve the attention of epidemiologists, as they present opportunities for new discoveries. Clusters of diseases with known etiologies are less worthwhile to pursue.

Other Analytical Techniques

A number of other methods have been used to analyze exposure–disease relations. Exposure measurements such as concentrations of air pollutants can be related to disease rates with linear regression models (Sunyer et al., 1993). If disease rates are low, then poisson regression models may be used (Liang & Zeger, 1986; Schwartz & Dockery, 1992; Zeger & Liang, 1986).

Many types of environmental measurements have natural temporal patterns that vary diurnally, weekly, and seasonally. These effects can confound the exposure of interest if they are not accounted for. Seasonal weather cycles and the seasonal patterns of viral diseases, for instance, can confound the effects of air pollutants, which may also vary seasonally (Lipfert, 1994). Time series analysis (Diggle, 1990) is a popular method for making such adjustments, and has been used extensively in studies of air pollution and disease (Perry et al., 1982; Pope, Dockery, Spengler, & Raizenne, 1991).

The effects of environmental agents on humans can also be assessed with studies of animals in contaminated environments. Studies in the fields of ecotoxicology and wildlife toxicology use designs similar to those of epidemiology (Giesy, Ludwig, & Tillitt, 1994; Myers et al., 1994). The results from such studies may be more relevant than laboratory studies, as animals are exposed to agents under the same environmental conditions as humans.

It has been suggested that these animal studies can be designed as sentinel systems for identifying new health hazards to humans and other species and for generating data for risk assessment. A sentinel species must have a measurable response to the agent in question, have a territory or home range that overlaps the area for which there is concern about exposure to humans, be easily captured, and have a sufficient population size and density to permit enumeration (NRC, 1991). Candidates for sentinel species include food animals, pets, fish, and other wildlife.

To date, animal sentinel systems have been used rarely, and there appears to be no effort to implement them. The reason is due, in part, to their cost and the effort required to document normal rates of disease for sentinel species and to standardize an ongoing data collection program. The use of animal sampling for dose estimates, however, will continue to be popular for particular environmental exposures.

SOURCES OF DATA FOR EPIDEMIOLOGIC STUDIES

The methodology chosen for an epidemiologic study is heavily influenced by the type of data available for measuring disease rates in the population of interest. Sources of these data vary in accuracy and availability (Centers for Disease Control and Prevention [CDC], 1990a, 1990b, 1992; Gable, 1990). Mortality records are the disease data most commonly used for studies in environmental epidemiology. They can be collected and coded uniformly and include demographic information that, when combined with census data, facilitate the computation of age-, race-, and gender-specific mortality rates.

In the United States, each state requires that all deaths within its boundaries be certified. Death certificates coded according to international standards are available on computer tapes from the National Center for Health Statistics (NCHS) of the CDC, or directly from most states. The NCHS also maintains the National Death Index to help researchers locate death certificates for subjects in epidemiologic studies who died on or after January 1, 1979 (CDC, 1992). Systems for death registration and the linkage of these data with other national and local records have been developed extensively in other countries (Lopez, 1992).

A death certificate may not accurately list all the diseases a decedent had, particularly if they were not associated with the immediate cause of death. Consequently, death-certificate data poorly reflect the true rates of many chronic diseases. Parkinson's disease, for example, is often not recorded as an underlying or contributing cause of death and mortality rates derived from death certificates may not be helpful in identifying etiologic agents in the environment. Potentially fatal diseases that are treatable are also underreported in mortality statistics. Childhood leukemia is one example. Decreases in leukemia mortality since the 1970s reflect successful treatment rather than reductions in environmental exposures. Mortality rates also may be biased by such factors as socioeconomic status and lack of access to medical facilities.

In most metropolitan and rural areas, deaths are investigated by a medical examiner or coroner (CDC, 1989). These investigations—particularly when conducted in metropolitan areas—are usually thorough and include toxicologic analyses. Medical examiners rarely investigate deaths from natural causes or from causes that were diagnosed before death. Their data, therefore, are not useful for research in the environmental causes of most chronic diseases. They are, however, extremely useful for studying acute poisonings, occupational injuries, intentional and unintentional injuries, and injuries resulting from natural and man-made disasters.

Morbidity data can be obtained from disease registries and surveillance systems that public health agencies maintain for a variety of diseases or conditions, such as spinal cord injuries and adverse reproductive outcomes (CDC, 1990a; Gable, 1990; Thacker & Berkelman, 1988). Cancer registries are the most common source of surveillance data in environmental epidemiology. These registries provide cancer incidence estimates and help identify subjects for case-control studies. Data from cancer registries are useful for studying treatable diseases such as childhood leukemia and breast cancer, because the incidence of these cancers is not accurately reflected by death certificates.

Cancer registries are maintained in most countries in Europe, North America, and Oceania, but only in some countries on other continents (Draper & Parkin, 1992; Shanmugaratnam, 1989; Swerdlow, 1992). In the United States, the Surveillance, Epidemiology, and End Results (SEER) program of the National Cancer Institute provides uniformly collected data for a selected group of states, metropolitan and rural areas, and territories (Ries et al., 1994). Elsewhere in the United States, cancer registries are maintained by individual states and other agencies; in 1993, 38 states had laws authorizing cancer registries (CDC, 1994). Most U.S. registries were started after the mid-1970s, and may not be useful for evaluating exposures from industries that were operating in the 1940s and 1950s. These registries will be useful, however, for assessing health risks from current and future exposures.

Hospital records for emergency room visits, inquiries to poison control centers, and regular admissions to hospitals may also be useful in studying acute injury and illness from industry and from disasters (American College of Emergency Physicians, 1988; Blanc & Olson, 1986). Data on regular hospital admissions—often called hospital discharge summaries—must be analyzed carefully, because many diseases are treated on an outpatient basis and would not be enumerated; multiple admissions for some diseases may also result in erroneously elevated rates (Boyle, 1989). Furthermore, as databases for hospital discharge summaries are designed primarily for analysis of hospital utilization and health-care costs, they may not be adequate for linking diagnoses to environmental exposures.

Data for surveillance of reproductive outcomes are also available. Many countries have computerized notification systems for birth defects and malformations diagnosed by physicians (Dolk & DeWals, 1992). There is also the International Clearing House for Birth Defects Monitoring Systems and a registry maintained by a consortium of European countries (Kline et al., 1989). In the absence of a surveillance system, birth records are useful sources of data for birth weights and congenital anomalies noted at birth, and some governmental jurisdictions collect additional data such as gestational age. The NCHS also maintains a database linking infant deaths with birth certificates (CDC, 1992).

Surveillance data for the health problems of workers exposed to toxic agents in the workplace are valuable because workers usually receive higher doses than the public, and occupational exposures are usually more easily quantified than environmental exposures. Reporting systems for occupational injuries, compensation and disability insurance claims, union records, and employer records are examples of occupational surveillance data (CDC, 1990a; Wegman, Levy, & Halperin, 1994). In the United States occupational data systems have been used to study injuries, diseases, and conditions resulting in disability compensation claims and for occupational exposure to ionizing radiation in the nuclear weapons industry.

Computerized health and environmental data can be linked with new systems for surveillance and research. To date, efforts to integrate sets of computerized data for toxic exposures, geographic boundaries, and disease have not been particularly successful (Curnen & Schoenfeld, 1983). Recently, a number of commercial software vendors have begun marketing geographic information systems with data files containing a variety of demographic and economic data for small areas defined by postal zip codes and census tracts. These data can be linked with health surveillance data and environmental measurements, thereby facilitating the rapid display of health effects for small areas with environmental contamination. As discussed previously, it is unlikely that these data systems will overcome the problems of exposure classification that plague studies of chronic diseases with long latent periods.

Specialized surveillance and survey systems have also been developed by many countries. In the United States databases are maintained on persons exposed to ionizing radiation from medical procedures, persons with blood disorders, the nutritional status of the general population, pregnancy outcomes and complications, and the fertility of different population groups. Surveillance systems for infectious diseases are also maintained by most countries.

Many special surveys on U.S. health status also provide data to the scientific community. For instance, each year the National Health Interview Survey (CDC, 1992) queries a representative sample of 50,000 households for information on illnesses, injuries, chronic conditions, socioeconomic status, and occupation. Such data could be combined with environmental data to examine relations between exposures and diseases, though the quality of exposure data for such studies would usually be low and the sample size too small to assess exposures from small geographic areas.

Health status for representative samples of the U.S. public has been determined periodically by physical examinations, medical records, and biochemical tests conducted by the U. S. Public Health Service and reported in the Health Examination Surveys, the National Health and Nutrition Examination Surveys (NHANES I, II, and III), and the Hispanic Health and Nutrition Examination Survey (CDC, 1992; Gable, 1990). Although these data include measurements of some pesticides in blood, the size of the study populations (for NHANES III, 40,000 persons; for the Hispanic HANES, 12,000 persons) and the difficulty in identifying exposures common to study participants limit the use of these data in environmental epidemiology.

Records of claims for national medical insurance plans are available for analysis in many countries, but coverage of these systems may be incomplete. Countries that provide health care through national systems—Canada, for example—can integrate a variety of computerized health data with data for environmental exposures for epidemiologic analysis. In the United States data from private insurance companies have not been helpful in assessing the effects of environmental exposures, but managed care plans have provided data for some recent studies (Krieger et al., 1994). Medicare covers most persons over 65 in the United States and may be useful for identifying subjects for case-control studies of environmental exposures (Lauderdale, Furner, Miles, & Goldberg, 1993). When surveillance data are unavailable, knowledge of diseases caused by particular agents and disease increases noted in exposed communities may help epidemiologists identify the types of new data needed to test hypotheses. Disease surveys conducted with interviews, physical examinations, and reviews of medical records from local physicians and hospitals have proved useful in some epidemiologic studies of environmental exposures. Analyses of tissue samples for microscopic pathology and chemical concentrations for groups exposed to toxic agents may also help clarify the effects of environmental exposures.

When data for diagnoses of cancer or other diseases are not available, when the time period between exposure and disease is shorter than the minimum latent period for a disease, or when the exposed population is small, epidemiologists might consider studying early evidence of disease. Biomarkers comprise a variety of evidence for exposure and structural and functional damage (Schulte & Perera, 1993; Garte, 1994), including structural changes in enzymes and DNA, concentrations of toxic chemicals or their metabolites in tissues, and direct or indirect evidence of structural damage to organelles or cells. Biomarkers may reflect the dose of a toxic agent, early disease caused by a toxic exposure, or both (Figure 10.3).

Many types of biomarkers have been used extensively in epidemiology. For instance, concentrations of toxic chemicals and their metabolites are routinely measured in blood and other tissues of study subjects; chromosomal abnormalities in peripheral lymphocytes are used to estimate doses from external exposures to ionizing radiation;

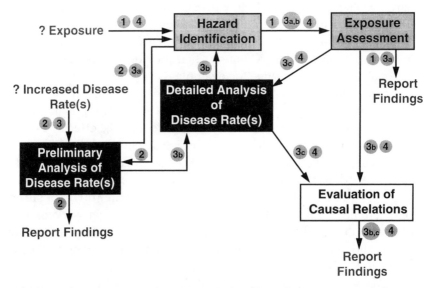

Figure 10.3   The spectrum of biological markers for exposure and disease in molecular epidemiology. From Schulte & Perera (1993), with permission.

and changes in molecular structure identify subtypes of bacteria and viruses in studies of epidemics of infectious diseases.

There has been a great deal of interest in using new techniques for detecting aberrant or variant molecular structures and employing immunologically based techniques for identifying specific molecules of interest (McMichael, 1994). There is particular interest in using these molecular biomarkers in studies of the epidemiology of cancer. The interest in molecular biomarkers is based on the assumption that they are more easily or reliably measured than traditional diagnostic tests, that they detect earlier stages of disease than traditional diagnostic tests, or that they detect evidence for individual susceptibilities to disease. These assumptions are based on the supposition that diseases are multi-stage processes and that, because only a portion of those with evidence of early biological damage will actually develop diagnosable disease, detection of this damage may improve the power of epidemiologic studies and expand our knowledge of the biological mechanisms of disease.

Although biomarkers have received a great deal of attention from environmental and occupational epidemiologists, they have yet to be applied widely in epidemiologic studies of cancer and other chronic diseases. The reasons for this include the lack of dose-response data relating biomarkers to specific toxic agents, the absence of data on the sensitivity and specificity of particular biomarkers, the cost of the analytical techniques necessary to identify and quantify biomarkers, and the fact that for many biomarkers, it is not clear whether they measure exposure, early disease, or both.

ASSESSING THE FEASIBILITY OF AN EPIDEMIOLOGIC STUDY

In evaluating links between environmental exposure and disease, epidemiologists are either provided with evidence of an exposure and asked to see if it increased disease rates, or to determine whether a disease cluster might be related to an environmental exposure. Although epidemiologic studies can clarify whether environmental exposures are related to one or more diseases in the exposed population, circumstances frequently prevent conclusive interpretation of their results (Rothman, 1990; Warner & Aldrich, 1988).

The weaknesses of epidemiologic methods are sometimes over-looked in planning studies and public agencies often have difficulty declining to conduct such studies even though they know, a priori, that methodologic limitations will prevent clear interpretation of their results. This has been particularly true for communities near industries and toxic waste sites.

In spite of these limitations, assessing environmental exposures with epidemiologic methods has become quite popular. This may be due to the assumption that successes in the epidemiologic analysis of acute infectious diseases can be repeated in studies of the relations between chronic diseases and environmental exposures (Neutra, 1990). This analogy may not be appropriate, as chronic diseases have long latent periods and environmental exposures have comparatively low relative risks. Infectious diseases, on the other hand, have short latent periods and exposures to infectious agents have high relative risks.

Before deciding to conduct an epidemiologic study, investigators should judge the proposed study design against the aforementioned criteria for causality and then decide whether the hypothesis for an exposure-disease relation can be tested with the proposed study design. The quality of the data selected to measure both exposure and disease should also be assessed during the planning stages of the study. As mentioned previously, imprecise measures of exposure may result in unexposed persons being misclassified as exposed and vice versa. A similar situation holds for incomplete or inaccurate data for disease classification. Misclassification errors usually bias the results of a study toward showing no relation between exposure and disease.

Surrogate measures for exposure and dose are sometimes help-ful. When crude exposure estimates are associated with disease, additional studies with more precise estimates are required before the relations will be accepted by the scientific community. However, finding no relation between disease and surrogate measures of exposure does not rule out an association.

An epidemiologic study cannot exclude a relation between exposure and disease if it has low statistical power—a common occurrence in studies of rare diseases in small populations. Many studies with low statistical power have been published recently, including analyses of disease rates in communities exposed to chemical wastes and nuclear facilities (Deane, Swan, Harris, Epstein, &

Neutra, 1989; Jablon, Hrubec, & Boice, 1991; Swan, Shaw, Harris, & Neutra, 1989), veterans exposed to radiation from atmospheric weapons tests (Robinette, Jablon, & Preston, 1985), and persons exposed to nonionizing electromagnetic radiation in the home (Monson, 1990; Verreault, Weiss, Hollenbach, Strader, & Daling, 1990). Each of these studies found no relation between exposure and disease, though each had little chance of detecting such a relation because of low statistical power.

When evaluating the feasibility of an epidemiologic study for an exposed community, investigators should determine whether previous epidemiologic studies for the same exposure–disease relation have been conducted with similar groups of exposed subjects. If so, more reliable data on community risk may be generated by accurately measuring exposure or dose in the community and estimating risk with dose–response data from the other studies.

CONCLUSION

When used sensibly, techniques of risk assessment and epidemiologic analysis can help investigators interpret the possible health effects from community exposure to toxic agents. Epidemiologic studies that are poorly designed or interpreted can misrepresent health risks to the public and lead to unnecessary expenditures of time and money. Risk assessments can also be misleading, particularly if they are based on data from only a few animal studies, if they use risk estimates extrapolated from the effects of extremely high doses, or if they involve incomplete analyses of the environmental processes responsible for human exposure.

Studies of communities exposed to toxic agents are superior to other approaches because their subjects come from populations that are actually at risk for diseases caused by the environmental exposures of interest. For instance, studies in occupational settings may be biased toward low estimates of risk because, as a condition of employment, workers are healthier than members of the community at large. Results from studies of the public are not subject to the selection bias introduced by this *"healthy worker effect,"* are not limited to disease risks for adult males, and are not contingent on extrapolating effects from high doses to those from low doses.

In contrast to studies of chemicals and radiation, epidemiologic studies of community exposures to infectious agents such as *Giardia lamblia* and hepatitis viruses have helped to eliminate and prevent health risks. Studies of chemical contamination of food and drugs have also been useful, primarily because large numbers of people were exposed to relatively high doses and because the toxic effects were acute in onset.

Successful epidemiologic analyses of public exposure to noninfectious agents in the environment include studies of residents of Mississippi exposed to DDT in contaminated fish (Kreiss et al., 1981), residents of Japanese villages exposed to methyl mercury in fish and shellfish (Tedeschi, 1982; Tokuomi et al., 1982), U.S. children and adults with heavy metal exposure from copper, lead, and zinc smelters (Baker et al., 1977; Brown, Pottern, & Blot, 1984), residents of a Turkish village exposed to erionite fibers (Baris et al., 1978, 1987), persons exposed to radioactive fallout from atmospheric weapons tests in the United States (Kerber et al., 1993; Stevens et al., 1990), Taiwanese villagers exposed to high concentrations of arsenic in ground water (Chen et al., 1988), and women exposed to woodsmoke in rural areas of the Third World (Sandoval et al., 1993).

REFERENCES

Aldrich, T. E., & Drane, J. W. (1993). Cluster 3.1: *Software system for epidemiologic analysis*. Springfield, VA: National Technical Information Service (Computer software).

Aldrich, T. E., Drane, J. W., & Griffith, J. (1993). Disease clusters. In T. E. Aldrich & J. Griffith (Eds.), *Environmental epidemiology and risk assessment*. New York: Van Nostrand Reinhold.

American College of Emergency Physicians. (1988). Report on the role of the emergency physician in occupational medicine. *Annals of Emergency Medicine, 17*, 1112-1114.

Ames, B. N., & Gold, L. S. (1990). Too many rodent carcinogens: Mitogenesis increases mutagenesis. *Science, 249*, 970-971.

Antenucci, J. C., Brown, K., Croswell, P. L., & Kevany, M. J. (1991). *Geographic information systems*. New York: Van Nostrand Reinhold.

Baker, E. L., Hayes, C. G., Landrigan, P. J., Handke, J. L., Leger, R. T., Housworth, W. J., & Harrington, J. M. (1977). A nationwide survey of heavy metal absorption in children living near primary copper, lead, and zinc smelters. *American Journal of Epidemiology, 106*, 261-273.

Baris, Y. I., Sahin, A., Ozesmi, M., Kerse, I., Ozen, E., Kolacan, B., Attinors, M., & Goktepeli, A. (1978). An outbreak of pleural mesothelioma and chronic fibrosing pleurisy in the village of Karain/Urgup in Anatolia. *Thorax, 33*, 181-192.

Baris, Y. I., Simonato, L., Artvinli, M., Pooley, F., Saracci, R., Skidmore, S., & Wagner, C. (1987). Epidemiological and environmental evidence of the health effects of exposure to erionite fibers: A four-year study in the Cappadocian region of Turkey. *International Journal of Cancer, 39*, 10-17.

Bertazzi, P. A., Pesatori, A. C., Consonni, D., Tironi, A., Landi, M. T., & Zocchetti, C. (1993). Cancer incidence in a population accidentally exposed to 2,3,7,8-tetrachlorodibenzo-para-dioxin. *Epidemiology, 4*, 398-406.

Blanc, P. D., & Olson, K. R. (1986). Occupationally-related illness reported to a regional poison control center. *American Journal of Public Health, 76*, 1303-1307.

Blot, W. J., & Fraumeni, J. F. (1982). Geographic epidemiology of cancer in the United States. In D. Schottenfeld & J. F. Fraumeni (Eds.), *Cancer epidemiology and prevention* (pp. 179-193). Philadelphia: Saunders.

Bolviken, B., & Bjorklund, A. (1990). Geochemical maps as a basis for geomedical investigations. In J. Lag. (Ed.), *Geomedicine* (pp. 75-106). Boca Raton, FL: CRC Press.

Boyle, P. (1989). Relative value of incidence and mortality data in cancer research. In P. Boyle, C. S. Muir, & E. Grundmann (Eds.), *Cancer mapping* (pp. 41-63). Berlin: Springer-Verlag.

Breslow, N. E., & Day, N. E. (1980). *Statistical methods in cancer research, Volume I—the analysis of case-control studies.* Lyon, France: International Agency for Research on Cancer.

Breslow, N. E., & Day, N. E. (1987). *Statistical methods in cancer research, (Volume II)—the design and analysis of cohort studies.* Lyon, France: International Agency for Research on Cancer.

Briggs, D. J. (1992). Mapping environmental exposure. In P. Elliott, J. Cuzick, D. English, & R. Stern (Eds.), *Geographical and environmental epidemiology: Methods for small-area studies* (pp. 158-176). Oxford: Oxford University Press.

Brown, L. M., Pottern, L. M., & Blot, W. J. (1984). Lung cancer in relation to environmental pollutants emitted from industrial sources. *Environmental Research, 34*, 250-261.

Brown, P. (1993). When the public knows better: Popular epidemiology challenges the system. *Environment,* October, 17-41.

Burmaster, D. E., & Harris, R. H. (1993). The magnitude of compounding conservativisms in superfund risk assessments. *Risk Analysis, 13*, 131-134.

Butterworth, B. E. (1990). Consideration of both genotoxic and nongenotoxic mechanisms in predicting carcinogenic potential. *Mutation Research, 239,* 117-132.

Calabrese, E. J., & Kostecki, P. T. (1992). *Risk assessment and environmental fate methodologies.* Boca Raton, FL: Lewis.

Caldwell, G. G. (1990). Twenty-two years of cancer cluster investigations at the Centers for Disease Control. *American Journal of Epidemiology, 132*(Suppl. No. 1), S43-S47.

Carstensen, B. (1989). Impact of cancer atlases on cancer epidemiology: Experience of the Danish Atlas of Cancer Incidence. In P. Boyle, C. S. Muir, & E. Grundmann (Eds.), *Cancer Mapping* (pp. 227-239). Berlin: Springer-Verlag.

Cate, S., Ruttenber, A. J., & Conklin, A. W. (1990). Feasibility of an epidemiologic study of thyroid neoplasia in persons exposed to radionuclides form the Hanford Nuclear Facility between 1944 and 1956. *Health Physics, 59,* 1-10.

Centers for Disease Control and Prevention. (1989). Death investigation —United States, 1987. *Morbidity and Mortality Weekly Report, 38,* 1-4.

Centers for Disease Control and Prevention. (1990a). Mandatory reporting of infectious diseases by clinicians and mandatory reporting of occupational diseases by clinicians. *Morbidity and Mortality Weekly Report, 39*(No. RR-9),

Centers for Disease Control and Prevention. (1990b). Guidelines for investigating clusters of health events. *Morbidity and Mortality Weekly Report, 39*(No. RR-11).

Centers for Disease Control and Prevention. (1992). *National Center for Health Statistics organization and activities* (Publication No. [PHS] 92-1200). Hyattsville, MD: Author.

Centers for Disease Control and Prevention. (1994). State cancer registries: Status of authorizing legislation and enabling regulations—United States, October 1993. *Morbidity and Mortality Weekly Report, 43,* 71-75.

Chen, C-J, Wu, M-M, Lee, S-S, Wand, J-D, Cheng, S-H, & Wu, S-Y. (1988). Atherogenicity and carcinogenicity of high-arsenic artesian well water. *Atherosclerosis, 8,* 452-460.

Cliff, A. D., & Haggett, P. (1990). *Atlas of disease distributions.* Cambridge, MA: Basil Blackwell.

Cohen, S. M., & Ellwein, L. B. (1990). Cell proliferation in carcinogenesis. *Science, 249,* 1007-1011.

Committee on Neurotoxicology and Models for Assessing Risk. (1992). *Environmental neurotoxicology.* New York: National Academy Press.

Curnen, M. G. M., & Schoenfeld, E. R. (1983). Standard information on environmental exposure linked to data on cancer patients, with a brief review of the literature. *Preventive Medicine, 12,* 242-261.

Dean, J. A., Dean, A. G., Burton, A. H., & Dicker, R. C. (1994). *Epi Info, version 6.* Stone Mountain, GA: USD, Inc. (Computer software).

Deane, M., Swan, S. H., Harris, J. A., Epstein, D. M., & Neutra, R. R. (1989). Adverse pregnancy outcomes in relation to water contamination, Santa Clara County, California, 1980-1981. *American Journal of Epidemiology, 129,* 894-904.

Decisioneering, Inc. (1993). *Crystal ball, version 3.0. Forecasting and risk analysis for spreadsheet users.* Denver: Author. (Computer software).

Devier, J. R., Brownson, R. C., Bagby, J. R., Carlson, G. M. & Crellin, J. R. (1990). A public health response to cancer clusters in Missouri. *American Journal of Epidemiology, 132*(Suppl. No. 1), S23-S31.

Diggle, P. J. (1990). *Time series: A biostatistical introduction.* Oxford: Clarendon Press.

Dockery, D. W., Pope, C. A., Zu, X., Spengler, J. D., Ware, J. G., Fay, M. F., Ferris, Jr., B. G., & Speizer, F. E. (1993). An association between air pollution and mortality in six U.S. cities. *New England Journal of Medicine, 329,* 1753-1759.

Dolk, H., & DeWals, P. (1992). Congenital anomalies. In P. Elliott, J. Cuzick, D. English, & R. Stern (Eds.), *Geographical and environmental epidemiology: Methods for small-area studies* (pp. 72-88). Oxford: Oxford University Press.

Draper, G. J., & Parkin, D. M. (1992). Cancer incidence data for children. In P. Elliott, J. Cuzick, D. English, & R. Stern (Eds.), *Geographical and environmental epidemiology: Methods for small-area studies* (pp. 63-71). Oxford: Oxford University Press.

Elliott, P., Cuzick, J., English, E., & Stern, R. (Eds.), *Geographical and environmental epidemiology: Methods for small-area studies.* Oxford: Oxford University Press.

Ellis, D. (1989). *Environments at risk: Case histories of impact assessment.* New York: Springer-Verlag.

Elwood, J. M. (1988). *Causal relationships in medicine: A practical system for critical appraisal.* New York: Oxford University Press.

English, D. (1992) Geographical epidemiology and ecological studies. In P. Elliott, J. Cuzick, D. English & R. Stern (Eds.), *Geographical and environmental epidemiology: Methods for small-area studies* (pp. 3-13). Oxford: Oxford University Press.

Enterline, P. E., & Henderson, V. L. (1987). Geographic patterns for pleural mesothelioma deaths in the United States, 1968-81. *Journal of the National Cancer Institute, 79,* 31-37.

Gable, C. B. (1990). A compendium of public health data sources. *American Journal of Epidemiology, 131,* 381-394.

Garte, S. J. (1994). *Molecular environmental biology.* Boca Raton, FL: Lewis.

Giesy, J. P., Ludwig, J. P., & Tillitt, D. E. (1994). Deformities in birds of the Great Lakes region. *Environmental Science and Technology, 28,* 128-134.

Goldstein, B. D., & Witz, G. (1992). Benzene. In M. Lippman (Ed.), *Environmental toxicants: Human exposures and their health effects* (pp. 76-97). New York: Van Nostrand Reinhold.

Goodman, R. A., Buehler, J. W., & Koplan, J. P. (1990). The epidemiologic field investigation: Science and judgement in public health practice. *American Journal of Epidemiology, 132,* 9-16.

Greenland, S., & Morgenstern, H. (1989). Ecological bias, confounding, and effect modification. *International Journal of Epidemiology, 18,* 269-274.

Hill, A. B. (1965). The environment and disease: Association or causation. *Proceedings of the Royal Society of Medicine, 58,* 295-300.

Hoffman, F. O., & Gardner, R. H. (1983). Evaluation of uncertainties in radiological assessment models. In J. E. Till & H. R. Meyer (Eds.), *Radiological assessment, a textbook on environmental dose analysis* (pp. 11-1—11-55). Washington, DC: U. S. Nuclear Regulatory Commission.

Hoffman, F. O., & Hammonds, J. S. (1992). An introductory guide to uncertainty analysis in environmental health and risk assessment (Publication No. ESD 3920; Report No. ES/ER/TM35). Oak Ridge, TN: Oak Ridge National Laboratory.

Hornung, R. W., & Meinhardt, T. J. (1987). Quantitative risk assessment of lung cancer in U. S. uranium miners. *Health Physics, 52,* 417-430.

Howe, G. M. (1989). Historical evolution of disease mapping in general and specifically of cancer mapping. In P. Boyle, C. S. Muir, & E. Grundmann (Eds.), *Cancer mapping* (pp. 1-21). Berlin: Springer-Verlag.

Huncharek, M. (1994). Asbestos and cancer: Epidemiological and public health controversies. *Cancer Investigation, 12,* 214-222.

International Agency for Research on Cancer. (1982). *Monographs on the evaluation of the carcinogenic risk of chemicals to humans, Vol. 29, some industrial chemicals and dyestuffs* (pp. 93-148). Lyons, France: Author

Jablon, S., Hrubec, Z., & Boice, J. D. (1991). Cancer in populations living near nuclear facilities: A survey of mortality nationwide and incidence in two states. *JAMA, 265,* 1403-1408.

Jenner, P., Marsden, C. D., Costall, B., & Naylor, R. J. (1986). MPTP and MPP+ induced neurotoxicity in rodents and the common marmoset as experimental models for investigating Parkinson's disease. In S. P. Markey, N. Castagnoli, A. J. Trevor, & I. J. Kopin (Eds.), *MPTP: a neurotoxin producing a parkinsonian syndrome* (pp. 45-68). New York: Academic Press.

Kerber, R. A., Till, J. E., Simon, S. L., Lyon, J. L., Thomas, D. C., Preston-Martin, S., Rallison, M. L., Lloyd, R. D., & Stevens, W. (1993). A cohort study of thyroid disease in relation to fallout from nuclear weapons testing. *JAMA, 270,* 2076-2082.

Kline, J., Stein, X., & Susser, M. (1989). *Conception to birth, epidemiology of prenatal development* (3rd ed.). New York: Oxford University Press.

Kociba, R. J. (1984). Evaluation of the carcinogenic and mutagenic potential of 2,3,7,8-TCDD and other chlorinated dioxins. In A. Poland & R. D. Kimbrough (Eds.), *Biological mechanisms of dioxin action, Banbury Report No. 18* (pp. 73-84). Cold Spring Harbor, NY: Cold Spring Harbor Laboratory.

Kreiss, K., Zack, M., Kimbrough, R. D., Needham, L. L., Smreak, A. L., & Jones, B. T. (1981). Cross-sectional study of a community with exceptional exposure to DDT. *JAMA, 245,* 1926-1930.

Krieger, N., Wolff, M. S., Hiatt, R. A., Rivera, M., Vogelman, J., Orentreich, N. (1994). Breast cancer and serum organochlorines: A prospective study among white, black, and asian women. *Journal of the National Cancer Institute, 86,* 589-599.

Landy, M. K., Roberts, M. J., & Thomas, S. R. (1990). *The Environmental Protection Agency: Asking the wrong questions* (pp. 188-189). New York: Oxford University Press.

Langston, J. W., Ballard, P. A., Tetrud, J. W., & Irwin, I. (1983). Chronic parkinsonism in humans due to a product of meperidine analog synthesis. *Science, 219,* 979-980.

Lauderdale, D. S., Furner, S. E., Miles, T. P., & Goldberg, J. (1993). Epidemiologic uses of medicare data. *American Journal of Epidemiology, 15,* 319-327.

Leung, H. W., & Paustenbach, D. J. (1989). Assessing health risks in the workplace: A study of 2,3,7,8-TCDD. In D. J. Paustenbach (Ed.), *The risk assessment of environmental and human health hazards: A textbook of case studies* (pp. 689-710). New York: Wiley.

Liang, K. Y., & Zeger, S. L. (1986). Longitudinal data analysis using generalized linear models. *Biometrika, 73,* 13-22.

Lipfert, F. W. (1994). *Air pollution and community health: A critical review and data sourcebook.* New York: Van Nostrand Reinhold.

Lopez, A. D. (1992). Mortality data. In P. Elliott, J. Cuzick, D. English, & R. Stern (Eds.), *Geographical and environmental epidemiology: Methods for small-area studies* (pp. 37-50). Oxford: Oxford University Press.

Mason, T. J., Fraumeni, J. F., Hoover, R., & Blot, W. J. (1981). *An atlas of mortality from selected diseases*. Washington, DC: U.S. Department of Health and Human Services.

Mausner, J. S., & Kramer, S. (1985). *Mausner & Bahn epidemiology—an introductory text*. Philadelphia: Saunders.

McMichael, A. J. (1994). Invited commentary—"molecular epidemiology": New pathway or new travelling companion. *American Journal of Epidemiology, 140*, 1-11.

Monson, R. R. (1990). Editorial commentary: Epidemiology and exposure to electromagnetic fields. *American Journal of Epidemiology, 131*, 774-775.

Morgenstern, H. (1982). Use of ecologic analyses in epidemiologic research. *American Journal of Public Health, 72*, 1336-1344.

Moskowitz, P. D., Pardi, R., DePhillips, M. P., & Meinhold, A. F. (1992). Computer models used to support cleanup decision-making at hazardous and radioactive waste sites. *Risk Analysis, 12*, 591-621.

Myers, M. S., Stehr, C. M., Olson, O. P., Johnson, L. L., McCain, B. B., Chan, S-L, & Varanasi, U. (1994). Relationships between toxicopathic hepatic lesions and exposure to chemical contaminants in English sole (*Pleuronectes vetulus*), starry flounder (*Platichthys stellatus*), and white croaker (*Genyonemus lineatus*) from selected marine sites on the Pacific coast, USA. *Environmental Health Perspectives, 102*, 200-215.

National Research Council, Committee on the Biological Effects of Ionizing Radiation (BEIR V). (1990). *The effects on populations of exposure to low levels of ionizing radiation*. Washington, DC: National Academy Press.

National Research Council, Committee on Animals as Monitors of Environmental Hazards. (1991). *Animals as sentinels of environmental health hazards*. Washington, DC: National Academy Press.

Neutra, R. R. (1990). Counterpoint from a cluster buster. *American Journal of Epidemiology, 132*, 1-8.

Nuckols, J. R., Berry, J. K., & Stallones, L. (1994). Defining populations potentially exposed to chemical waste mixtures using computer-aided mapping and analysis. In R. S. H. Yang (Ed.), *Toxicology of chemical mixtures: Case studies, mechanisms, and novel approaches*. San Diego: Academic Press.

Office of Technology Assessment, United States Congress (1990). Neurotoxicity: *Identifying and controlling poisons of the nervous system* (Publication No. OTA-BA-436). Washington, DC: U.S. Government Printing Office.

Paustenbach, D. J. (1989). A survey of health risk assessment. In D. J. Paustenbach (Ed.), *The risk assessment of environmental and human health hazards: A textbook of case studies* (pp. 27-124). New York: Wiley.

Perry, G. B., Hyman, C., Dickey, D. W., Jones, R. H., Kinsman, R. A., Morrill, C. G., Spector, S. L., & Weiser, P. C. (1982). Effects of particulate air pollution on asthmatics. *American Journal of Public Health, 73,* 50-54.

Pickle, L. W., Mason, T. J., Howard, N., Hoover, R., & Fraumeni, J. F. (1987). *Atlas of U.S. cancer mortality among whites: 1950-1980.* Washington, DC: U.S. Department of Health and Human Services, U. S. Government Printing Office.

Pope, C. A., Dockery, D. W., Spengler, J. D., Raizenne, M. E. (1991). Respiratory health and PM_{10} pollution: A daily time series analysis. *American Review of Respiratory Disease, 144:* 1123-1128.

Ries, L. A. G., Miller, B. A., Hankey, B. F., Kosary, C., Harris, A., & Edwards, B. K. (1994). *Cancer statistics review, 1973-1991.* Bethesda, MD: National Cancer Institute.

Robinette, C. D., Jablon, S., & Preston, T. L. (1985). *Studies of participants in nuclear tests* (Report No. DOE/EV/01577). Washington, DC: Medical Follow-up Agency, National Research Council.

Rothman, K. J. (1982). Causation and causal inference. In D. Schottenfeld & J. F. Fraumeni. (Eds.), *Cancer epidemiology and prevention* (pp. 15-22). Philadelphia: W.B. Saunders.

Rothman, K. J. (1986). *Modern epidemiology.* Boston: Little, Brown.

Rothman, K. J. (Ed.). (1988). *Causal inference.* Chestnut Hill, MA: Epidemiology Resources, Inc..

Rothman, K. J. (1990). A sobering start for the cluster busters' conference. *American Journal of Epidemiology, 132*(Suppl., No. 1), S6-S13.

Ruttenber, A. J. (1993). Assessing environmental health risks, part I. *Chemtech, 23:* 53-59.

Ruttenber, A. J. (1995). Evaluating health risks in communities near nuclear facilities. In J. P. Young & R. S. Yalow (Eds.). *Radiation and public perception: Benefits and risks.* Washington, DC: American Chemical Society.

Sandoval, J, Salas, J., Martinez-Guerra, M. L., Gomez, A., Martinez, C., Portales, A., Palomar, A., Villegas, M., & Barrios, R. (1993). Pulmonary arterial hypertension and cor pulmonale associated with chronic domestic woodsmoke inhalation. *Chest, 103,* 12-20.

Savitz, D. A., Wachtel, H., Barnes, F. A., John, E. M., & Tvrdik, J. G. (1988). Case-control study of childhood cancer and exposure to 60-HZ magnetic fields. *American Journal of Epidemiology, 128,* 21-38.

Schulte, P. A., & Perera, F. P. (1993). *Molecular epidemiology.* San Diego: Academic Press.

Schlesselman, J. J. (1982). *Case-control studies: Design, conduct, analysis* (pp. 144-158). New York: Oxford University Press.

Schwartz, J., & Dockery, D. (1992). Particulate air pollution and daily mortality in Steubenville, Ohio. *American Journal of Epidemiology, 135,* 12-19.

Selikoff, I. J., Hammond, E. C., & Seidman, H. (1979). Mortality experience of insulation workers in the United States and Canada, 1943-1976. *Annals of New York Academy of Science, 330,* 91-116.

Selikoff, I. J., & Lee, D. H. K. (1978). *Asbestos and disease.* New York: Academic Press.

Shanmugaratnam, K. (1989). Availability and completeness of cancer registration worldwide. In P. Boyle, C. S. Muir, & E. Grundmann (Eds.), *Cancer mapping* (pp. 28-33). Berlin: Springer-Verlag.

Shimizu, Y., Schull, W. J., & Kato, H. (1990). Cancer risk among atomic bomb survivors, the RERF life span study. *JAMA, 264,* 601-604.

Shleien, B., Ruttenber, A. J. & Sage, M. (1991). Epidemiologic studies of cancer in populations near nuclear facilities. *Health Physics, 61,* 699-713.

Sielken, R. L. (1987). Quantitative cancer risk assessments for 2,3,7,8-tetrachlorodibenzo-p-dioxin (TCDD). *Food Chemistry and Toxicology, 25,* 257-267.

Statistics and Epidemiology Research Corporation. (1993). *EGRET SIZ: Sample size and power for nonlinear regression models, Version 1.* Seattle: Author (Computer software).

Stevens, W., Thomas, D. C., Lyon, J. L., Till, J. E., Kerber, R. A., Simon, S. L., Lloyd, R. D., Abd Elghany, N., & Preston-Martin, S. (1990). Leukemia in Utah and radioactive fallout from the Nevada Test Site. *JAMA, 264,* 585-591.

Sunyer, J., Saez, M., Murillo, C., Castellsague, J., Martinez, F., & Anto, J. M. (1993). Air pollution and emergency room admissions for chronic obstructive pulmonary disease: A 5-year study. *American Journal of Epidemiology, 137,* 701-705.

Susser, M. (1988). Falsification, verification and causal inference in epidemiology: Reconsideration in the light of Sir Karl Popper's philosophy. In K. J. Rothman (Ed.), *Causal inference* (pp. 33-57). Chestnut Hill, MA: Epidemiology Resources Inc.

Swan, S. H., Shaw, G., Harris, J. A., & Neutra, R. R. (1989). Congenital cardiac anomalies in relation to water contamination, Santa Clara, County, California, 1981-1983. *American Journal of Epidemiology, 129,* 885-893.

Swerdlow, A. J. (1992). Cancer incidence data for adults. In P. Elliott, J. Cuzick, D. English, & R. Stern (Eds.), *Geographical and environmental epidemiology: Methods for small-area studies* (pp. 51-62). Oxford: Oxford University Press.

Taylor, D. R. F. (1991). *Geographic information systems: The microcomputer and modern cartography.* New York: Pergamon Press.

Tedeschi, L. G. (1982). The Minamata disease. *American Journal of Forensic Medicine and Pathology, 3,* 335-338.

Thacker, S. B., & Berkelman, R. L. (1988). Public health surveillance in the United States. *Epidemiology Reviews, 10,* 164-190.

Tokuomi, H., Uchino, M., Imamura, S., Yamanaga, H., Nakanishi, R., & Ideta, T. (1982). Minamata disease (organic mercury poisoning): Neuroradiologic and electrophysiologic studies. *Neurology, 32,* 1369-1375.

U. S. Environmental Protection Agency. (1988). *Superfund exposure assessment manual* (Publication No. EPA-540-1-88- 001). Washington, DC: Author.

U. S. Environmental Protection Agency. (1989a). *Risk assessment guidance for Superfund (Vol.II). Environmental evaluation manual, interim final* (Publication No. EPA-540-1-89-001). Washington, DC: Author.

U. S. Environmental Protection Agency. (1989b). *Ecological assessments of hazardous waste sites: A field and laboratory reference document* (Publication No. EPA-600-3-89-013). Washington, DC: Author.

U. S. Environmental Protection Agency. (1989c). *Risk assessment guidance for Superfund (Vol. 1): Human health evaluation manual. Part A* (Publication No. EPA-540-1-002). Washington, DC: Author.

U. S. Environmental Protection Agency. (1993a). *Health effects assessment summary tables: Annual update* (Publication No. OHEA ECAO-CIN-909). Washington, DC: Author.

U. S. Environmental Protection Agency. (1993b). Draft report: Principles of neurotoxicity risk assessment. *Federal Register, 58,* 41556-41599.

Upton, A. C. (1988). Epidemiology and risk assessment. In L. Gordis (Ed.), *Epidemiology and health assessment* (pp. 19-36). New York: Oxford University Press.

Verreault, R., Weiss, N. S., Hollenbach, K. A., Strader, C. H., & Daling, J. R. (1990). Use of electric blankets and risk of testicular cancer. *American Journal of Epidemiology, 131,* 759-773.

Wachtel, H., Barnes, F. A., John, E. M., & Tvrdik, J. G. (1988). Case-control study of childhood cancer and exposure to 60-HZ magnetic fields. *American Journal of Epidemiology, 128,* 21-38.

Wakeford, R., Binks, K., & Wilkie, D. (1989). Childhood leukaemia and nuclear installations. *Journal of the Royal Statistical Society, 152,* 61-86.

Wald, N. J., & Doll, R. (1985). *Interpretation of negative epidemiological evidence for carcinogenicity.* Lyon, France: International agency for Research on Cancer.

Warner, S. C., & Aldrich, T. E. (1988). The status of cancer cluster investigations undertaken by state health departments. *Public Health Briefs, 78,* 306-307.

Wegman, D. H., Levy, B. S., & Halperin, W. E. (1994). Recognizing occupational disease. In B. S. Levy & D. H. Wegman (Eds.), *Occupational health: Recognizing and preventing work-related disease* (pp. 639-649). Boston: Little, Brown.

Williams, S. (1990). Neglected neurotoxins. *Science, 248,* 958.

Zeger, S. L., & Liang, K. Y. (1986). Longitudinal data analysis for discrete and continuous outcomes. *Biometrics, 42,* 121-130.

SUGGESTED READINGS

Aldrich, T. E., & Griffith, J. (1993). *Environmental epidemiology and risk assesment.* New York: Van Nostrand Reinhold.

Armstrong, B. K., White, E., & Saracci, R. (1992). *Principles of exposure measurement in epidemiology.* New York: Oxford University Press.

Boyle, P., Muir, C. S., & Grundmann, E. (Eds.), *Cancer mapping.* Berlin: Springer-Verlag.

Calabrese, E. J., & Kostecki, P. T. (1992). *Risk assessment and environmental fate methodologies.* Boca Raton, FL: Lewis.

Cutter, S. L. (1993). *Living with risk.* London: Edward Arnold.

Elliott, P., Cuzick, J., English, D., & Stern, R. (Eds.). (1992). *Geographical and environmental epidemiology: Methods for small-area studies.* New York: Oxford University Press.

Gordis, L. (Ed.). (1988). *Epidemiology and risk assessment.* New York: Oxford University Press.

Kolluru, R. V. (Ed.). (1994). *Environmental strategies handbook.* New York: McGraw-Hill.

Lag, J. (Ed.), *Geomedicine.* Boca Raton, FL: CRC Press.

Lipfert, F. W. (1994). *Air pollution and community health: A critical review and data sourcebook.* New York: Van Nostrand Reinhold.

National Research Council. (1991). *Human exposure assessment for airborne pollutants: Advances and opportunities.* Washington, DC: National Academy Press.

National Research Council. (1991). *Environmental epidemiology volume I: Public health and hazardous wastes.* Washington, DC: National Academy Press.

Paustenbach, D. J. (Ed.). (1989). *The risk assessment of environmental and human health hazards: A textbook of case studies.* New York: Wiley.

Rappaport, S. M., & Smith, T. J. (1991). *Exposure assessment for epidemiology and hazard control.* Chelsea, MI: Lewis.

Schulte, P. A., & Perera, F. P. (1993). *Molecular epidemiology.* San Diego: Academic Press.

U. S. Environmental Protection Agency (EPA). (1988). *Superfund exposure assessment manual* (Publication No. EPA-540-1-88- 001). Washington, DC: Author.

U. S. Environmental Protection Agency. (1989). *Risk assessment guidance for Superfund (Vol.II). Environmental evaluation manual, interim final* (Publication No. EPA-540-1-89-001). Washington, DC: Author.

U. S. Environmental Protection Agency. (1989). *Ecological assessments of hazardous waste sites: A field and laboratory reference document* (Publication No. EPA-600-3-89-013). Washington, DC: Author.

U. S. Environmental Protection Agency. (1989). *Risk assessment guidance for Superfund (Vol. I): Human health evaluation manual. Part A* (Publication No. EPA-540-1-002). Washington, DC: Author.

U. S. Environmental Protection Agency. (1992). *Guidance for data useability in risk assessment* (Parts A & B, Publication No. 9285.7-09A & B). Washington, DC: Author.

U. S. Environmental Protection Agency. (1993). *Health effects assessment summary tables: Annual update* (Publication No. OHEAECA O-CIN-909). Washington, DC: Author.

Index

Springer Publishing Company

ALTERNATIVE HEALTH PRACTITIONER

The Journal of Complementary and Natural Care

Carolyn Chambers Clark, EdD, RN, ARNP, FAAN, Editor

With health care professionals, the federal government, and the public seeking more information on noninvasive, natural methods of care, there is a growing need for a single publication that can serve as a comprehensive, interdisciplinary resource for alternative medicine. This journal also serves as a forum for traditional health care practitioners who are looking to complement their practice with alternative methods.

This peer-reviewed journal offers a refreshingly new and practical way to stay informed about research, reports of new methodologies, case studies, practice issues, and news of policy developments from the Office of Alternative Medicine of the National Institutes of Health.

Alternative Health Practitioner encompasses issues, interests, and applications that cut across a wide range of disciplines — from sources of funding, obtaining grants, running an efficient practice, and obtaining third-party reimbursement to reviews of new books, information about audiovisual resources, and research abstracts.

SAMPLE ARTICLES

Departments
- News from NIH/OAM
- Spotlight on Alternative Practices
- Healing: Personal to Planetary
- Grants/Funding
- Practice Issues
- Research Abstracts
- Nutrition/Lifestyle Change

Articles
- Alternative to What? — *J. Gilkeson*
- A Theory for Alternative Health Practitioners — *C. O. Helvie*
- Alternatives to Antibiotics — *S. Burch*
- Alternative Health and Spiritual Practices — *R. Schaub*
- Therapeutic Touch: Foundations and Current Knowledge — *D. F. Wilson*
- Grant Writing: The Uncertain Road to Funding — *C. S. Zagury*
- Imagery in Health Care — *B. G. Schaub*
- Collaborative Practice: Empowered by Inner Work — *L. E. Wilkins*

	Domestic		Outside US	
Individual:	$36 / 1 yr	$ 62 / 2 yrs	$40 / 1 yr	$ 74 / 2 yrs
Institutional:	$70 / 1 yr	$109 / 2 yrs	$79 / 1 yr	$119 / 2 yrs

536 Broadway, New York, NY 10012-3955 • (212) 431-4370 • Fax (212) 941-7842

Springer Publishing Company

FORTHCOMING

INTERNATIONAL PERSPECTIVES IN ENVIRONMENT, DEVELOPMENT, AND HEALTH
Toward a Sustainable World

Gurinder S. Shahi, MD, PhD, MBBS, MPH, **Barry S, Levy,** MD, MPH, **Al Binger,** PhD, **Tord Kjellstrom,** MD, and **Robert Lawrence,** MD

A collaborative initiative of the World Health Organization, the United Nations Development Programme, and the Rockefeller Foundation, this comprehensive text examines health and development issues on a global scale. The volume addresses the broad range of approaches necessary to deal with environment- and development-related concerns across various fields of endeavor and geographical regions. Following the Introductory Overview, the book systematically approaches the topic through a conceptual framework, reviewing approaches and methodologies, policy considerations, international case studies, diverse opinions and perspectives, and finally outlining research and intervention priorities. The book includes international contributions from all five continents.

Topics include: Epidemiology, Comparative Health Risk Assessment, Environmental Risk Transition, Population Growth, Sanitation, Food Security, Lifestyle, Poverty and Global Economics, Gender, Species Extinction, Climate Change, Vector-Borne Diseases, Coastal Management, Military Impact, Global Migration and Hazardous Industries, Workers' Health, Urban and Rural Planning, Child Development, GIS, LEAD, and INCLEN.

1996   480pp   0-8261-9190-8   hard $59.95 prepub.

536 Broadway, New York, NY 10012-3955 • (212) 431-4370 • Fax (212) 941-7842